根管治疗后的牙体修复

主编 [美]乔奇·佩尔迪高
主译 梁景平

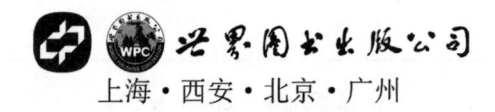

世界图书出版公司
上海·西安·北京·广州

图书在版编目(CIP)数据

根管治疗后的牙体修复 /（美）乔奇·佩尔迪高主编；
梁景平译. —上海：上海世界图书出版公司,2019.7
ISBN 978-7-5192-6308-9

Ⅰ.①根… Ⅱ.①乔… ②梁… Ⅲ.①牙体-修复术
Ⅳ.①R781.05

中国版本图书馆 CIP 数据核字(2019)第 102275 号

Translation from the English language edition：
Restoration of Root Canal-Treated Teeth
An Adhesive Dentistry Perspective
edited by Jorge Perdigão
Copyright © Springer International Publishing Switzerland 2016
This Springer imprint is published by Springer Nature
The registered company is Springer International Publishing AG
All Rights Reserved

书　　名	根管治疗后的牙体修复 Genguan Zhiliao Hou de Yati Xiufu
主　　编	［美］乔奇·佩尔迪高
主　　译	梁景平
责任编辑	胡　青
装帧设计	南京展望文化发展有限公司
出版发行	上海世界图书出版公司
地　　址	上海市广中路88号9-10楼
邮　　编	200083
网　　址	http://www.wpcsh.com
经　　销	新华书店
印　　刷	杭州恒力通印务有限公司
开　　本	787mm×1092mm　1/16
印　　张	17.5
字　　数	270千字
印　　数	1-2200
版　　次	2019年7月第1版　2019年7月第1次印刷
版权登记	图字09-2018-048号
书　　号	ISBN 978-7-5192-6308-9/R·501
定　　价	180.00元

版权所有　翻印必究
如发现印装质量问题，请与印刷厂联系
（质检科电话：0571-88914359）

主译简介

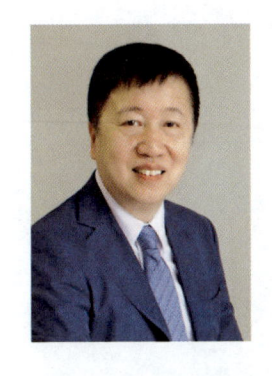

梁景平　教授，主任医师，博士生导师，现为上海交通大学医学院附属第九人民医院牙体牙髓病科主任，中华口腔医学会牙体牙髓病学专业委员会副主任委员，上海口腔医学会牙体牙髓病学专业委员会名誉主委，主攻牙体牙髓发病和预防机制研究，口腔微生物与全身疾病的关系，发表论文百余篇，其中 SCI 50 多篇，主编临床根管治疗学等专著，担任卫生部规划教材牙体牙髓病学编委，高等院校研究生规划教材龋病学、牙体牙髓病学副主编，培养硕士博士 50 余名。先后获得教育部科技进步一等奖，华夏医学科技进步二等奖、中华口腔医学科技进步二等奖等奖项。

译者名单

主译 梁景平

译者 （按姓氏拼音排序）

顾申生　黄正蔚　姜　葳

梁景平　刘　斌　孙　喆

唐子圣　朱来宽

译者序

根管治疗后的牙体修复一直是临床医师关注的重点，也是保证根管治疗成功的关键之一。本书多位作者，分别来自不同的国家，以循证医学为依据，站在牙科黏结修复学的角度，从临床病例收集、诊断，治疗计划的制订，材料的性能，临床操作步骤以及根管治疗后不同牙体修复方式的使用寿命等多方面，以专业角度给予了见解和指导，是一本非常有价值的临床治疗参考书籍。

在本书翻译过程中，我科十余位医师经过反复多次的修改，尤其在专业用词方面反复斟酌、反复查询和讨论，并经交互式审稿，花费了一年余时间才完成。希望尽可能达到"信、达、雅"的境界。现在译稿出版在即，如释重负，但我们也看到，鉴于我们的知识、能力、水平和文化背景，尤其是语言文字表达水平有限，难免在翻译过程中出现错误、疏忽，尤其是在牙体黏结修复方面，牵涉到化学知识、力学知识、口腔修复美学等知识，使我们更是感到力不从心，如能得到各位专家、同行的批评指正，这也是我们的荣幸、不胜感激！

梁景平
2018 年 10 月

序　言

我阅读过很多牙科学的教材，在这些教材中，各个独立单元的作者都讲到，共同编写一本书是多么令人感到烦恼的一件事。不过在编写这本书的过程中，我并没有遇到什么难题，我十分幸运能够邀请到这么多有才能的同行，虽然他们来自不同的国家，如巴西、加拿大、芬兰、德国、葡萄牙、韩国和美国，也有着不同的牙科教育背景，但他们都说着共同的"牙科语言"。

我从1985年毕业开始就一直担任本科生的临床牙科学教学工作。出于教授基于循证医学的根管治疗后牙体修复需要，编写这本教材的想法开始在我脑海中形成，以供明尼苏达大学的牙科学学生和所有参加我讲座的同道们参考。这本书背后的构思蓝图并非是撰写一本关于根管治疗后修复的百科全书，我们的目的在于对包括诊断、治疗计划、材料性能、临床步骤与根管治疗后牙体修复寿命这些不同方面给出专业的见解，最终的目标就是让临床操作者们能够根据已有的证据制订方案。

我们真诚希望读者们都可以从这本书中有所收获。

乔奇·佩尔迪高（Jorge Perdigão）
于美国明尼阿波利斯

致 谢

致敬所有我在葡萄牙、美国和比利时这 40 年的职业生涯中帮助过我的人,感激我从你们那里学到的一切。在此,我必须由衷地感谢我在里斯本大学牙科学院的导师——Humberto Ferreira da Costa 教授。

我也诚挚地感谢我的父亲 Adelino 和我的母亲 Arlete,感谢他们的谦卑、诚实和努力的工作,使我成为家里第一个完成中等教育或大学预科的成员。

我也感谢我的同事 Dr. Andressa Ballarin 和 Dr. Guilherme C. Lopes,他们有着卓越的设计技术。除了作为全职牙医和母亲外,Andressa 还抽时间制作了本书的图 1-1 和图 1-2。

最后也是最重要的,特别要感谢我的同事 Dr. Ana Sezinando 和 Dr. Elen Borges。

我们感激不尽!

目 录

1 根管治疗后修复的牙体牙髓学考量 ⋯⋯⋯⋯⋯⋯⋯⋯⋯⋯ 1
  1.1 前言 ⋯⋯⋯⋯⋯⋯⋯⋯⋯⋯⋯⋯⋯⋯⋯⋯⋯⋯⋯⋯⋯⋯ 1
  1.2 冠修复对根管治疗成功的影响 ⋯⋯⋯⋯⋯⋯⋯⋯⋯⋯⋯⋯ 2
  1.3 全冠修复的时机和原因 ⋯⋯⋯⋯⋯⋯⋯⋯⋯⋯⋯⋯⋯⋯⋯ 4
     1.3.1 前牙 ⋯⋯⋯⋯⋯⋯⋯⋯⋯⋯⋯⋯⋯⋯⋯⋯⋯⋯⋯⋯ 4
     1.3.2 后牙 ⋯⋯⋯⋯⋯⋯⋯⋯⋯⋯⋯⋯⋯⋯⋯⋯⋯⋯⋯⋯ 4
     1.3.3 肩领 ⋯⋯⋯⋯⋯⋯⋯⋯⋯⋯⋯⋯⋯⋯⋯⋯⋯⋯⋯⋯ 4
  1.4 其他修复方式的选择 ⋯⋯⋯⋯⋯⋯⋯⋯⋯⋯⋯⋯⋯⋯⋯⋯ 6
     1.4.1 牙尖覆盖的汞合金 ⋯⋯⋯⋯⋯⋯⋯⋯⋯⋯⋯⋯⋯⋯ 6
     1.4.2 牙尖覆盖复合材料 ⋯⋯⋯⋯⋯⋯⋯⋯⋯⋯⋯⋯⋯⋯ 8
  1.5 桩修复的原则和操作技巧 ⋯⋯⋯⋯⋯⋯⋯⋯⋯⋯⋯⋯⋯⋯ 8
     1.5.1 桩预备的时机 ⋯⋯⋯⋯⋯⋯⋯⋯⋯⋯⋯⋯⋯⋯⋯⋯ 8
     1.5.2 桩的长度 ⋯⋯⋯⋯⋯⋯⋯⋯⋯⋯⋯⋯⋯⋯⋯⋯⋯⋯ 9
     1.5.3 修复的并发症和应对措施 ⋯⋯⋯⋯⋯⋯⋯⋯⋯⋯⋯ 10
  1.6 冠方微渗漏 ⋯⋯⋯⋯⋯⋯⋯⋯⋯⋯⋯⋯⋯⋯⋯⋯⋯⋯⋯ 13
  1.7 牙体牙髓学中使用暂时封闭材料的指征 ⋯⋯⋯⋯⋯⋯⋯⋯ 15

2 根管治疗过程对根管形态和机械性能的影响 ⋯⋯⋯⋯⋯⋯⋯ 23
  2.1 根管牙本质的机械和结构特性 ⋯⋯⋯⋯⋯⋯⋯⋯⋯⋯⋯⋯ 23
  2.2 根管治疗引起牙齿易折的可能因素 ⋯⋯⋯⋯⋯⋯⋯⋯⋯⋯ 25
     2.2.1 牙根未完全形成的年轻恒牙 ⋯⋯⋯⋯⋯⋯⋯⋯⋯⋯ 26
     2.2.2 牙髓治疗通道的预备 ⋯⋯⋯⋯⋯⋯⋯⋯⋯⋯⋯⋯⋯ 27
     2.2.3 根管预备：根管成形时管周牙本质的压力分布及其对垂直型根折的作用 ⋯⋯⋯⋯⋯⋯⋯⋯⋯⋯⋯⋯⋯⋯⋯ 27

2.2.4 牙髓治疗过程中牙本质的丧失 …………………… 30
2.3 根管冲洗、根管封药和根管充填材料对根管牙本质机械性能的影响 …………………………………………… 30
2.4 根管治疗后患牙的潮湿状态对根管抗折能力的影响 …… 31
2.5 不同的根管锥度对根管壁压力分布的影响 ……………… 32
2.6 根管治疗过程中温度升高及桩道制备对根折发生的影响 ………………………………………………………… 33

3 根管治疗后的牙体修复：制订治疗计划的思路 …………… 41
3.1 引言 ………………………………………………………… 41
3.2 诊断 ………………………………………………………… 42
 3.2.1 评估牙髓状态 ……………………………………… 42
 3.2.2 牙髓/牙周病变 …………………………………… 43
 3.2.3 牙吸收 ……………………………………………… 43
 3.2.4 牙周评估 …………………………………………… 45
3.3 牙体修复 …………………………………………………… 46
 3.3.1 剩余牙体组织的评估 ……………………………… 47
 3.3.2 牙本质肩领 ………………………………………… 47
 3.3.3 牙本质和牙釉质完整性 …………………………… 48
3.4 根管治疗后牙齿的预后 …………………………………… 50
 3.4.1 前牙根管治疗后的存留率 ………………………… 51
 3.4.2 后牙根管治疗后的存留率 ………………………… 51
 3.4.3 邻面接触点的重要性 ……………………………… 52
 3.4.4 固定局部义齿和可摘局部义齿 …………………… 52
3.5 辅助外科手术 ……………………………………………… 53
 3.5.1 生物学宽度 ………………………………………… 53
 3.5.2 冠延长术 …………………………………………… 54
3.6 缺失牙的修复方案选择 …………………………………… 56
 3.6.1 固定局部义齿 ……………………………………… 56
 3.6.2 可摘局部义齿 ……………………………………… 57
 3.6.3 口腔骨内种植体 …………………………………… 58

3.7　总结 ··· 58

4　纤维增强牙科材料在根管治疗后牙齿修复中的应用 ············ 65
　　4.1　关于牙科纤维增强复合材料的介绍 ···················· 65
　　4.2　纤维增强复合材料的结构和特点 ························ 66
　　　　4.2.1　纤维的长度和方向 ·································· 67
　　　　4.2.2　纤维类型 ·· 68
　　　　4.2.3　黏结性能 ·· 70
　　　　4.2.4　纤维增强复合材料的水解稳定性 ················ 71
　　4.3　纤维增强复合材料在根管治疗后牙齿修复中的应用 ··· 73
　　　　4.3.1　单向纤维增强复合材料 ···························· 73
　　　　　　4.3.1.1　预成纤维增强树脂桩 ······················ 73
　　　　　　4.3.1.2　个性化纤维增强树脂桩 ··················· 75
　　　　4.3.2　短而不连续的纤维增强复合材料在根管治疗后牙齿
　　　　　　　修复中的应用 ·· 78

5　纤维加强型树脂桩修复根管治疗后牙齿的生物力学原则 ······ 87
　　5.1　桩系统的力学特性和桩-牙本质相互作用对修复后牙齿的
　　　　压力/张力 ··· 87
　　5.2　桩的长度对根管治疗后牙齿的力学特性分析 ·········· 89
　　5.3　前牙和后牙纤维桩的生物力学性能 ····················· 90
　　5.4　解剖型纤维桩修复根管治疗后的薄弱牙齿 ············ 90
　　5.5　固化步骤的影响 ··· 92
　　5.6　肩领设计对牙髓治疗后修复牙齿生物力学行为的影响 ··· 93
　　5.7　冠修复对纤维桩修复后牙齿的生物力学行为的影响 ···· 95
　　5.8　纤维桩修复之外：根管治疗后牙齿嵌体冠整体黏结
　　　　修复 ·· 95

6　纤维加强型树脂桩（纤维桩） ································· 101
　　6.1　前言 ··· 101
　　6.2　预成纤维桩的总则 ······································· 104

6.3 桩的设计 ………………………………………… 105
　6.3.1 桩的长度 …………………………………… 105
　6.3.2 桩的厚度 …………………………………… 106
　6.3.3 桩的形态 …………………………………… 107
6.4 纤维桩的构成 …………………………………… 107
6.5 为什么是纤维桩? ……………………………… 111
　6.5.1 纤维桩和金属桩的比较 …………………… 111
　6.5.2 纤维桩和氧化锆桩的比较 ………………… 113
6.6 纤维桩的表面处理 ……………………………… 114
6.7 常见的观点 ……………………………………… 115
　6.7.1 桩能加固残留的牙齿结构 ………………… 115
　6.7.2 桩的合适程度对固位的影响 ……………… 116
　6.7.3 冠部的修复对根管治疗后牙齿的临床成功率起着最重要的作用 …………………… 117
　6.7.4 宽大的桩道可以使用宽大的桩从而可以获得比较好的桩固位 …………………… 117
　6.7.5 透明的纤维桩可以传导光来固化根管内的水门汀 …………………………………… 117
　6.7.6 凸凹纤维桩的固位能力比光滑桩好 ……… 118
　6.7.7 根管封闭剂的类型影响根管牙本质的黏结 … 118
　6.7.8 固化前桩的表面必须使用硅烷溶液涂布到桩的表面 ………………………………… 118
　6.7.9 由于纤维桩在咬合情况下可以弯曲,所以根管内纤维桩的使用不能提供充分的封闭效果 … 119
6.8 纤维桩的优缺点 ………………………………… 120
6.9 可修复性 ………………………………………… 121
　6.9.1 所有的龋坏组织去除了吗? ……………… 123
　6.9.2 有足够的肩领来支撑基础吗? …………… 124
　6.9.3 牙周状态评估了吗? ……………………… 125
　6.9.4 剩余冠部洞壁的最小数目是什么? ……… 125
　　　6.9.4.1 前牙 ………………………………… 126

目 录

　　　　　6.9.4.2　后牙 ………………………………………… 127
　6.10　临床研究 ……………………………………………………… 127
　6.11　总结 …………………………………………………………… 129

7 根管牙本质黏结：一项具有挑战性的任务 …………………………… 137
　7.1　牙根内的解剖 …………………………………………………… 138
　　7.1.1　牙根解剖 ………………………………………………… 138
　　7.1.2　牙本质基质 ……………………………………………… 138
　7.2　玷污层 …………………………………………………………… 139
　　7.2.1　根管治疗来源的玷污层 ………………………………… 139
　　7.2.2　二次玷污层 ……………………………………………… 139
　7.3　根管治疗过程中的化学预备 …………………………………… 141
　　7.3.1　次氯酸钠和其他氧化性溶液 …………………………… 141
　　7.3.2　EDTA ……………………………………………………… 141
　　7.3.3　氯己定 …………………………………………………… 142
　　7.3.4　氢氧化钙 ………………………………………………… 142
　　7.3.5　根管封闭剂 ……………………………………………… 142
　7.4　黏结剂之间的不相容性 ………………………………………… 143
　7.5　聚合时光照强度不够 …………………………………………… 144
　7.6　术者的经验 ……………………………………………………… 146
　7.7　C因素 …………………………………………………………… 146

8 延长根管壁牙本质黏结寿命的方法 …………………………………… 153
　8.1　引文 ……………………………………………………………… 153
　8.2　与根管壁牙本质黏结老化相关的影响因素 …………………… 154
　　8.2.1　聚合物网络的降解 ……………………………………… 154
　　　　8.2.1.1　酸蚀-冲洗（ER）黏结系统 ………………………… 154
　　　　8.2.1.2　自酸蚀（SE）黏结系统 …………………………… 157
　　　　8.2.1.3　自黏结树脂水门汀 ………………………………… 157
　　8.2.2　胶原纤维的降解 ………………………………………… 159
　8.3　如何提升树脂-牙本质黏结的稳定性 ………………………… 161

8.3.1 提高树脂渗入脱矿或未脱矿牙本质的能力 ……… 162
　　8.3.1.1 使用金刚砂车针预备根管 ………………… 162
　　8.3.1.2 使用液体型酸蚀剂 …………………………… 162
　　8.3.1.3 用力涂布黏结剂 ……………………………… 163
　　8.3.1.4 多层黏结技术 ………………………………… 163
8.3.2 提高黏结层聚合物的强度 ……………………………… 164
　　8.3.2.1 疏水性树脂覆盖 ……………………………… 164
　　8.3.2.2 乙醇湿黏结 …………………………………… 164
　　8.3.2.3 提高根管内树脂的聚合程度 ……………… 165
　　8.3.2.4 使用含有草酸的脱敏剂 …………………… 166
8.3.3 提高胶原纤维的抗酶解能力 …………………………… 166
　　8.3.3.1 氯己定 ………………………………………… 166
　　8.3.3.2 EDTA ………………………………………… 167
　　8.3.3.3 交联剂 ………………………………………… 168
　　8.3.3.4 苯扎氯铵 ……………………………………… 169
8.4 自黏结树脂水门汀 …………………………………………… 169
8.5 总结 ………………………………………………………………… 169
　8.5.1 玷污层的预备 ……………………………………………… 170
　8.5.2 磷酸酸蚀 …………………………………………………… 170
　8.5.3 在黏结剂中添加酶抑制剂 …………………………………… 172
　8.5.4 去除多余的水分 …………………………………………… 172
　8.5.5 乙醇黏结技术 ……………………………………………… 172
　8.5.6 涂布黏结剂 ………………………………………………… 173
　8.5.7 黏结剂的光固化 …………………………………………… 174
　8.5.8 涂布树脂黏结剂 …………………………………………… 174
　8.5.9 树脂水门汀的光固化 ……………………………………… 174

9 用于黏结纤维桩的黏固剂材料的选择 …………………………… 185
9.1 简介 ………………………………………………………………… 185
9.2 影响纤维桩黏结强度和固位的因素 ……………………………… 186
　9.2.1 预备后桩道的清洁程度 ……………………………………… 186

目录

9.2.2	根管充填的封闭剂的选择	188
9.2.3	桩道预备后的最终冲洗	189
9.2.4	纤维桩的预处理	192
9.2.5	桩的贴合度及树脂水门汀层的厚度	195
9.3	纤维桩黏结的黏结剂和系统	196
9.3.1	针对根管内黏结系统的选择：酸蚀-冲洗 vs 自酸蚀	196
9.3.2	自黏结树脂水门汀对纤维桩的黏结效果	198
9.3.3	桩-核系统	200
9.4	结论	201
9.5	总结	202

10 临时修复体 …… 209

10.1	简介	209
10.2	材料	210
10.2.1	定制临时修复体的材料	212
10.2.1.1	聚甲基丙烯酸甲酯(PMMA)	213
10.2.1.2	聚甲基丙烯酸乙酯(PEMA)	214
10.2.1.3	复合树脂	214
10.2.1.4	用于 CAD/CAM 的材料	217
10.2.2	用于预成型的临时修复材料	217
10.2.2.1	赛璐珞冠	218
10.2.2.2	牙色树脂冠	218
10.2.2.3	金属冠	218
10.2.2.4	Protemp™冠	219
10.2.3	临时黏结材料	221

11 铸造桩与核 …… 225

11.1	介绍	225
11.2	铸造桩&核的适应证	226
11.3	影响铸造桩&核长期成功的因素	229

11.3.1　保留健康的牙体结构 …………………………………… 229
　　　11.3.2　铸造桩&核的长度 …………………………………… 230
　　　11.3.3　根管预备过程中操作者的临床专业知识 …………… 231
　　　11.3.4　铸造桩&核和冠的黏固/黏结技术 ………………… 231
　11.4　预制铸造桩&核的临床过程和后续的全冠修复 ………… 231
　　　11.4.1　应用EZ桩和自固化树脂的直接模型技术 ………… 233
　　　11.4.2　间接印模技术 ……………………………………… 235
　11.5　黏固/黏结铸造桩&核以及全冠修复体 ………………… 237
　11.6　总结 ………………………………………………………… 238

12　临床过程 ………………………………………………………… 243
　12.1　自黏结黏固技术 …………………………………………… 243
　12.2　传统黏固技术 ……………………………………………… 244

根管治疗后修复的牙体牙髓学考量

1

布赖恩·D.巴斯尼斯(Brian D. Barsness)
萨曼莎·哈里斯·罗奇(Samantha Harris Roach)

摘 要

　　本章通过牙体牙髓医师的专业角度探讨根管治疗后的牙齿如何修复,同时为达成良好的修复目标提供临床指导。从传统的概念看来,根管治疗和修复通常被认为是两个独立的阶段。然而,从长期预后来看,由于这两部分都会对牙齿的保存疗效产生影响,那么在实施具体的治疗前就有必要将这两个部分结合在一起考虑。由于无论是治疗的时机,还是根管和修复材料的选择,抑或是修复方案的制订方面都有多重选择,临床医师在治疗计划的制订阶段常会发现很难做出决定。本章内容有材料特性、修复方案设计、桩的使用和并发症的应对,同时探讨它们对预后的影响。此外,治疗的顺序、技术方法、减少冠部微渗漏的策略也会在本章中详细阐述。

1.1 前言

　　非手术的牙体牙髓治疗有两重目标:生物目标和机械目标。根管治疗的生物学目标是去除感染组织并清除根管内的细菌及其产物如内毒素等。治疗的成功与否,是否治愈和发挥功能,很大程度上取决于治疗后牙齿的冠方及根方封闭。

　　同样,一些研究表明在评估根管治疗的长期预后时,冠修复与根管治疗本身的质量有着同等的重要性。这些研究突出了根管治疗后冠修复的重要地位。在制订根管治疗计划的同时就应当明确咬合修复方案,于是问题就上升到如何才能更好地修复根管治疗后的患牙。

虽然近年来对牙体牙髓治疗的研究趋向于在开髓和预备中尽量保存牙体组织，但事实上，仍然会有部分牙体组织丧失。此外，根管治疗过程中使用的材料也会降低牙本质的完整性。在许多情况下，由于龋齿或既往的修复，需要根管治疗的牙齿都有术前牙体组织丧失，从而增加根管治疗及后续修复的复杂性。

本章是从牙体牙髓医师的专业角度探讨根管治疗后的牙齿如何修复，同时为达成良好的修复目标提供临床指导。

1.2 冠修复对根管治疗成功的影响

现有的研究普遍认为根管治疗的预后与根管消毒以及根充材料的长期密封性有关。根据一些前瞻性研究的统计结果表明，术前无根尖周病损的患牙，其初次根管治疗的成功率超过90%，而有根尖周病损的患牙则降至80%以下。因此，根管治疗术的预后在根充不足或伴有根尖周病损的情况下下降明显。

虽然完善的根管充填可以提供良好的冠方封闭，然而不良的冠方修复体随着时间的延长，依然可以为细菌提供进入的通道，造成再感染，从而导致根管治疗及修复的最终失败。关于哪个因素对治疗预后的影响最大一直存在争论，究竟是根管治疗的完善程度还是冠方修复体呢？或者它们同等重要？雷（Ray）和特罗佩（Trope）（1995）早期所做的一项研究提出了一个发人深省的观点，从影像学统计来看，良好冠修复比良好的根管充填能更有效地保护牙齿。不过在这一问题上，特朗斯塔德（Tronstad）（2000）等人提出了相反的观点，他们认为根管充填质量是决定预后最为重要的因素，而良好的冠修复只是一个在此基础上的促进因素，可提高10%的治疗成功率。如果根管充填质量欠佳，那么冠修复的质量对预后没有任何意义。

在吉伦（Gillen）等人已发表的一项系统回顾中，比较了冠修复质量和根管充填质量对治疗成功的影响，他们的发现证明各方面的因素均会影响到治疗的结局。完善的根管治疗以及冠修复可以促进根尖周病变的愈合，完善的根管充填但不完善的冠修复，或者不完善的根管治疗伴有完善的冠修复均会导致治疗的失败，两者之间并无统计学差异。

由于治疗和评价准则的差异，因此对造成不良治疗结局的危险因素的评价有着相当大的难度。大样本量的流行病学调查有助于人群间评估，从而影响临床决策的制订和影响临床结局。萨勒拉比(Salehrabi)和罗斯坦(Rotstein)(2004)在一项研究中回顾了1 126 288位患者，他们在8年前进行过初次根管治疗，从这项8年的随访中发现，97%的患牙得以保存下来，而在拔除的患牙中，有85%是由于未进行永久性的冠修复。

从这些研究来看根管治疗后的冠修复十分必要，那么修复体的失败与不良治疗结局是否具有相关性呢？维里(Vire)(1991)将失败的根管治疗患牙依照修复来源、牙周来源或牙体来源的进行分类，发现有冠修复的患牙(平均存留时间87个月)比未行冠修复的牙齿(平均存留时间50个月)存留时间长。有趣的是，在116颗治疗后失败的牙齿中，59.4%是由于修复体的失败，主要是由冠折引起的。

伊克巴尔(Iqbal)等人(2003)进行的一项回顾分析，比较了影响已修复的根管治疗后牙齿根尖周状态的因素。这项研究的特点是作者列举了修复学因素、殆学因素、牙体牙髓因素，以及牙周因素与根管治疗后患牙根尖病损愈合的关系。研究发现以下3个因素与根尖病损的延迟愈合存在显著相关：咬合早接触；不良的根管充填；冠边缘不密合。良好的根管充填和密合的修复体边缘有助于治疗的预后，而咬合早接触与根管治疗的失败密切相关。

为了探讨永久修复、修复材料以及牙位的影响，某学者(2010)进行了一项前瞻性研究，该研究评估了初次和二次根管治疗的存活率。572个患者接受了初次根管治疗，642个患者接受的是根管再治疗。对这些患者在2～4年间每年进行随访。存活率的判断基于牙是否存留以及回访时是否有功能，患牙被拔除则被认为治疗失败。研究发现，4年存活率在初次根管治疗和再次根管治疗中分别为95.4%、95.2%。修复因素也会显著增加拔牙风险，比如只做了临时冠，桩核冠，缺乏邻间接触点以及游离端的牙齿。

总体来说，牙体牙髓和修复治疗的复杂性给临床医师增加了很多考虑因素。如前文中列举的那样，对于材料学、生物力学、治疗时机的充分考虑在根管治疗和后期修复中相当重要。充分考虑到这些因素后，相信根管治疗后的牙齿经过合适的冠方修复也可以使用很多年。

1.3 全冠修复的时机和原因

根管治疗后的患牙是否需要全冠修复很大程度上取决于牙齿的类型，剩余牙体组织以及牙齿所承受的殆力。

1.3.1 前牙

在一项体外研究中，特拉伯特（Trabert）等人发现对于未行全冠修复的牙齿来说，是否做过根管治疗的牙齿抗折能力并无统计差异。在一项基于临床的回顾性研究中，索伦森（Sorensen）和马丁诺夫（Martinoff）（1984）纳入1 273颗根管治疗牙齿，发现前牙的长期预后，无论是上颌还是下颌，有无金属桩的全冠与简单的封闭开髓孔相比并无统计学差异。不过，近期一些研究表明，纤维桩似乎可以增加抗折力。在大部分病例中，前牙可以从舌侧进行树脂修复。修复这些牙齿时，牙胶充填的平面需要位于釉牙本质界以下，树脂可以直接充填在牙胶上方。对于前牙，全冠仅在牙体大面积缺损以及出于某些美学因素考量时才是必要的。

1.3.2 后牙

在索伦森和马丁诺夫的这项研究中，还发现对于前磨牙和磨牙来讲，全冠对长期成功率的增加有显著的促进作用。根管治疗后的后牙未行牙尖覆盖的修复导致长期预后下降的原因可能是牙尖产生了偏移。当进行MO或MOD洞型预备的牙齿承受殆力时，牙尖的移动要大于完整的牙齿。即便保留了边缘嵴，相近的牙尖仍然很脆弱。这种类型的牙尖偏移从牙齿内部产生应力，可能会造成灾难性的冠折。基于这些发现，作者建议对所有根管治疗后的后牙进行全冠修复。唯一可以例外的是下颌第一前磨牙。当下颌第一前磨牙的舌尖未发育时，它不需要承受对颌牙尖所施加的力，因此仅仅对开髓孔进行封闭也是可以的。

1.3.3 肩领

如果根管治疗后冠修复是必需的，那么牙医们也必须考量剩余牙体组织到牙槽骨的距离,这是为了遵守生物学宽度且为冠边缘留下空间。保留完整的冠方及根方牙体组织对于优化修复后牙齿的生物力学性能是至关重要的,因为在冠预备时可以形成肩领的特征。索伦森和恩格尔曼(Engelman)(1990)提出肩领效应是从冠方牙本质延伸到预备的肩台的一个360°环,可以作为牙体组织的延伸从而增加抗折性能(图1-1)。

根管治疗后牙体修复的考量包括维持一个良好的冠方封闭、保护剩余牙体组织、恢复功能和美观。罗森(Rosen)(1961)定义冠外"支撑"的概念,即一个肩领,应尽可能地延伸到桩核的龈方,完全环绕牙颈部,可用来预防根折。罗森等人(1996)用76颗拔除的上颌侧切牙以金肩领的方式修复,冠方用一个桩穿过,直到折断发生。这个肩领结构显著降低了根折的发生。利伯

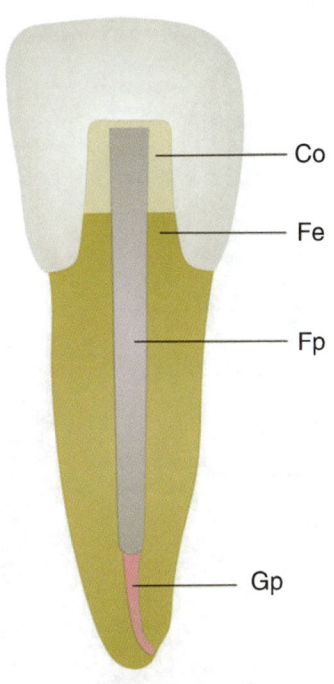

图1-1 根管治疗后牙齿放置纤维桩、核及冠的示意图
Co—核;Fe—肩领效应;Gp—剩余牙胶;Fp—纤维桩。

曼(Libman)和尼科尔斯(Nicholls)(1995)报道增加肩领的长度可以增加抗折力,但是仅增加桩的长度并不能增加抗折力。肩领设计中一个重要的考虑因素是对生物学宽度的影响。一些学者提出冠边缘到牙槽骨至少要留下3 mm,以避免对牙周结缔组织的冠部附着产生冲击。因此,除肩领的高度,至少在牙槽骨上方留有3 mm的牙体组织,这是一个有效的修复体所必需的尺寸(图1-2)。

有时,临床医师会建议对一些没有足够牙体组织的患牙进行冠延长,以获得有效的肩领高度和足够的生物学宽度。在一些病例中,冠延长意味着牺牲牙周骨组织。这种情况中,正畸牵引是更为合理的选择。然而,这一步骤需要治疗过程中留有更长的长度,临床医师需要决定是否预备环绕的肩领。这一问题在朱洛斯基(Juloski)等人的一篇回顾了62篇文献的综述中得到探讨,他们发现如果临床的情况不允许360°的肩领,那么预备一个不完全的肩领也是相对可行的选择。此外,肩领的存在降低了

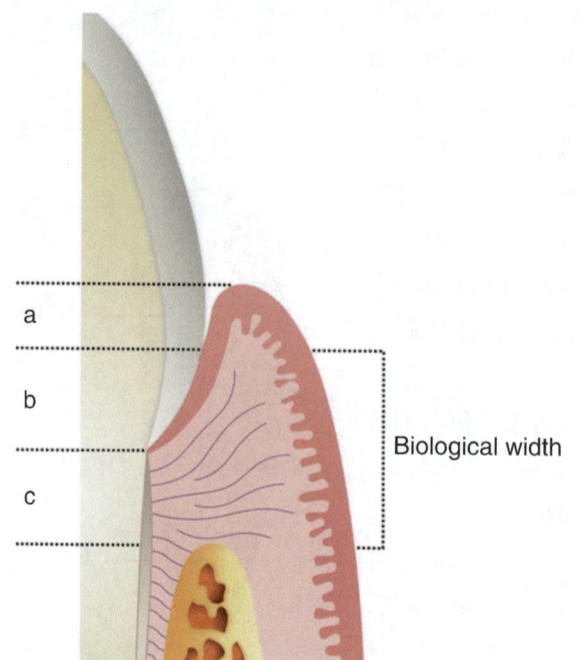

图 1-2 生物学宽度
a. 龈沟上皮；b. 结合上皮；
c. 结缔组织。

桩核系统、黏冠材料和最后修复体对根管治疗后牙齿的影响。这一研究还发现正畸牵引比冠延长术预后好。

1.4 其他修复方式的选择

1.4.1 牙尖覆盖的汞合金

虽然后牙全冠修复是最为常见的选择，银汞合金复合体覆盖牙尖的修复方式也是一种不错的选择(图 1-3)。这种类型的修复适用于承担不了全冠费用，或者冠部到牙槽嵴的牙体组织不够，无法维持足够的生物学宽度和肩领。用这种方法修复时，所有牙尖降低 2 mm，用汞合金覆盖。此外，如果髓室高度小于 4 mm，汞合金需要进入根管 2~4 mm 来增加修复体的抗折性。蒙代利(Mondelli)(1998)等人也发现牙尖覆盖的汞合金修复比未行牙尖修复的患牙抗折性能要好，虽然这种修复的预后不如全冠修复。斯迈尔斯(Smales)和霍桑(Hawthorne)(1997)还发现汞合金牙

1 根管治疗后修复的牙体牙髓学考量

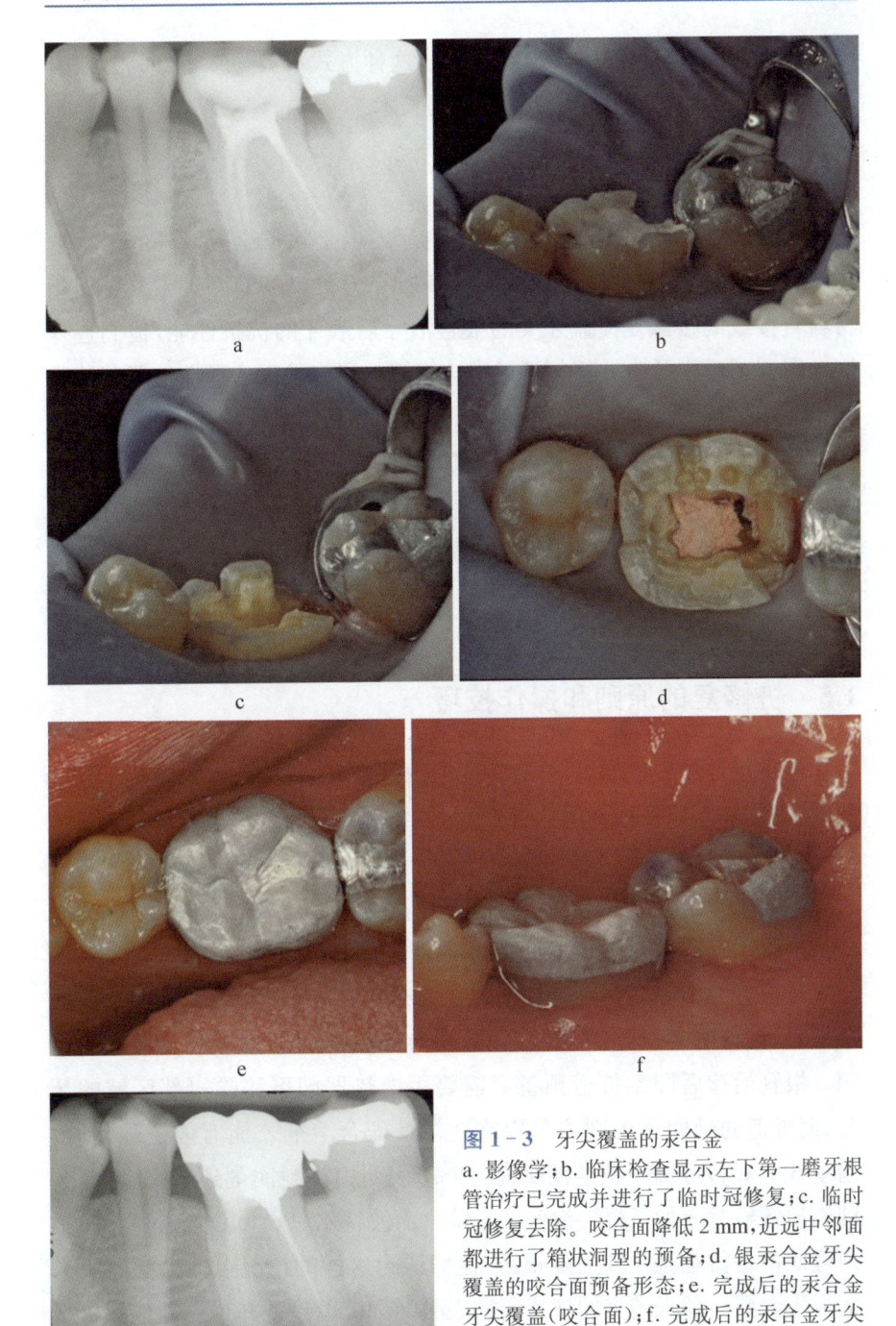

图1-3 牙尖覆盖的汞合金
a. 影像学;b. 临床检查显示左下第一磨牙根管治疗已完成并进行了临时冠修复;c. 临时冠修复去除。咬合面降低2 mm,近远中邻面都进行了箱状洞型的预备;d. 银汞合金牙尖覆盖的咬合面预备形态;e. 完成后的汞合金牙尖覆盖(咬合面);f. 完成后的汞合金牙尖覆盖(舌面);g. 影像学显示汞合金牙尖覆盖。注意汞合金进入远中根管以增加抗力。

尖修复的平均存活率为 14.6 年。因此，这种方式不失为一个好的过渡方案，直到患者有能力行全冠修复或冠延长术。

1.4.2　牙尖覆盖复合材料

与汞合金类似，复合树脂材料覆盖牙尖也是除了全冠以外的一个选择。在一项实验室研究中，普洛蒂诺（Plotino）等（2008）测试了复合树脂材料直接或间接修复覆盖牙尖的根管治疗后磨牙的抗折性能，他们选择性地覆盖了近中牙尖并修复了近中边缘嵴。研究发现选择性地覆盖牙尖并不能增加抗力。然而，在一项对于根管治疗后前磨牙的体外实验中，蒙代利等人发现牙尖全覆盖是可以增加抗折能力的。因此，将全部牙尖降低 2 mm 进行复合材料覆盖至少对于前磨牙来说是一个很好的选择，兼顾了美观需求。不过有一项综述表明，汞合金后牙牙尖覆盖的长期预后优于树脂复合体，这仍然只能作为一种过渡修复方式。

1.5　桩修复的原则和操作技巧

当决定要放置桩时，操作者需要考虑桩修复的时机、方案设计（长度、宽度、锥度等），以及最佳的放置位置。

1.5.1　桩预备的时机

根管治疗后修复的顺序很明确，在进行了暂时的修复后，进一步确保冠方及根方封闭的完整性。其中的一个难点就是桩的预备。当明确要放置桩时，预备的时机是需要考虑的，因为这涉及冠部微渗漏及根方的封闭。根管治疗后即刻桩道预备只需要用携热器即可移除冠部区域的牙胶，而桩道的延期预备则需采用旋转器械配合溶剂才能有效去除牙胶。迪基（Dickey）等的一项早期研究（1982）表明由于封闭剂还未完全固化，即刻预备显著增加了根尖渗漏的风险。而波特尔（Portell）等人（1982）报道延期预备很难将牙胶去除干净，他们认为这样的情况可能会导致更大的根尖渗漏。越来越多的现代研究表明即刻桩道预备并且立即放置桩核可以显著减少根尖渗漏。得益于材料与技术的发展，如热牙胶连续波回填技术以及一些树脂类封闭剂的应用，临床医师似乎更应该考虑即刻预备而非延期预备了。

1.5.2 桩的长度

桩放置的长度取决于机械要求和根方封闭的要求(保留足够用于根方封闭的牙胶)。使用染料加压渗透实验的体外研究表明,当根方保留的牙胶尺寸小于 5 mm 时,其根尖封闭效果要显著差于完整的根管充填。此外,如果根尖剩余牙胶少于 3 mm,那根尖封闭将被破坏。波特尔等(1982)发现剩余牙胶达到 7 mm 根尖渗漏明显较少。因此桩道预备时需要保留足够的根管充填材料。

有些也会碰到一些两难的情况,比如遇到冠根比很小的牙齿,保存足够的牙胶就意味着牺牲桩的长度。马维克 Mavec 等(2006)提出一个特别的方法,结合使用根管内玻璃离子屏障来帮助较少根尖渗漏,在这项体外研究中,对于那些只能保留根尖区 3 mm 根充材料的患牙根管内,他们放置了 1 mm 厚度的玻璃离子,结果发现这一方案显著降低了根尖封闭被破坏的可能(图 1-4)。

除了保留足够的牙胶以外,另一个需要考虑的因素是桩与根管形态是否匹配或者"形态一致性"。这一概念的提出是为了让桩与根管最大程度的契合,以分散应力。基申(Kishen)等(2004)认为根的稳固不只是依

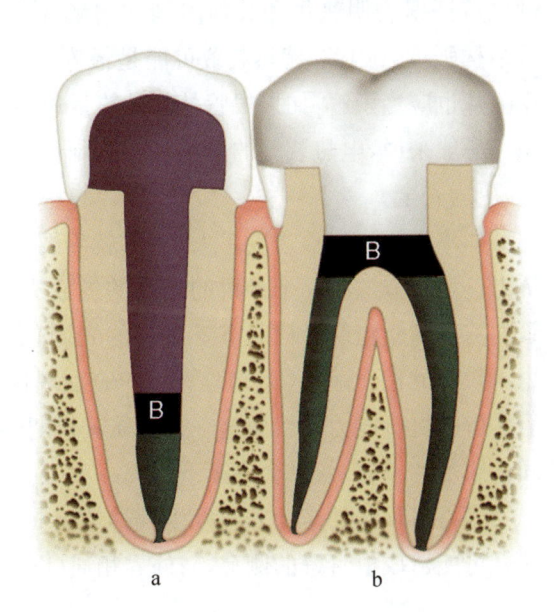

图 1-4 根管内及根管口屏障示意图
a. 根管治疗后行全冠修复示例,可见桩、核以及根管内屏障(B);
b. 根管治疗后行牙尖覆盖修复示例以及根管口屏障(B)。

靠牙本质壁的厚度,还需要尽可能保留弹性模量较外部矿化的牙本质低的内部牙本质。这在大尺寸桩道预备时十分重要,此时为了将桩放入,会将椭圆形的根管预备成圆柱形,从而去除了过多的内部牙本质。选择一个与根管形态接近的可以尽可能少的移除内部牙本质,然而形态一致性就比较差。巴特尔(Büttel)等(2009)报道了用纤维桩修复以及直接树脂冠修复的牙齿不受桩尺寸和长度的影响。这意味着过度桩预备不利于增加根管抗折性。

1.5.3 修复的并发症和应对措施

虽然在部分情况下推荐使用桩,然而桩道的预备对后续修复步骤也会带来一定的风险。包括根管系统的再污染、根管壁穿孔,以及降低牙本质抗力导致根折等,这些都会影响到牙齿的长期预后。

造成根折的一个重要的因素就是桩预备过程中降低了牙本质壁的厚度。在一项临床试验中,科恩(Cohen)等(2003)发现91%的根折是由于不合适的桩设计(太宽或者太大),这意味着过度地去除了很多牙本质。因此,在预备桩道的空间时,医师要尽可能地保守操作,以避免对根管的过度扩大。相对于旋转器械的器械预备,利用氯仿等溶剂以及携热设备移除牙胶,可避免额外移除牙本质或者破坏根尖封闭。不过也有证据表明氯仿和其他溶剂在溶解牙胶的同时也会降低牙本质的微结构强度。因此,携热装置可能是最安全的去除牙胶的方法。但是临床医师也应当了解,如果根管外部的热量过高,同样会影响到牙周支持组织。一般来说,电热装置的温度需要控制在200℃以内,间断加热(间隔4秒)更为安全。

如果根管已经被过度扩大了,那就需要用树脂加强系统加强牙本质抗力。这种方法将一个平滑的透光的桩放进过度扩大的根管内,桩与根管间隙由树脂包绕。树脂靠桩透过的光固化。然后将桩去除,再放置一个永久性的桩。萨柏(Saupe)等(1996)发现这一方法可以增加根管治疗后牙齿的抗折能力。然而这一方法随着长期的咬合力以及树脂与牙本质间黏结剂的减弱,效果会逐渐下降。

当桩道预备的车针方向发生偏移或者桩放置在了薄弱牙本质壁处,那就可能造成根管壁的侧穿,与外界相通(图1-5)。在一项影像学实验

1 根管治疗后修复的牙体牙髓学考量

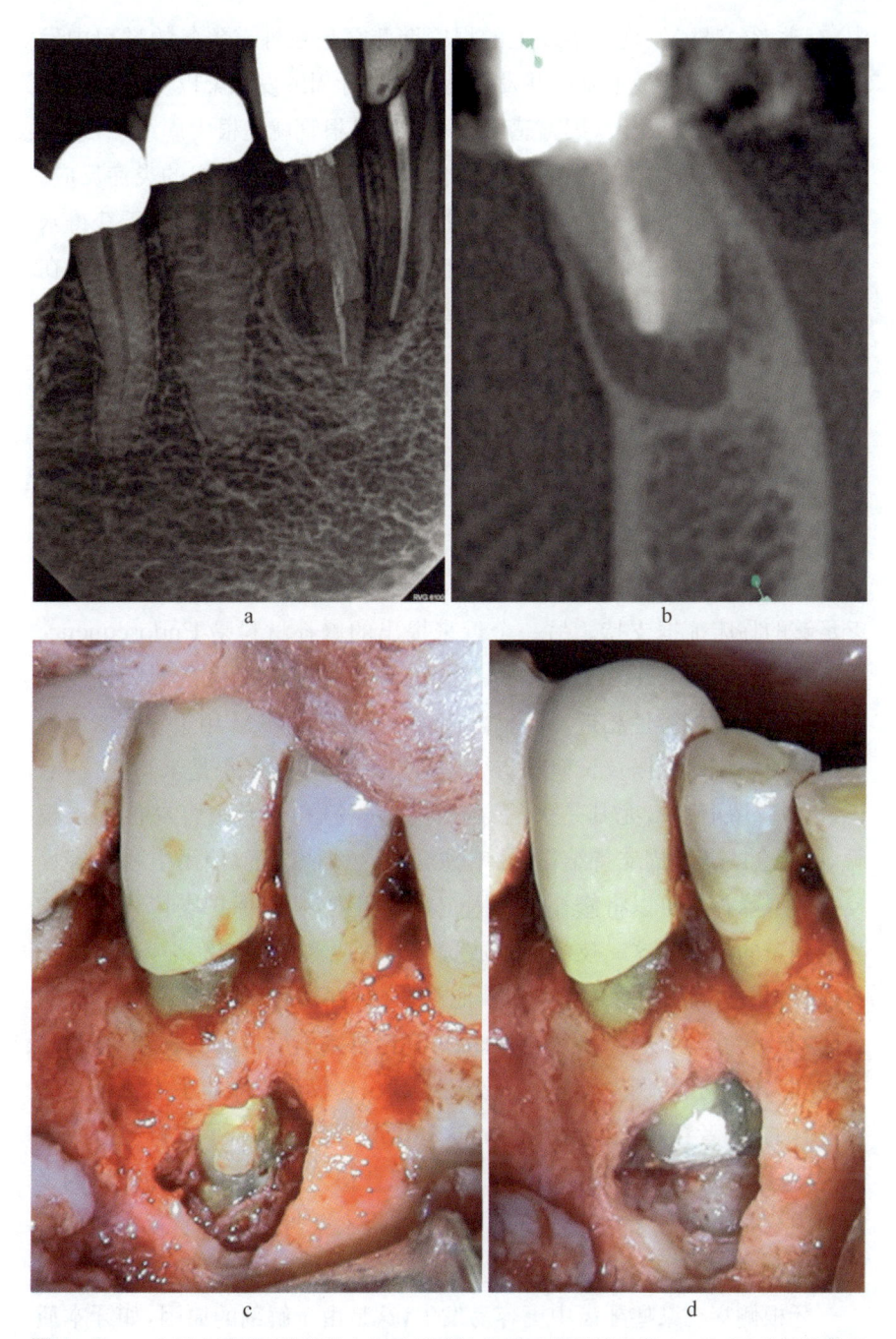

图 1-5 a. 右下尖牙的影像学检查显示纤维桩放置于根管近中侧；b. CBCT 显示桩从根管的颊侧穿孔；c. 术中图显示桩从根管的近颊侧穿孔；d. 术中图示穿孔的修复以及根管倒充填。

中,有学者(1989)发现一半以上的根管壁侧穿是在桩道预备的过程中发生的。根管壁侧穿最主要的并发症是潜在的牙周继发感染以及支持组织的丧失,最终导致拔牙。细菌感染的来源不是根管就是根尖周组织,或者两者都有,造成根尖周病损的无法愈合并导致牙周支持组织的炎症反应。这种反应可以是化脓、囊肿、瘘管和骨吸收。修补穿孔的目的在于获得永久的封闭,防止细菌及其产物从根管内进入牙周组织。如果穿孔很小,在骨平面以上或是修补及时,那么牙周组织愈合的可能性还是比较大的。

修补穿孔的材料包括汞合金、牙胶、磷酸三钙、氧化锌丁香酚、超级EBA、牙本质片、Cavit、羟基磷灰石、玻璃离子水门汀和MTA。现阶段,MTA是使用最为广泛的穿孔修补材料,这得益于体外实验对其封闭性能和生物相容性的证明。病例研究也证实其临床应用的有效性。Biodentine (Septodont,USA)是一种硅酸钙基材料,近来也被提出可以作为穿孔修复材料。虽然体外实验证明 Biodentine 生物相容性良好,但是目前还缺乏足够的临床证据支持。另一个近来提出的修补材料是 Endosequence Root Repair Material (ERRM),最初的研究发现 ERRM 的封闭性能好于MTA,生物相容性相近。但目前而言,还缺乏 ERRM 用于穿孔修复的大量临床病例研究以及长期随访结果的支持,所以效果仍是未知。

在一些病例中,尤其是大的穿孔修复过程中,材料很容易被推出根管,可能会改变牙周支持结构,影响愈合。这种情况下,使用生物相容性良好的屏障材料可以将修补材料固定在牙齿内,从而保护支持骨组织和牙周韧带的健康。这一技术包括放置一片可吸收的凝胶海绵,这块海绵可以将根管外部封闭。MTA和其他修补材料可以紧贴凝胶海绵形成的屏障,而不会超出根管外。凝胶海绵可在修补数周后自行吸收。

在大的穿孔病例中,穿孔可造成骨吸收,这仅仅依靠非手术修补是无法愈合的;或者穿孔位置无法进入,这种情况下就需要行手术修复。一般来说,手术修补包括翻瓣术,必要时去骨以获得入路。去除穿孔区域的炎性组织,用MTA等材料修补穿孔区域,获得永久封闭。在上颌窦区域可能还需行引导组织再生术,以促进穿孔区域的愈合以及促进骨组织再生。

牙根侧穿在某些牙齿中更容易发生,这是由于解剖的原因,如牙本质厚度,根管的形态和外部牙根的形状。下颌中切牙一般为扁形牙根,颊舌侧牙本质厚而近远中牙本质薄。如果采用圆形的桩预备,就容易造成近远中壁的侧穿。上颌前磨牙为双根,颊根的根分叉区域牙本质较薄,因此腭根更适合放置桩。同样地,如果上颌磨牙必须要放置桩,那么腭根将是比较好的选择;然而,腭根根尖的弯曲也是在治疗过程中需要充分考虑的。桩以及桩预备的车针并不会随根管弯曲而弯曲,因此在弯曲的内侧区域极容易发生根管壁的穿孔。在下颌磨牙中,穿孔的"危险区域"是近中根的远中区域,根分叉以下。因此,在这些牙齿中,建议桩放置于远中根。不过,近来的研究表明,下颌第一磨牙近中根和远中根的分叉区域牙本质极薄,所以即便是在远中根管,预备时也应尽量少去除牙体组织。

此外,桩的设计也会增加牙根折裂的风险。有螺纹的桩会在牙本质上产生更多应力,造成更大的折裂风险,因此螺纹桩只适用于牙本质壁较厚的牙齿。

1.6 冠方微渗漏

由于时间限制或者患者疗程安排上的冲突,很多时候医师无法在根管治疗完成后直接进行永久性冠修复。但是为了提供一个良好的环境有助于根管治疗后愈合,我们必须确保冠方和根方结构有足够的密闭。如果根管空间充填不严密,那么微生物,或者其产物就会引发炎症反应,甚至形成永久性的病变。有很多种途径可以使得根管在充填后再次受到微生物及其毒性产物的污染。根管治疗结束后未行永久性的冠修复,而只是使用临时性修复就可能会造成微渗漏的发生。氧化锌丁香油材料,比如 Cavit(3M ESPE)等虽有良好的封闭性能,但它们的有效封闭时间是很有限的。此外,冠修复体的折断,或者牙齿折裂导致根充材料的暴露,桩预备造成的根方封闭不足也是微渗漏发生的原因。预防桩预备和冠修复过程中根管系统再污染的一个方法就是治疗过程中使用橡皮障。在高德芬(Goldfein)等人的一项回顾性研究中发现,桩放置的过程中如果未使用橡皮障,随访发现其成功率仅为 73.6%,而使用了橡皮障的成功率则为 93.3%,两者之间有着显著的统计学差异。

冠方微渗漏对临床结局有影响已经不是很新鲜的话题了。埃里森(Allison)等人发现冠方封闭不佳会造成最终的治疗失败。随后几年,斯旺森(Swanson)和麦迪逊(Madison)(1987)进行的体外染料渗透实验表明牙胶暴露于人工唾液仅仅3天,大部分牙齿即会发生明显的微渗漏。实验中微渗漏的程度在第3天和第8周相似,说明微渗漏的发生相当快速且严重。之后的研究更为强调了冠部微渗漏的重要性。一些学者发现50%的单根牙在治疗后19天或42天时微生物会污染整个根管,感染进展的速度取决于微生物的种类。在另一个实验中,马古拉(Magura)等人检测了根管充填后唾液的渗透情况,发现牙胶暴露如果达到3个月以上,在最终修复前即应当重新进行根管治疗。因此,足够的冠方封闭对预防微渗漏的重要性已得到充分的证明,对冠部微渗漏的关键时间点应当进行充分的讨论。

  鉴于桩核冠修复的材料选择日益增多,选择何种材料可以最大程度上保证冠根复合体封闭的完整性,这是个挑战。巴奇卡(Bachicha)等人早期进行过一项研究,旨在探究不锈钢桩系统和碳纤维桩系统,分别用不同水门汀进行黏结,包括磷酸锌、玻璃离子、Panavia-21和C&B Metabond。对这个实验的液体渗透模型进行的统计学分析显示,磷酸锌水门汀的微渗漏显著高于其他材料。在另一项实验中,弗里曼(Freeman)等人提高了机械压力,测试拥有最小肩领高度及3种桩系统的全铸造冠修复,包括牙本质黏结复合树脂核(Coltene)黏合的惰性不锈钢(ParaPost)、牙本质黏结复合树脂黏结的螺纹(Flexi-Post)(EssentialDental Systems Inc.)以及由磷酸锌黏合的常规铸造桩核。研究发现桩核修复的牙齿,在预备阶段的失败是很难在临床上发现的,然而结果却可以造成修复体与牙齿之间产生一直延伸到桩空隙间的微渗漏。实验的几种桩核系统均无法避免这一问题。但增加肩领的长度可显著增强了抗力,抵抗额外的10 000次压力实验。

  使用根管内屏障来预防根管再污染是一种修复学的考量,并获得了很多文献的支持。这一措施不仅仅是为了应对临时冠修复的失败,也是出于对多根管牙齿根管形态的考虑。就像桑德斯(Saunders)提到的那样,完整而严密的冠封闭是十分必要的,因为磨牙的髓室底存在很多副根管。这会导致根分叉区微渗漏的发生。根管口多余的封闭剂和牙胶应当被去除且由修复材料充满。在一项关于微渗漏的体外研究中,一些学者在根管治疗后多根牙的根管口放置一层1 mm厚的Vitrabond(一种树脂玻璃离子水门汀衬底,3M ESPE),可以在两年内100%保持根管湿度。

治疗60天后，用Vitrabond封闭后的根管可有效防止两种类型细菌由根尖通过根充材料引起的微渗漏。另一项实验中，马洛尼（Maloney）等人研究了1 mm或2 mm厚度的玻璃离子屏障在预防冠部微渗漏中的作用。发现使用1 mm或2 mm屏障均可有效降低微渗漏。

1.7　牙体牙髓学中使用暂时封闭材料的指征

对根管治疗后牙齿的临时修复是治疗及后期修复中一个重要且基本的步骤。主要的目标是为后续的治疗提供一个良好的环境，便于再进入髓室。一般是使用一种甚至多种临时修复材料，加上在根管口放置一个无菌棉球或海绵屏障。最常用的3种暂时封闭材料是IRM（Dentsply Caulk），Cavit（3M ESPE）和T.E.R.M（DentsplyMaillefer）。材料的选择、剩余牙体组织的考虑以及预计修复的时间是临时封闭前考虑的重点。

中间修复材料（IRM）由氧化锌粉末和丁香油组成，丁香油的添加增加了材料的抗压强度、耐磨性与硬度。这些使得IRM有足够的强度修复边缘嵴和抵抗咬合力。然而，IRM的封闭性似乎不如市面上其他的暂时封闭材料。

Cavit由氧化锌、硫酸钙、硫酸锌、乙二醇乙酸酯、聚醋酸乙烯树脂、聚氯酯、三乙醇胺、色素等组成，水分含量高，可提供一个充分的流动封闭且在后续治疗中易于去除。皮萨诺（Pisano）等人提出了Cavit能够提供有效封闭所需要的材料厚度。在他们的实验中，3.5 mm的充填厚度在85%的样本中可提供90天的有效封闭。相比之下，IRM和Super EBA只在65%的样本中有用。但Cavit一个显著的缺陷是相对较差的磨损特性和抗断裂性能，无法很好地修复边缘嵴。

结合Cavit的封闭优势和IRM优越的抗磨损特性，一项三明治技术应运而生。通过这项技术，先在棉球上放置3.5 mm Cavit以防止渗漏，再在顶部放置IRM来增加磨损特性和抗断裂性能（图1-6）。

T.E.R.M.是一种新型的暂时封闭材料。它是一种光固化树脂，含有氨基甲酸乙酯二甲基丙烯酸酯聚合物、不透射线的无机填料、有机聚合填料、颜料和引发剂。据汉森（Hansen）和蒙哥马利（Montgomery）报道，在一项长达5周的热循环微渗漏实验中，T.E.R.M.的表现优于IRM。

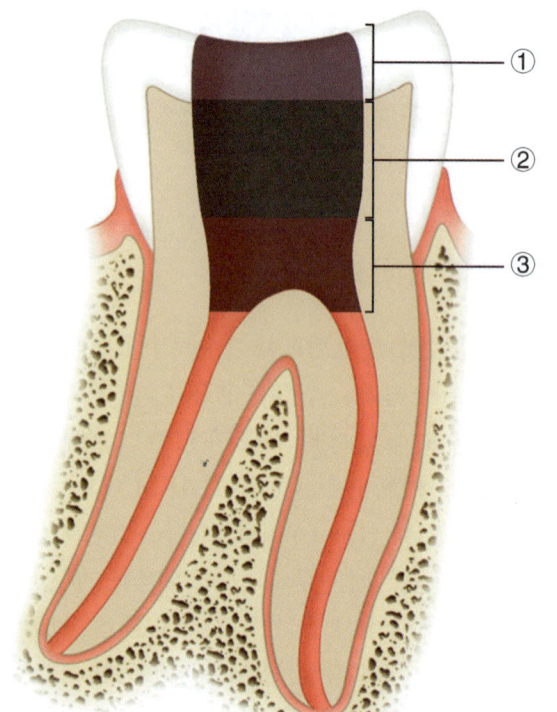

图 1-6 临时修复的"三明治技术"
① IRM（Dentsply）；② 约为 3.5 mm 厚度的 Cavit(3MESPE)；③ 干棉球衬里。

T.E.R.M.填充 1、2、3 mm 厚度时，封闭效果等同于 IRM 充填 4 mm，这表明当充填深度无法达到 4 mm 时，T.E.R.M.更有用。

虽然体外实验的结果令人信服，但是目前仍缺乏在体模型试验的比较研究。更有力的证据需要通过更多的临床研究获得，如某学者用一项临床实验比较了 Cavit、IRM 和 T.E.R.M.的细菌微渗漏，他们将 51 颗需根管治疗的牙齿开髓后随机封上这 3 种材料中的其中一种，厚度为 4 mm，3 周后进行需氧菌和厌氧菌的检测。14 个 T.E.R.M.样本中有 4 个检测出阳性结果，而 18 个 IRM 样本中仅有 1 个。Cavit 没有检测出微渗漏。这个实验证明，在实验期间 Cavit 的封闭性能显著好于 T.E.R.M 等暂封材料。

结束语

根管治疗后牙齿的远期预后不仅仅取决于根管系统内的无菌，还取决于是否具有高质量的冠方修复，以及是否能维持根管长期的无菌化。

为了保护根管系统不受污染，同时尽可能保留冠方及根部牙本质，以确保持久的健康和牙齿的稳固，在临床决策中，医师需要综合考虑患牙是否已行全冠修复，是否需放置桩，又或者在永久性修复前是否需采用临时冠修复这些因素。

（黄正蔚　译）

参考文献

Abramovitz S, Lev R, Tamse A, Metzger Z (2001) The unpredictability of seal after post space preparation: a fluid transport study. J Endod 27: 292-295.

AlAnezi AZ, Jiang J, Safavi KE, Spangberg LSW, Zhu Q (2010) Cytotoxicity evaluation of endosequence root repair material. Oral Surg Oral Med Oral Pathol Oral Radiol Endod 109: e122-e125.

Allison DA, Weber CR, Walton RE (1979) The influence of the method of canal preparation on the quality of apical and coronal obturation. J Endod 10: 298-304.

Arens D, Torabinejad M (1996) Repair of furcal perforations with mineral trioxide aggregate: two case reports. Oral Surg Oral Med Oral Pathol Oral Radiol Endod 82: 84-88.

Bachicha WS, DiFiore PM, Miller DA, Lautenschlager EP, Pashley DH (1998) Microleakage of endodontically treated teeth restored with posts. J Endod 24: 703-708.

Balla R, Lomonaco C, Skribner J, Lin L (1991) Histological study of furcation perforations treated with tricalcium phosphate, hydroxylapatite, amalgam and Life. J Endod 17: 234-238.

Bargholz C (2005) Perforation repair with mineral trioxide aggregate: a modified matrix concept. Int Endod J 38: 59-69.

Barkhorder RA, Stark MM (1990) Sealing ability of intermediate restorations and cavity design used in endodontics. Oral Surg Oral Med Oral Pathol 69: 99-101.

Beach C, Calhoun J, Bramwell D, Hutter J, Miller G (1996) Clinical evaluation of bacterial leakage of endodontic temporary filling materials. J Endod 22: 459-462.

Benenati FW, Roane JB, Biggs JT, Simon JH (1986) Recall evaluation of iatrogenic root perforations repaired with amalgam and gutta-percha. J Endod 12: 161-166.

Berutti E, Fedon G (1992) Thickness of cementum/dentin in mesial roots of mandibular first molars. J Endod 18: 545-548.

Bogaerts P (1997) Treatment of root perforations with calcium hydroxide and SuperEBA cement: a clinical report. Int Endod J 30: 210-219.

Bone J, Moule AJ (1986) The nature of curvature of palatal canals in maxillary molar teeth. Int Endod J 19: 178-186.

Bramante CM, Berbert A (1987) Root perforations dressed with calcium hydroxide or zinc oxide and eugenol. J Endod 13: 392-395.

Buchanan LS (2007) Continuous wave of condensation technique for enhanced precision. Endod Ther 7: 23-24.

Büttel L, Krastl G, Lorch H, Naumann M, Zitzmann NU, Weiger R (2009) Influence of post fit and post length on fracture resistance. Int Endod J 42: 47-53.

Chailertvanitkul P, Saunders WP, Saunders EM, MacKenzie D (1997) An evaluation of microbial coronal leakage in the restored pulp chamber of root-canal treated multi-rooted teeth. Int Endod J 30: 318-322.

Cohen S, Blanco L, Berman L (2003) Vertical root fractures clinical and radiographic

diagnosis. J Am Dent Assoc 134: 434 - 441.
Daoudi MF, Saunders WP (2002) In vitro evaluation of furcal perforation repair using mineral trioxide aggregate or resin modified glass ionomer cement with and without the use of the operating microscope. J Endod 28: 512 - 515.
de Chevigny C, Dao TT, Basrani BR, Marquis V, Farzaneh M, Abitbol S, Friedman S (2008) Treatment outcome in endodontics: the Toronto study - phase 4: initial treatment. J Endod 34: 258 - 263.
Dean JW, Lenox RA, Lucas FL, Culley WL, Himel VT (1997) Evaluation of a combined surgical repair and guided tissue regeneration technique to treat recent root canal perforations. J Endod 23: 525 - 532.
Demarchi MGA, Sato EFL (2002) Leakage of interim post and cores used during laboratory fabrication of custom posts. J Endod 28: 328 - 329.
Dickey DJ, Harris GZ, Lemon RR, Luebke RG (1982) Effect of post space preparation on apical seal using solvent techniques and Peeso reamers. J Endod 8: 351 - 354.
Eriksson AR, Albrektsson T (1983) Temperature threshold levels for heat-induced bone tissue injury: a vital-microscopic study in the rabbit. J Prosthet Dent 50: 101 - 107.
Felton DA, Webb EL, Kanoy BE, Dugoni J (1991) Threaded endodontic dowels: effect of post design on incidence of root fracture. J Prosthet Dent 65: 179 - 187.
Fennis WM, Kuijs RH, Kreulen CM, Roeters FJ, Creugers NH, Burgersdijk RC (2002) A survey of cusp fractures in a population of general dental practices. Int J Prosthodont 15: 559 - 563.
Freeman MA, Nicholls JI, Kydd WL, Harrington GW (1998) Leakage associated with load fatigue- induced preliminary failure of full crowns placed over three different post and core systems. J Endod 24: 26 - 32.
Fugazatto PA, Parma-Benfenait S (1984) Pre-prosthetic periodontal considerations. Crown length and biologic width. Quintessence Int 12: 1247 - 1256.
Fuss Z, Abramovitz I, Metzger Z (2000) Sealing furcation perforations with silver glass ionomer cement: an in vitro evaluation. J Endod 26: 466 - 468.
Fuss Z, Trope M (1996) Root perforations: classification and treatment choices based on prognostic factors. Endod Dent Traumatol 12: 255 - 264.
Gillen BM, Looney SW, Gu LS, Loushine BA, Weller RN, Loushine RJ, Pashley DH, Tay FR (2011) Impact of the quality of coronal restoration versus the quality of root canal fillings on success of root canal treatment: a systematic review and meta-analysis. J Endod 37: 895 - 902.
Gluskin AH, Radke RA, Frost SL, Watanabe LG (1995) The mandibular incisor: rethinking guidelines for post and core design. J Endod 21: 33 - 37.
Goerig AC, Mueninghoff LA (1983) Management of the endodontically treated tooth. Part II: technique. J Prosthet Dent 49: 491 - 497.
Goldfein J, Speirs C, Finkelman M, Amato R (2013) Rubber dam use during post placement influences the success of root canal-treated teeth. J Endod 12: 1481 - 1484.
Grecca FS, Rosa AR, Gomes MS, Parolo CF, Bemfica JR, Frasca LC, Maltz M (2009) Effect of timing and method of post space preparation on sealing ability of remaining root filling material: in vitro microbiological study. J Can Dent Assoc 75: 583.
Hagemeier MK, Cooley RL, Hicks JL (1990) Microleakage of five temporary endodontic restorative materials. J Esthet Dent 2: 166 - 169.
Hakki SS, Bozkurt SB, Ozcopur B, Purali N, Belli S (2012) Periodontal ligament fibroblast response to root perforations restored with different materials — a laboratory study. Int Endod J 45: 240 - 248.
Hansen EK, Asmussen E, Christiansen NC (1990) In vivo fractures of endodontically treated posterior teeth restored with amalgam. Endod Dent Traumatol 6: 49 - 55.
Hansen SR, Montgomery S (1993) Effect of restoration thickness on the sealing ability of

TERM. J Endod 9: 448-452.

Harris SP, Bowles WR, Fok A, McClanahan SB (2013) An anatomical investigation of the man-dibular first molar using micro-computed tomography. J Endod 39: 1374-1378.

Heydecke G, Butz F, Strub JR (2001) Fracture strength and survival rate of endodontically treated maxillary incisors with approximal cavities after restoration with different post and core systems: an in-vitro study. J Dent 29: 427-433.

Holland R, Filho JA, de Souza V, Nery MJ, Bernabe PF, Junior ED (2001) Mineral trioxide aggregate repair of lateral root perforations. J Endod 27: 281-284.

Hunter AJ, Feiglin B, Williams JF (1989) Effects of post placement on endodontically treated teeth. J Prosthet Dent 62: 166-172.

Iqbal MK, Johansson AA, Akeel RF, Bergenholtz A, Omar R (2003) A retrospective analysis of factors associated with the periapical status of restored, endodontically treated teeth. Int J Prosthodont 16: 31-38.

Jeevani E, Jayaprakash T, Bolla N, Vemuri S, Sunil CR, Kalluru RS (2014) Evaluation of sealing ability of MM-MTA, endosequence, and biodentine as furcation repair materials: UV spectrophotometric analysis. J Conserv Dent 17: 340-343.

Juloski J, Radovic I, Goracci C, Vulicevic ZR, Ferrari M (2012) Ferrule effect: a literature review. J Endod 38: 11-19.

Kane JJ, Burgess JO, Summitt JB (1990) Fracture resistance of amalgam coronal-radicular restorations. J Prosthet Dent 63: 607-613.

Kishen A, Kumar GV, Chen NN (2004) Stress-strain response in human dentine: rethinking fracture predilection in postcore restored teeth. Dent Traumatol 20: 90-100.

Kovarik RE (2009) Restoration of posterior teeth in clinical practice: evidence for choosing amalgam versus composite. Dent Clin N Am 53: 71-76.

Krishan R, Paqué F, Ossareh A, Kishen A, Dao T, Friedman S (2014) Impacts of conservative endodontic cavity on root canal instrumentation efficacy and resistance to fracture assessed in incisors, premolars, and molars. J Endod 40: 1160-1166.

Kvinnsland I, Oswald RJ, Halse A, Gronningsaeter AG (1989) A clinical and roentgenological study of 55 cases of root perforation. Int Endod J 22: 75-84.

Lammertyn PA, Rodrigo SB, Brunotto M, Crosa M (2009) Furcation groove of maxillary first premolar, thickness and dentin structures. J Endod 35: 814-817.

Libman WJ, Nicholls JI (1995) Load fatigue of teeth restored with cast post and cores and complete crowns. Int J Prosthodont 8: 155-161.

Linn J, Messer HH (1994) Effect of restorative procedures on the strength of endodontically treated molars. J Endod 20: 479-485.

Magura ME, Kafrawy AH, Brown CE, Newton CW (1991) Human saliva coronal microleakage in obturated root canals: an in vitro study. J Endod 17: 324-331.

Main C, Mirzayan N, Shabahang S, Torabinejad M (2004) Repair of root perforations using mineral trioxide aggregate: a long-term study. J Endod 30: 80-83.

Malkondu Ö, Karapinar Kazandağ M, Kazazoğlu E (2014) A review on biodentine, a contemporary dentine replacement and repair material. Biomed Res Int 2014: 160951.

Maloney SM, McClanahan SB, Goodell GG (2005) The effect of thermocycling on a colored glass ionomer intracoronal barrier. J Endod 31: 526-528.

Marquis VL, Dao T, Farzaneh M, Abitbol S, Friedman S (2006) Treatment outcome in endodontics — the Toronto study. Phase III: initial treatment. J Endod 32: 299-306.

Martin JA, Bader JD (1997) Five-year treatment outcomes for teeth with large amalgams and crowns. Oper Dent 22: 77-78.

Mavec JC, McClanahan SB, Minah GE, Johnson JD, Blundell RE (2006) Effects of an intracanal glass ionomer barrier on coronal microleakage in teeth with post space. J Endod 32: 120-122.

Mente J, Hage N, Pfefferle T, Koch MJ, Geletneky B, Dreyhaupt J, Martin N, Staehle HJ

(2010) Treatment outcome of mineral trioxide aggregate: repair of root perforations. J Endod 36: 208-213.

Mondelli RF, Barbosa WF, Mondelli J, Franco EB, Carvalho RM (1998) Fracture strength of weakened human premolars restored with amalgam with and without cusp coverage. Am J Dent 11: 181-184.

Mondelli RF, Ishikiriama SK, de Oliveira FO, Mondelli J (2009) Fracture resistance of weakened teeth restored with condensable resin with and without cusp coverage. J Appl Oral Sci 17: 161-165.

Mori GG, Teixeira LM, de Oliveira DL, Jacomini LM, da Silva SR (2014) Biocompatibility evaluation of biodentine in subcutaneous tissue of rats. J Endod 40: 1485-1488.

Nakata TT, Bae KS, Baumgartner JC (1998) Perforation repair comparing mineral trioxide aggregate and amalgam using an anaerobic bacterial leakage model. J Endod 24: 184-186.

Naoum HJ, Chandler NP (2002) Temporization for endodontics. Int Endod J 35: 964-978.

Nayyar A, Walton RE, Leonard LA (1980) An amalgam coronal-radicular dowel and core technique for endodontically treated posterior teeth. J Prosthet Dent 43: 511-515.

Ng Y-L, Mann V, Gulabivala K (2010) Tooth survival following non-surgical root canal treatment: a systematic review of the literature. Int Endod J 43: 171-189.

Panitvisai P, Messer HH (1995) Cuspal deflection in molars in relation to endodontic and restorative procedures. J Endod 21: 57-61.

Petersson K, Hasselgren G, Tronstad L (1985) Endodontic treatment of experimental root perforations in dog teeth. Endo Dent Traumatol 1: 22-28.

Pisano DM, DiFiore PM, McClanahan SB, Lautenschlager EP, Duncan JL (1998) Intraorifice sealing of gutta-percha obturated root canals to prevent coronal microleakage. J Endod 24: 659-662.

Plotino G, Buono L, Grande N, Lamorgese V, Somma F (2008) Fracture resistance of endodontically treated molars restored with extensive composite resin restorations. J Prosthet Dent 99: 225-232.

Portell FR, Bernier WE, Lorton L, Peters DD (1982) The effect of immediate versus delayed dowel space preparation on the integrity of the apical seal. J Endod 8: 154-160.

Ray HA, Trope M (1995) Periapical status of endodontically treated teeth in relation to the technical quality of the root filling and the coronal restoration. Int Endod J 28: 12-18.

Rosen H (1961) Operative procedures on mutilated endodontically treated teeth. J Prosthet Dent 11: 973-986.

Rosen H, Partida-Rivera M (1996) Iatrogenic fracture of roots reinforced with a cervical collar. Oper Dent 11: 46-50.

Rotstein I, Cohenca N, Teperovich E, Moshonov J, Mor C, Roman I, Gedalia I (1999) Effect of chloroform, xylene, and halothane on enamel and dentin micro-hardness of human teeth. Oral Surg Oral Med Oral Pathol Oral Radiol Endod 87: 366-368.

Salehrabi R, Rotstein I (2004) Endodontic treatment outcomes in a large population in the USA: an epidemiological study. J Endod 30: 846-850.

Sathorn C, Palamara JEA, Palamara D, Messer HH (2005) Effect of root canal size and external root surface morphology on fracture susceptibility and pattern: a finite element analysis. J Endod 31: 288-292.

Saunders WP, Saunders EM (1994) Coronal leakage as a cause of failure in root canal therapy: a review. Endod Dent Traumatol 10: 105-108.

Saupe WA, Gluskin AH, Radke RA (1996) A comparative study of fracture resistance between morphological dowel and cores and a resin reinforced dowel system in the intraradicular restoration of structurally compromised roots. Quintessence Int 27: 483-491.

Schmage P, Ozcan M, McMullan-Vogel C, Nergiz I (2005) The fit of tapered posts in root canals luted with zinc phosphate cement: a histological study. Dent Mater 21: 787-793.

Schwartz RS, Robbins JW (2004) Post placement and restoration of endodontically treated teeth: a literature review. J Endod 30: 289-301.

Silver GK, Love RM, Purton DG (1999) Comparison of two vertical condensation obturation techniques: Touch'n Heat modified and System B. Int Endod J 32: 287-295.

Sinai IH, Romea DJ, Glassman G, Morse DR, Fantasia J, Furst ML (1989) An evaluation of tricalcium phosphate as a treatment for endodontic perforations. J Endod 15: 399-403.

Smales RJ, Hawthorne WS (1997) Long-term survival of extensive amalgams and posterior crowns. J Dent 25: 225-227.

Solano F, Hartwell G, Appelstein C (2005) Comparison of apical leakage between immediate versus delayed post space preparation using AH Plus Sealer. J Endod 31: 752-754.

Sorensen JA, Engelman MJ (1990) Ferrule design and fracture resistance of endodontically treated teeth. J Prosthet Dent 63: 529-536.

Sorensen JA, Martinoff JT (1984) Intracoronal reinforcement and coronal coverage. J Prosthet Dent 51: 780-784.

Starr CB (1990) Amalgam crown restorations for posterior pulpless teeth. J Prosthet Dent 63: 614-619.

Swanson K, Madison S (1987) An evaluation of coronal microleakage in endodontically treated teeth. Part 1. Time periods. J Endod 13: 56-59.

Tjan AHL, Whang SB (1985) Resistance to root fracture of dowel channels with various thicknesses of buccal dentin walls. J Prosthet Dent 53: 496-500.

Torabinejad M, Ung B, Kettering JD (1990) In vitro bacterial penetration of coronally unsealed endodontically treated teeth. J Endod 16: 566-569.

Trabert KC, Caput AA, Abou-Rass M (1978) Tooth fracture — a comparison of endodontic and restorative treatments. J Endod 4: 341-345.

Tronstad L, Asbjornsen K, Doving L, Petersen I, Eriksen HM (2000) Influence of coronal restorations on the periapical health of endodontically treated teeth. Endod Dent Traumatol 16: 218-221.

Tsesis I, Fuss Z (2006) Diagnosis and treatment of accidental root perforations. Endod Topics 13: 95-107.

Vire DE (1991) Failure of endodontically treated teeth: classification and evaluation. J Endod 17: 338-342.

White JD, Lacefield WR, Chavers LS, Eleazer PD (2002) The effect of three commonly used endodontic materials on the strength and hardness of root dentin. J Endod 28: 828-830.

Wong R, Cho F (1997) Microscopic management of procedural errors. Dent Clin N Am 41: 455-480.

根管治疗过程对根管形态和机械性能的影响

2

卡洛斯·何塞·苏亚雷斯(Carlos José Soares)
安西尼斯·凡尔路易斯(Antheunis Versluis)
达拉尼·坦比罗恩(Daranee Tantbirojn)
惠昂-凯恩尔·金(Hyeon-Cheol Kim)
克里斯尼克科夫·维瑞西莫(Crisnicaw Veríssimo)

摘 要

根管治疗过程中根管冲洗剂的使用、根管封药、根管封闭材料、治疗过程中温度升高,以及根管锥度的增加,均可引起牙齿结构的变化,并可能导致根管承受压力的分布状态发生改变,这些变化会使根管发生折裂的概率增加。本章将着重讨论根管治疗过程引起的根管牙本质机械性能的改变和根管形态的变化。

2.1 根管牙本质的机械和结构特性

牙齿是人体中唯一的一部分位于颌骨内,一部分位于颌骨外部的矿化器官。为了减少在行使功能时的折裂和磨损,牙齿由高度矿化的组织构成,其组织的成分和微形态决定了牙齿具有十分优良的物理和机械性能。牙冠由人体最硬的组织——牙釉质所包裹,牙釉质由92%~96%的无机物,1%~2%的有机物和占重量比3%~4%的水分组成。因为牙釉质的高度矿化成分,使其具有较高的弹性模量和较低的抗拉强度,因此,牙釉质虽然很硬但是也较易碎裂。研究发现,牙釉质的机械性能依赖于对其施加的压力类型和方向,以及釉柱的方向。

釉牙本质界是位于牙釉质和牙本质之间的生物学连接部位,可以分散牙齿的应力以及避免牙釉质裂纹的进一步蔓延。釉牙本质界具有较大的韧性和弹性,可保护牙齿在行使功能时最大限度地避免折裂,以维持釉质的完整性。牙本质是牙齿的重要组成部分,具有优异的结构特性。位

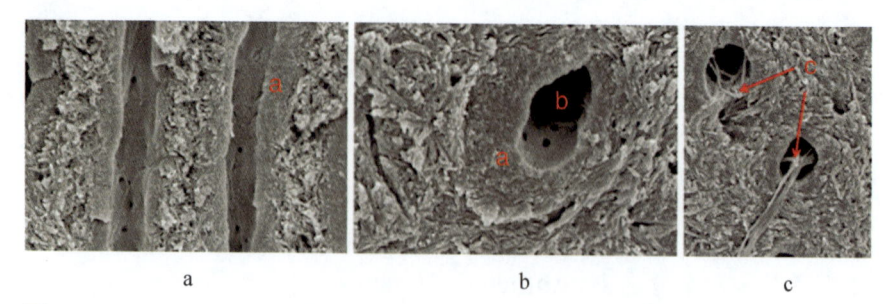

图 2-1 扫描电镜下的牙本质结构
a. 管周牙本质；b. 牙本质小管；c. 胶原纤维。

于冠部的牙本质小管自牙髓向釉牙本质界方向发散，位于根部的牙本质小管自牙髓向牙骨质方向发散。牙本质是含水混合物，由 70% 无机物、18% 有机物和占重量比 12% 的水，共同形成矩阵结构，因分布在牙齿的部位不同，其特性和结构也有所差异。相比牙釉质，牙本质中的胶原蛋白弹性较低；且由于矿物质含量较低，牙本质的硬度也较低。牙本质小管由高度矿化的管周牙本质和 I 型胶原纤维构成的管间牙本质小管复合物所包绕（图 2-1）。牙本质小管、管周牙本质和管间牙本质的作用依其结构组成和部位的不同有显著差异，这些成分上的差异对牙本质的拉伸强度有很大影响。

人类牙列的主要功能是通过切、咬等生物力学的过程，准备和传递食物，这个过程建立在牙齿介导的咀嚼力的传递之上。牙列的主要功能是机械性的，这一点众所周知，但仅仅是在过去的几十年中，科学家才认识到这种机械特性是以分层的微结构为单位的。搞清楚牙本质的机械学行为和其结构之间的内在关系，为科学家们制订如何恢复牙齿功能和提高牙体修复技术的策略提供了一个方向。

牙本质的最大弹性强度范围变化很大，取决于牙齿的位置和深度。索雷斯（Soares）等研究发现，当力垂直作用于牙本质小管的排列方向时，其具有更高的弹性强度。这可能是由于牙本质小管是由一层一层的矿化胶原纤维横向堆积包绕的。

牙齿有支持、转移压力和产生最大咀嚼力的天性。牙釉质、冠部牙本质和根部牙本质共同发挥协同作用，形成一个完善的器官系统，使之有能力支持巨大的咀嚼压力（图 2-2）。根部牙本质是牙列—咀嚼肌—颌骨这一系统的重要组成部分，对其完整性起到了重要作用。人类的根部牙本

2 根管治疗过程对根管形态和机械性能的影响 25

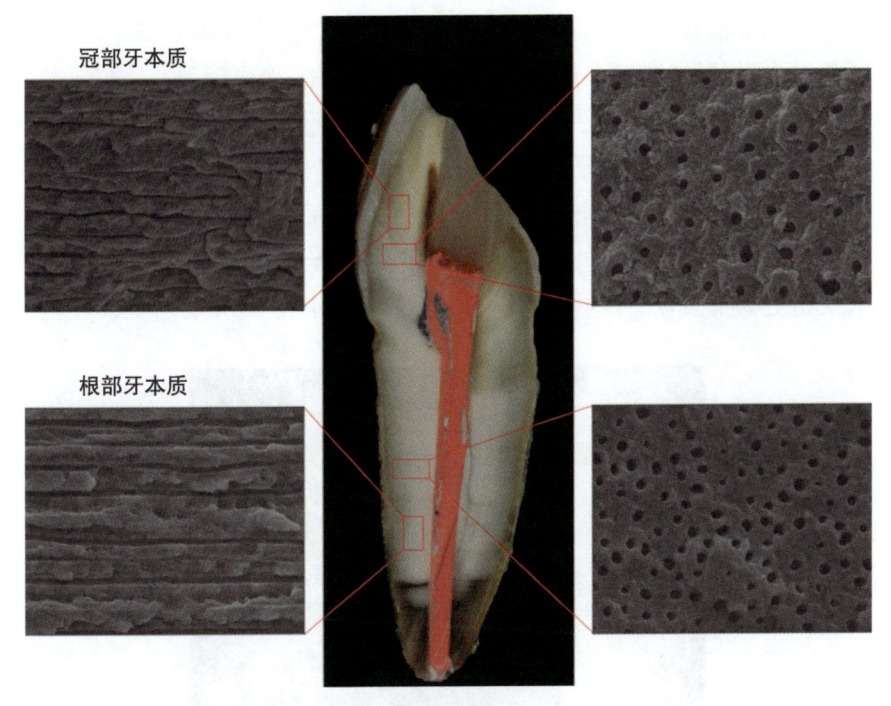

图 2-2 扫描电镜下冠部和根部牙本质小管（垂直和平行于牙本质小管方向）

质较冠部牙本质有较高的弹性强度和更显著的非弹性形变能力。当牙齿被龋或不良修复体破坏后，往往需要通过根管治疗来保持牙齿的完整以及冠修复的稳定性。

2.2 根管治疗引起牙齿易折的可能因素

摔倒、打架、交通事故、癫痫发作等突发创伤，喉镜的不当使用，以及长期反复的压力过大导致的牙齿疲劳等，均可引起牙折。当压力作用于牙齿时，会使牙齿微结构发生形变，这是牙齿发挥正常作用的前提条件，但当压力过大，超出牙齿的弹性形变限度，牙折就可能会发生了。

牙髓治疗是临床上的常规治疗手段，一般是在牙髓发生不可逆的感染或坏死后，以保存患牙为目的的一种治疗方式。牙髓治疗的过程包括去除牙髓组织和感染的牙本质壁等，这些步骤包括根管的机械预备和化学预备，然后这些操作有可能使分布在牙齿上的力发生变化，增加了牙折的发病率。

临床上根管治疗后的牙齿发生牙折非常常见,常常需要拔牙。牙本质机械力学特性的变化,是牙齿更易发生牙折的一个可能因素(图2-3)。牙本质胶原对其机械特性的变化影响,胶原纤维网状结构的变化,可能是治疗后牙齿"变脆"的重要原因。牙髓治疗后成熟的胶原纤维网状结构减少,不成熟结构增多,这会降低牙本质的强度;而牙髓失去活力也会影响牙本质的水分含量。此外,治疗过程中医师的操作原因也有可能导致牙齿变得更易折裂,尽管这些原因大部分是可控的。

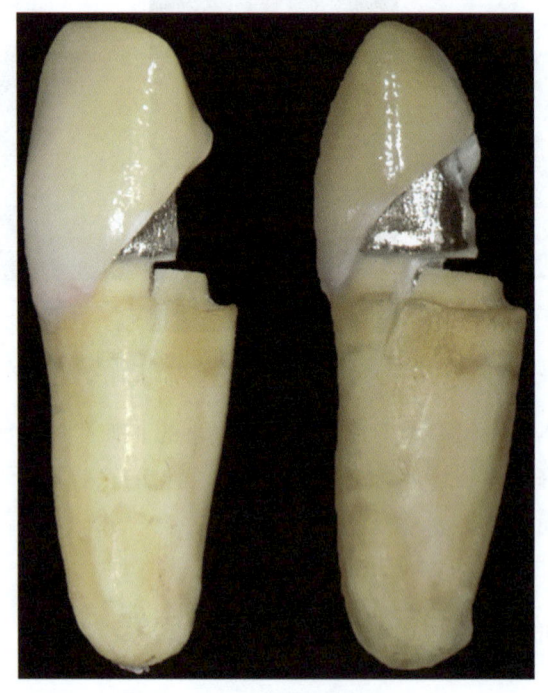

图 2-3 经过牙髓治疗后的齿牙本质更易发生折裂

2.2.1 牙根未完全形成的年轻恒牙

牙根未完全形成的牙齿,如果发生牙髓疾病或坏死,往往会影响牙根的进一步发育,导致牙根发育停止,根尖孔敞开。根管治疗后,年轻恒牙由于根管宽大、牙本质壁薄,使其变得更加脆弱。临床中纤维桩的使用,可以减少因牙根发育不完全所导致的根管机械性能不良。有限元分析结果证明,牙髓治疗后的患牙,在修复过程中如不使用纤维桩,仅进行复合树脂充填修复或其他修复方式修复,其根部牙本质受到的压力明显大于那些使用纤维桩的患牙(图2-4)。使用桩的修复方式相比而言具有更大的抗折能力。

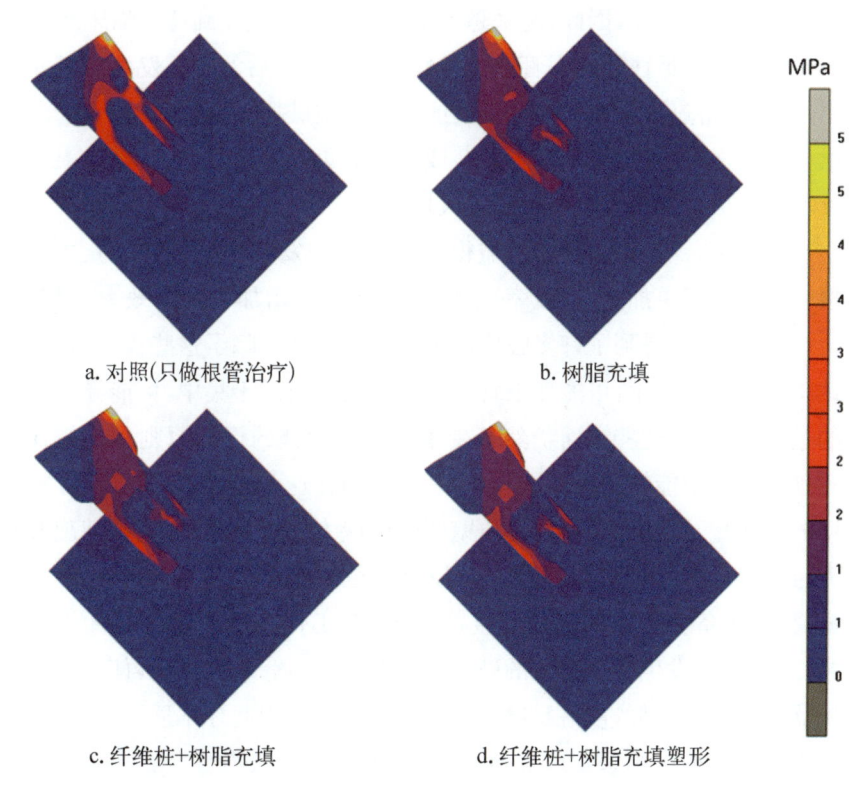

a. 对照(只做根管治疗)　　　b. 树脂充填

c. 纤维桩+树脂充填　　　d. 纤维桩+树脂充填塑形

图 2-4　不同修复方式时,范式等效应力在牙根未完成患牙的分布情况

2.2.2　牙髓治疗通道的预备

牙髓治疗中,通道预备的作用实际上有很大的争议。一些研究结果表明,髓腔通道制备过程中导致的牙体组织丧失很可能增加牙折的发生率,这些学者认为相对保守的通道制备后,牙根的形变也较小。研究者一致认为,根管预备和充填后,特别是根管桩制备后,牙根会逐步发生变形。

2.2.3　根管预备:根管成形时管周牙本质的压力分布及其对垂直型根折的作用

尽管牙髓治疗的成功率可达到97%,但很多患牙在治疗完成后的数年中，仍可能被拔除。最常见的拔牙原因便是垂直型根折，垂直型根折的主要因素，是因龋破坏的牙体组织过大以及在牙髓治疗及修复过程中根管预备过大。垂直型根折是根管治疗最令人头疼的并发症，因为往往意味着患牙必须拔除，因此，越来越多的研究者开始关注到这个临床问题。

垂直型根折往往在根管治疗及修复治疗完成后的数年发生。研究表明，根管预备过程会使管周牙本质的完整性被破坏，这可能使根管壁产生微小的缺损，这些部位则有可能会成为压力集中的区域，从而导致根管治疗术后根折及根裂发生的风险大大增加。

近年来，镍钛机用旋转器械得到了长足的发展，这些器械的出现，使根管预备过程更加舒适，效率也更高，因其大大增加了切削效率，缩短了治疗时间，因此得到了许多临床医师的认可。然而除了这些优势以外，镍钛旋转器械的使用，可能使根管牙本质壁的应力过于集中，可能导致根管的过度预备等，这些方面仍然备受争议。根管锉的设计原则是希望在根管预备过程中能够起到清洁和成形作用，而在这个过程中，器械与牙本质壁的多次短暂接触，会使牙本质壁所受的应力集中，使根管壁被切削和扩大，这很可能会引起牙本质微裂、裂纹甚至缺损。阿多诺（Adorno）等报道，根管预备会降低牙根的强度，特别是在工作长度超过普通牙齿的时候，还有可能发生根尖部位的破坏。比尔（Bier）等研究发现，使用多种镍钛器械品牌的器械进行根管预备后的根管，均会引起牙本质裂纹及缺损，而在手用器械中则未发现缺损；这种牙本质壁的缺损直接影响到患牙在修复完成之后的强度，因为牙齿在行使咀嚼功能后，重复的咬𬌗力会作用于牙本质裂产生的部位，从而导致垂直型根折的发生。

有限元分析结果也证实了镍钛预备器械与牙本质裂及垂直型根折发生之间存在潜在关系。金（Kim）等的研究比较了镍钛器械预备后的弯曲根管，在根尖部不同横截面和轴面所受的压力。结果发现，使用镍钛器械进行根管预备（特别是预备重度弯曲的根管）时，大锥度或/和硬度较大的产品设计，其产生的压力会超过根尖牙本质所能承受的弹性强度（图2-5）。

另一方面，有研究显示，在根管预备初始，用于根管冠部敞开的镍钛预备系统，相较于GG钻，产生牙本质裂纹的可能性较小。

近年来镍钛器械的设计得到了改进，使用旋转往复运动代替了持续性的旋转运动。这种设计也用在单支锉根管预备系统中，大大提高了临床操

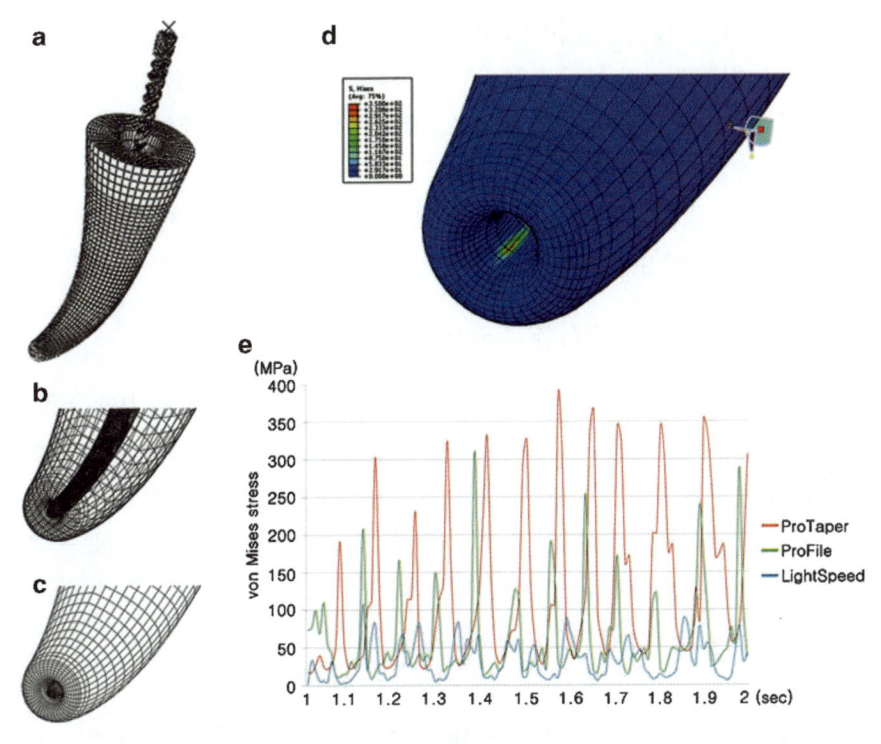

图 2-5　不同根管预备器械产生应力集中的有限元分析
a-c. 根管和器械的有限元模型；d. 模拟根管成形过程中，范式等效应力在根尖牙本质的分布；e. 模拟根管成形过程中，产生最大范式等效应力的部位，其循环应力的分布。

作效率和舒适度，并有相关研究发表。研究表明，尽管无论使用旋转往复运动器械或是持续性旋转器械进行根管预备，均会引起牙本质壁的破坏，但新的设计可明显减少这种破坏。镍钛手用器械及 K 锉在根管的任一水平均未引起牙本质壁破坏；ProTaper 旋转器械较 ProTaper 手用器械及 Waveone 预备系统，产生的根尖破坏更大。另有研究表明，Waveone 根管预备器械与 ProTaper F2 相比，产生的牙本质微裂更小，也更不易发生牙根折裂。一般来说，制造器械所用的合金是否对牙本质壁具有更小的破坏，是在选择材料时的一个重要考量因素。还有一些研究认为，使用往复旋转器械时，牙本质微裂的产生与根管预备没有显著关系。

近年来，自调节式的根管锉应运而生，这是一种全新的设计——这种锉没有内核，而用网格样的结构取而代之，可使弯曲根管的根尖部牙本质在根管预备过程中所受的应力更小，从而保护根尖部牙本质的完整性，降低牙本质微裂的发生率。

和初次进行根管治疗相比,根管再治疗会导致更多的牙本质破坏,因此,在评估根管再治疗的效果时,治疗过程对根管壁的潜在破坏应该加以考虑,术者的这种意识,会使其在治疗过程中注意避免可控的风险,从而会减少牙折发生的可能性。

尽管根管预备对牙本质的确切影响尚有争议,但是不同的器械设计对根尖牙本质微裂产生的作用大小不同,这一点得到了研究者的广泛认可。

2.2.4 牙髓治疗过程中牙本质的丧失

根管治疗过程中,部分根管壁牙本质的丧失会影响根管压力的分布。在一些病例中,由于髓腔入口以及根管的过度预备,甚至会导致根管口呈喇叭口样敞开,这种根管的牙本质壁非常薄,以至于难以承受咬𬌗力,从而更易引起应力疲劳和根折,这类牙齿的修复难度也更大,被认为是一个挑战。在第5章中,我们会详细介绍如何使用玻璃纤维桩来调整根管壁表面的应力分布,使其接近完好的牙齿。

2.3 根管冲洗、根管封药和根管充填材料对根管牙本质机械性能的影响

根管治疗成功与否取决于感染是否彻底去除以及根管系统是否清洁干净。根管在完善的清洁和成形后,使用生物相容性好、性能稳定的充填材料进行三维充填是根管治疗的主要目的。进行根管化学及机械预备过程中使用的材料,可能会影响牙本质的胶原蛋白结构,从而影响牙本质的机械性能。次氯酸钠(NaOCl)和EDTA是根管治疗过程中常用的药物,萨利赫(Saleh)和埃特曼(Ettman)(1999)评估了多种根管治疗药物对根管牙本质微硬度的影响,当使用3% H_2O_2、5% NaOCl和17% EDTA冲洗根管后,牙本质的微硬度均有所下降。EDTA相较于NaOCl和H_2O_2,牙本质硬度降低得更多。这些药物也改变了牙本质的机械性能,如弹性和韧性模量。格里戈拉托斯(Grigoratos)等(2001)使用三点抗挠强度量表评价了使用3%和5%的NaOCl以及$Ca(OH)_2$之后的牙本质弹性模量和韧性模量。结果发现,NaOCl的使用同时降低了牙本质的弹性模量和韧性强度,而$Ca(OH)_2$则只降低了牙本质的韧性强度。长时间使用高

浓度的 EDTA 和 NaOCl 可能会增加根折的发生风险。因此，临床医师应该注意，在根管充填之前，必须将根管内的冲洗药物去除干净。

根管充填材料必须具有放射线阻射、易操作、抗菌、可与根管壁稳定、紧密的结合等特性。目前临床上最常用的根充材料仍然是牙胶尖，牙胶尖的使用可以为根管治疗后的患牙提供一些支持，使其抵抗根折的能力增加。在根管再治疗的病例中，因为需要去除感染和原有的根充材料，往往会对根管牙本质壁的机械性能产生不良影响。根管治疗失败的标志包括持续的根尖感染和根管治疗后的一系列症状，这是表示患牙需要进一步治疗的指征。在根管再治疗过程中，根管和冠部牙本质暴露于牙胶溶解剂中，这些溶解牙胶的材料可能会改变牙本质表面的化学组成，从而影响其与再次根充的材料和修复体之间的相互作用。研究表明，在使用二甲苯和橙油溶解牙胶尖后，根管壁和玻璃纤维桩之间的黏结强度未见明显变化；而使用桉树油时，则会显著降低根上 1/3 和根中 1/3 纤维桩与根管牙本质壁之间的黏结强度。

2.4 根管治疗后患牙的潮湿状态对根管抗折能力的影响

根管治疗过程中，大量液体的使用使得髓腔及其邻近的牙本质小管黏滞性增加，这也会使根管在受力时应力的分布发生改变。另一方面，根管治疗后，牙本质会发生脱水，牙体结构的部分丧失以及牙本质小管的脱水被公认为根管治疗后患牙脆性增加的最主要因素。冠部牙本质的含水量约为 13.2%，而在单位面积内，冠部牙本质含有的牙本质小管数目是根部牙本质的 2 倍。因此，拥有更少牙本质小管的根部牙本质，其含水量更低。随着年龄的增长，会有更多根尖部牙本质小管堵塞，从而造成牙本质小管的有机物含量降低，进一步降低其含水量。在牙齿发育过程中，靠近牙骨质的透明牙本质层是最先形成的，随后向冠部延伸，透明牙本质的矿物质含量最高，因此韧性较低。根管治疗后的牙齿，其含水量较活髓牙降低（根管钙化的牙齿较活髓牙的含水量少 9%），根管治疗后水分的减少会增加牙本质裂的发生率，而这些牙本质的裂纹则可能引起根折。这便可以解释为什么根管治疗后牙齿强度会大大降低。与此同时，根管治疗后患牙的抗剪切力和韧性的降低也是其易发生根折的因素。

2.5　不同的根管锥度对根管壁压力分布的影响

根管治疗后的牙齿所受的压力与其抵抗根折的能力密切相关，因为当其所受压力大于牙本质壁所能承受的机械强度时，根折便会发生。如果不考虑牙本质本身的强度，根管所能承受的压力往往由3个因素决定：根管的形变物性，比如弹性模量；根管的几何形态以及根管的承重限度。根管能承受的最大压力除了受根管治疗后牙本质特性改变的影响，也受根管形态和根管治疗过程中所受的外力的影响。根管受到两种力的作用：①是根管治疗过程中根管壁所受的内力；②是行使咀嚼功能时所受的外力。在不同外力的作用下，根管的锥度对于根管压力分布有不同影响。

当根管充填时，根管内壁所受的压力最大，外壁所受的压力相对较小。大锥度根管比小锥度根管，根管壁表面积更大（图2-6）。因此，在密合度和分散度相同的条件下，大锥度根管在根管充填时，所受的压力可以分散至更大的根管壁面积。但与此同时，根管在进一步扩大时，管壁的厚度会相应减小，从而降低根管在受到外力时的抵抗能力。根充时施加在根管横断面上的力，最佳根管内径和牙根的比例是0.3~0.6。根管外壁所受的压力会随根管径的增加而增加，对于非圆形根管，比如扁根的薄壁部分，根管内壁所受的力会更大。

在行使功能过程中，由于根管受到了侧向咀嚼力，其受力最显著的部位会发生相应弯曲，这会改变压力在牙齿上的分布。牙齿在咀嚼过程中，受力最大的部位是根上1/3的根部外侧壁，大锥度根管较小锥度根管所受的压力更大，主要是由于在根管预备过程中，大锥度使得根管口和根管的牙本质结构丧失更多，但是锥度对于根管受力的影响有限，研究表明，当牙齿某部位由于受力发生弯曲时，根管的中心并未受力。因此，去除必要的牙本质，建立根管直线通路对根管受力基本无影响。

综合考虑多种因素，我们可以得出结论，在根管治疗过程中，使用大锥度根管预备器械无疑会去除大量的牙本质，这会使牙齿变得相对脆弱，但其实对根折发生的影响并不是非常大。牙髓治疗后患牙发生根折的更主要原因是受到的局部压力增加，有些压力在根管预备以及充填过程中已经施加到牙齿上了。根管治疗后牙齿在根尖部的压力分布状态是最关

2　根管治疗过程对根管形态和机械性能的影响　　33

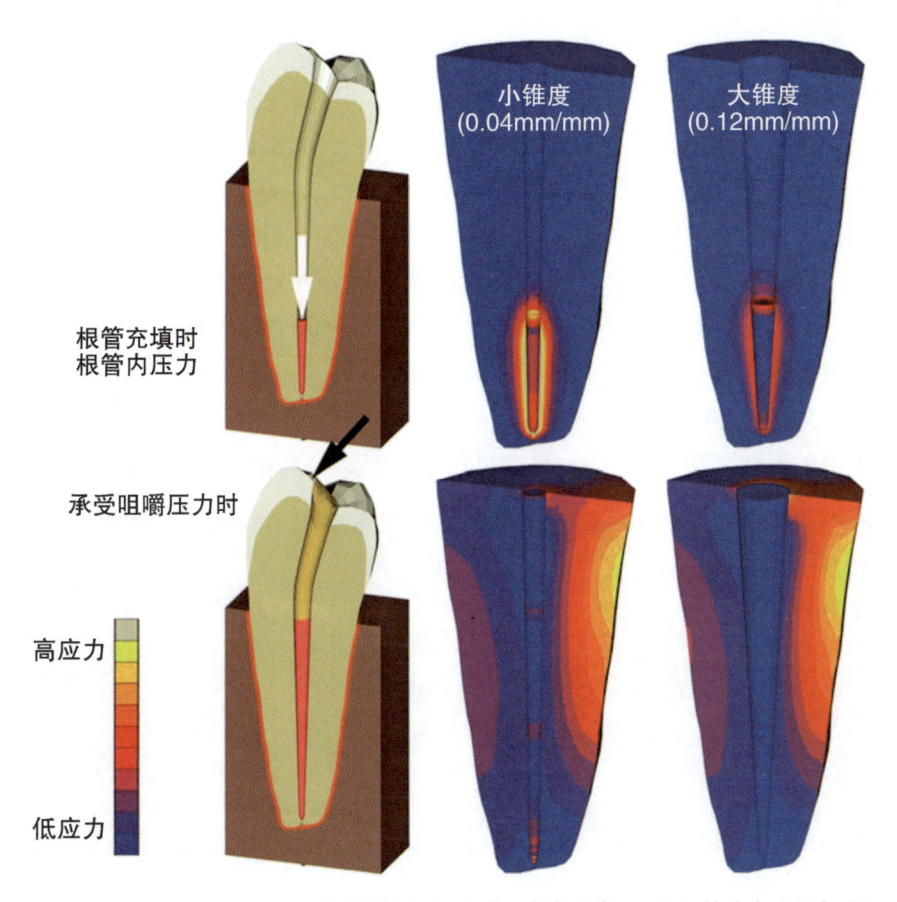

图 2-6　根的应力分布(改良范式等效应力)取决于载荷的类型：在根管治疗过程中，根管壁所受的应力最大；在咀嚼载荷作用下，根外表面所受的应力最大。在根管充填时，大锥度根管预备所受的应力通常低于小锥度根管预备，但在承受咀嚼压力时则相反

键的，小锥度根管尤其重要，小锥度根管在根尖部受到的压力更大，因此更易引起牙本质裂，特别是在根尖 1/3 处。尽管大锥度器械在进行根管预备时，根管也存在不完全光滑的状态，但相较于小锥度根管而言，大锥度根管预备器械可以使根管清洁得更彻底、根管壁更光滑；而且，大锥度器械预备根管后可以为后续根管桩的制备预留更大的空间。

2.6　根管治疗过程中温度升高及桩道制备对根折发生的影响

前面的章节我们讲到过，根折通常先发生在根管壁内侧，然后慢慢向牙根表面发展，根管治疗操作过程可能会引起根管壁微小裂纹的产生，之后可能会发展为根裂。如果牙齿的冠部组织余留很少，根管治疗后往往需要打根管桩以确保压力分布平衡，使牙齿可以正常行使功能。这些后续的治疗步骤，如冠部充填体的去除、根充材料的去除、桩道的制备等会产热，从而对牙齿及其邻近组织造成破坏，甚至会造成骨的破坏和吸收。此外，受热可使牙本质发生收缩，这可能是牙齿颈部发生折断的一个影响因素。

高温会对骨组织和牙周组织造成破坏，骨组织对47°以上的高温很敏感，如果将牙周组织暴露在43°温度下，会导致蛋白质的变性，通常认为，当温度升高超过10°时，会对牙齿的支持组织造成破坏。

阿曼达（Amade）等测量了根管治疗前到根管桩制备完成后，牙本质表面的温度变化（图2-7），根充过程中需要大量的聚合力才能使根充材

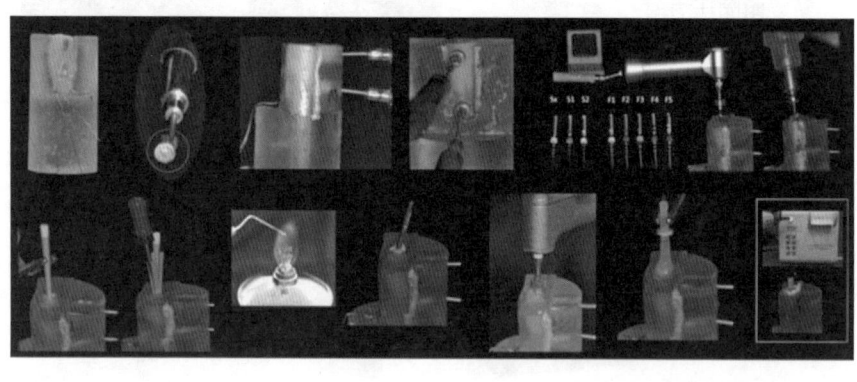

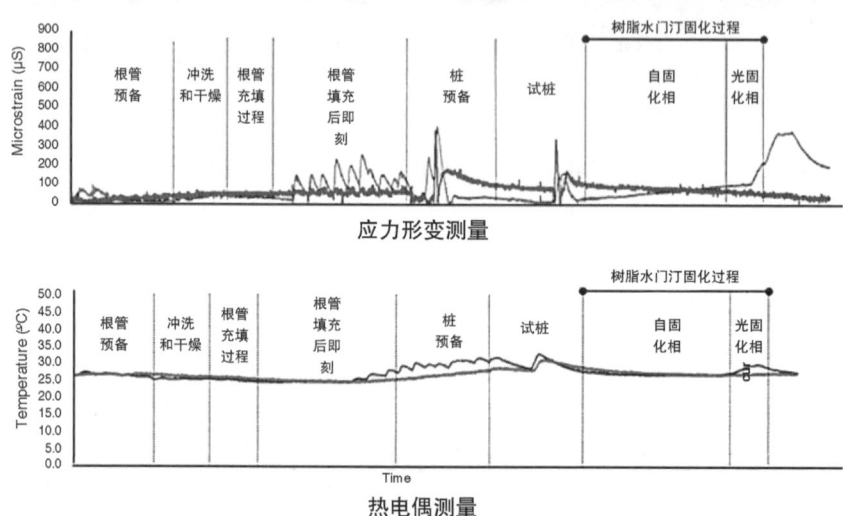

图2-7　牙髓治疗和玻璃纤维桩固过程中根部牙本质的应变及升温测量（红线：颈部1/3，绿线：根尖1/3）

料密合,在使用大锥度器械进行根管预备时,颈部牙本质受到的切削更大,这个研究可以解释为什么颈部牙本质的收缩率要大于根尖部的牙本质。大锥度器械的使用以及术者在进行根管充填时的操作与牙颈部根管壁的接触时间和面积都更大。在根管治疗过程中,去除封闭材料和预备桩道间隙是产热最多的步骤,去除封闭材料时,牙颈部的温度显著升高,可达3.0~7.8℃,这个温度变化还是低于会对组织产生破坏的临界温度10℃;而当为纤维玻璃桩进行桩道制备时,会产生高达10.8~14℃的温度变化,超出了避免组织破坏的临界温度。在桩道制备过程中,有一些因素可能影响到产热情况,比如扩孔钻的类型、操作时力的大小、扩孔钻和根管壁的摩擦、钻头的状态(新或旧)等。冲洗可以降低桩道预备过程中的温度升高,且术者在操作时应使用较新的钻头以使得在切削牙本质时的摩擦力较小,从而降低产热;另外,操作过程中应间断使用冲洗液冲洗以避免温度升高过快。

(梁景平　姜葳　译)

参考文献

Abou El Nasr HM, Abd El Kader KG (2014) Dentinal damage and fracture resistance of oval roots prepared with single-file systems using different kinematics. J Endod 40: 849–851.

Adorno CG, Yoshioka T, Suda H (2009) The effect of root preparation technique and instrumentation length on the development of apical root cracks. J Endod 35: 389–392.

Amade ES, Novais VR, Roscoe MG, Azevedo FM, Bicalho AA, Soares CJ (2013) Root dentin strain and temperature rise during endodontic treatment and post rehabilitation. Braz Dent J 24: 591–598.

Arslan H, Karatas E, Capar ID, Ozsu D, Doğanay E (2014) Effect of ProTaper Universal, Endoflare, Revo-S, HyFlex coronal flaring instruments, and Gates Glidden drills on crack formation. J Endod 40: 1681–1683.

Ashwinkumar V, Krithikadatta J, Surendran S, Velmurugan N (2014) Effect of reciprocating file motion on microcrack formation in root canals: an SEM study. Int Endod J 47: 622–627.

Barreto MS, Moraes Rdo A, Rosa RA, Moreira CH, Só MV, Bier CA (2012) Vertical root fractures and dentin defects: effects of root canal preparation, filling, and mechanical cycling. J Endod 38: 1135–1139.

Bier CA, Shemesh H, Tanomaru-Filho M, Wesselink PR, Wu MK (2009) The ability of different nickel-titanium rotary instruments to induce dentinal damage during canal preparation. J Endod 35: 236–238.

Blum JY, Cohen A, Machtou P, Micallef JP (1999) Analysis of forces developed during mechanical preparation of extracted teeth using Profile NiTi rotary instruments. Int Endod J 32: 24–31.

Brauer DS, Hilton JF, Marshall GW, Marshall SJ (2011) Nano- and micromechanical

properties of dentine: investigation of differences with tooth side. J Biomech 44: 1626 - 1629.
Brito-Junior M, Pereira RD, Verissimo C, Soares CJ, Faria-e-Silva AL, Camilo CC, Sousa-Neto MD (2014) Fracture resistance and stress distribution of simulated immature teeth after apexification with mineral trioxide aggregate. Int Endod J 47: 958 - 966.
Bürklein S, Tsotsis P, Schäfer E (2013) Incidence of dentinal defects after root canal preparation: reciprocating versus rotary instrumentation. J Endod 39: 501 - 504.
Carter JM, Sorensen SE, Johnson RR, Teitelbaum RL, Levine MS (1983) Punch shear testing of extracted vital and endodontically treated teeth. J Biomech 16: 841 - 848.
Carvalho RM, Fernandes CA, Villanueva R, Wang L, Pashley DH (2001) Tensile strength of human dentin as a function of tubule orientation and density. J Adhes Dent 3: 309 - 314.
Chatvanitkul C, Lertchirakarn V (2010) Stress distribution with different restorations in teeth with curved roots: a finite element analysis study. J Endod 36: 115 - 118.
Chen G, Fan W, Mishra S, El-Atem A, El-Atem A, Schuetz MA, Xiao Y (2012) Tooth fracture risk analysis based on a new finite element dental structure models using micro-CT data. Comput Biol Med 42: 957 - 963.
Coelho CS, Biffi JC, Silva GR, Abrahão A, Campos RE, Soares CJ (2009) Finite element analysis of weakened roots restored with composite resin and posts. Dent Mater J 28: 671 - 678.
Craig RG, Peyton FA (1958) Elastic and mechanical properties of human dentin. J Dent Res 37: 710 - 718.
De-Deus G, Silva EJ, Marins J, Souza E, Neves Ade A, Gonçalves Belladonna F, Alves H, Lopes RT, Versiani MA (2014) Lack of causal relationship between dentinal microcracks and root canal preparation with reciprocation systems. J Endod 40: 1447 - 1450.
Driscoll CO, Dowker SE, Anderson P, Wilson RM, Gulabivala K (2002) Effects of sodium hypochlorite solution on root dentine composition. J Mater Sci Mater Med 13: 219 - 223.
Eltit F, Ebacher V, Wang R (2013) Inelastic deformation and microcracking process in human dentin. J Struct Biol 183: 141 - 148.
Eriksson AR, Albrektsson T (1983) Temperature threshold levels for heat-induced bone tissue injury: a vital-microscopic study in the rabbit. J Prosthet Dent 50: 101 - 107.
Estrela C, Guedes OA, Pereira-Júnior W, Esponda L, Cruz AG (2009) Diagnosis of endodontic failure. In: Endodontic science. Artes Médicas, São Paulo, pp. 883 - 915.
Fuss Z, Lustig J, Katz A, Tamse A (2001) An evaluation of endodontically treated vertical root fractured teeth: impact of operative procedures. J Endod 27: 46 - 48.
Giannini M, Soares CJ, de Carvalho RM (2004) Ultimate tensile strength of tooth structures. Dent Mater 20: 322 - 329.
Grigoratos D, Knowles J, Ng YL, Gulabivala K (2001) Effect of exposing dentine to sodium hypochlorite and calcium hydroxide on its fl exural strength and elastic modulus. Int Endod J 34: 113 - 119.
Guedes OA, Chaves GS, Alencar AH, Borges AH, Estrela CR, Soares CJ, Estrela C (2014) Effect of gutta-percha solvents on fiberglass post bond strength to root canal dentin. J Oral Sci 56: 105 - 112.
Gutmann JL (1992) The dentin-root complex: anatomic and biologic considerations in restoring endodontically treated teeth. J Prosthet Dent 67: 458 - 467.
Gwinnett AJ (1992) Structure and composition of enamel. Oper Dent Suppl 5: 10 - 17.
Habelitz S, Marshall SJ, Marshall GW Jr, Balooch M (2001) Mechanical properties of human dental enamel on the nanometre scale. Arch Oral Biol 46: 173 - 183.
Harvey TE, White JT, Leeb IJ (1981) Lateral condensation stress in root canals. J Endod 7: 151 - 155.
Helfer AR, Melnick S, Schilder H (1972) Determination of the moisture content of vital and pulpless teeth. Oral Surg Oral Med Oral Pathol 34: 661 - 670.

Heulsmann M, Peters OA, Dummer PMH (2005) Mechanical preparation of root canals: shaping goals, techniques and means. Endod Topics 10: 30–76.

Holcomb JQ, Pitts DL, Nicholls JI (1987) Further investigation of spreader loads required to cause vertical root fracture during lateral condensation. J Endod 13: 277–284.

Kim HC, Cheung GS, Lee CJ, Kim BM, Park JK, Kang SI (2008) Comparison of forces generated during root canal shaping and residual stresses of three nickel-titanium rotary files by using a three-dimensional finite-element analysis. J Endod 34: 743–747.

Kim HC, Kwak SW, Cheung GS, Ko DH, Chung SM, Lee W (2012) Cyclic fatigue and torsional resistance of two new nickel-titanium instruments used in reciprocation motion: Reciproc versus WaveOne. J Endod 38: 541–544.

Kim HC, Lee MH, Yum J, Versluis A, Lee CJ, Kim BM (2010) Potential relationship between design of nickel-titanium rotary instruments and vertical root fracture. J Endod 36: 1195–1199.

Kim HC, Sung SY, Ha JH, Solomonov M, Lee JM, Lee CJ, Kim BM (2013) Stress generation during self-adjusting file movement: minimally invasive instrumentation. J Endod 39: 1572–1575.

Kinney JH, Marshall SJ, Marshall GW (2003) The mechanical properties of human dentin: a critical review and re-evaluation of the dental literature. Crit Rev Oral Biol Med 14: 13–29.

Kinney JH, Nalla RK, Pople JA, Breunig TM, Ritchie RO (2005) Age-related transparent root dentin: mineral concentration, crystallite size, and mechanical properties. Biomaterials 26: 3363–3376.

Lam PP, Palamara JE, Messer HH (2005) Fracture strength of tooth roots following canal preparation by hand and rotary instrumentation. J Endod 31: 529–532.

Lee BS, Hsieh TT, Chi DC, Lan WH, Lin CP (2004) The role of organic tissue on the punch shear strength of human dentin. J Dent 32: 101–107.

Lertchirakarn V, Palamara JE, Messer HH (2003) Patterns of vertical root fracture: factors affecting stress distribution in the root canal. J Endod 29: 523–528.

Lin CP, Douglas WH (1994) Structure–property relations and crack resistance at the bovine dentin-enamel junction. J Dent Res 73: 1072–1078.

Liu R, Hou BX, Wesselink PR, Wu MK, Shemesh H (2013) The incidence of root microcracks caused by 3 different single-file systems versus the ProTaper system. J Endod 39: 1054–1056.

Marshall GW Jr, Marshall SJ, Kinney JH, Kinney JH, Balooch M (1997) The dentin substrate: structure and properties related to bonding. J Dent 25: 441–458.

Mjör IA (1972) Human coronal dentine: structure and reactions. Oral Surg Oral Med Oral Pathol 33: 810–823.

Nalla RK, Kinney JH, Ritchie RO (2003) Effect of orientation on the in vitro fracture toughness of dentin: the role of toughening mechanisms. Biomaterials 24: 3955–3968.

O'Brien WJ (1987) Dental materials and their selection, 2nd edn. Quintessence Publishing Co., Chicago.

Perdigao J (2010) Dentin bonding-variables related to the clinical situation and the substrate treatment. Dent Mater 26: E24–E37.

Peters OA (2004) Current challenges and concepts in the preparation of root canal systems: a review. J Endod 30: 559–567.

Pitts DL, Matheny HE, Nicholls JI (1983) An in vitro study of spreader loads required to cause vertical root fracture during lateral condensation. J Endod 9: 544–550.

Ratih DN, Palamara JE, Messer HH (2007) Temperature change, dentinal fluid flow and cuspal displacement during resin composite restoration. J Oral Rehabil 34: 693–701.

Reeh ES, Messer HH, Douglas WH (1989) Reduction in tooth stiffness as a result of endodontic and restorative procedures. J Endod 15: 512–516.

Renovato SR, Santana FR, Ferreira JM, Souza JB, Soares CJ, Estrela C (2013) Effect of calcium hydroxide and endodontic irrigants on fibre post bond strength to root canal dentine. Int Endod J 46: 738-746.

Rundquist BD, Versluis A (2006) How does canal taper affect root stresses? Int Endod J 39: 226-237.

Saleh AA, Ettman WM (1999) Effect of endodontic irrigation solutions on microhardness of root canal dentine. J Dent 27: 43-46.

Salehrabi R, Rotstein I (2004) Endodontic treatment outcomes in a large patient population in the USA: an epidemiological study. J Endod 30: 846-850.

Santos-Filho PC, Verissimo C, Raposo LH, Noritomi PY, Marcondes Martins LR (2014) Influence of ferrule, post system, and length on stress distribution of weakened root-filled teeth. J Endod 40: 1874-1878.

Sathorn C, Palamara JE, Messer HH (2005) A comparison of the effects of two canal preparation techniques on root fracture susceptibility and fracture pattern. J Endod 31: 283-287.

Sauk JJ, Norris K, Foster R, Moehring J, Somerman MJ (1988) Expression of heat stress proteins by human periodontal ligament cells. J Oral Pathol 17: 496-499.

Saunders EM, Saunders WP (1989) The heat generated on the external root surface during post space preparation. Int Endod J 22: 169-173.

Schafer E, Lau R (1999) Comparison of cutting efficiency and instrumentation of curved canals with nickel-titanium and stainless-steel instruments. J Endod 25: 427-430.

Schafer E, Schulz-Bongert U, Tulus G (2004) Comparison of hand stainless steel and nickel titanium rotary instrumentation: a clinical study. J Endod 30: 432-435.

Schmidt KJ, Walker TL, Johnson JD, Nicoll BK (2000) Comparison of nickel-titanium and stainless- steel spreader penetration and accessory cone fit in curved canals. J Endod 26: 42-44.

Shemesh H, Roeleveld AC, Wesselink PR, Wu MK (2011) Damage to root dentin during retreatment procedures. J Endod 37: 63-66.

Shin CS, Huang YH, Chi CW, Lin CP (2014) Fatigue life enhancement of NiTi rotary endodontic instruments by progressive reciprocating operation. Int Endod J 47: 882-888.

Silva GR, Santos-Filho PC, Simamoto-Junior PC, Martins LR, Mota AS, Soares CJ (2011) Effect of post type and restorative techniques on the strain and fracture resistance of flared incisor roots. Braz Dent J 22: 230-237.

Soares CJ, Castro CG, Neiva NA, Soares PV, Santos-Filho PC, Naves LZ, Pereira PN (2010) Effect of gamma irradiation on ultimate tensile strength of enamel and dentin. J Dent Res 89: 159-164.

Soares CJ, Santana FR, Silva NR, Pereira JC, Pereira CA (2007) Influence of the endodontic treatment on mechanical properties of root dentin. J Endod 33: 603-606.

Soares CJ, Soares PV, de Freitas Santos-Filho PC, Castro CG, Magalhaes D, Versluis A (2008) The influence of cavity design and glass fiber posts on biomechanical behavior of endodontically treated premolars. J Endod 34: 1015-1019.

Stanford JW, Weigel KV, Paffenbarger GC, Sweeney WT (1960) Compressive properties of hard tooth tissues and some restorative materials. J Am Dent Assoc 60: 746-756.

Tamse A, Fuss Z, Lustig J, Kaplavi J (1999) An evaluation of endodontically treated vertically fractured teeth. J Endod 25: 506-508.

Tamse A (2006) Vertical root fractures in endodontically treated teeth: diagnostic signs and clinical management. Endod Topics 13: 84-94.

Tang W, Wu Y, Smales RJ (2010) Identifying and reducing risks for potential fractures in endodontically treated teeth. J Endod 36: 609-617.

Tidmarsh BG (1976) Restoration of endodontically treated posterior teeth. J Endod 2: 374-375.

Tronstad L (1973) Ultrastructural observations on human coronal dentin. Scand J Dent Res 81:

101 - 111.
Tsesis I, Rosen E, Tamse A, Taschieri S, Kfir A (2010) Diagnosis of vertical root fractures in end-odontically treated teeth based on clinical and radiographic indices: a systematic review. J Endod 36: 1455 - 1458.
Urabe I, Nakajima S, Sano H, Tagami J (2000) Physical properties of the dentin-enamel junction region. Am J Dent 13: 129 - 135.
Vasiliadis L, Darling AI, Levers BGH (1983) The amount and distribution of sclerotic human root dentin. Arch Oral Biol 28: 645 - 649.
Versluis A, Messer HH, Pintado MR (2006) Changes in compaction stress distributions in roots resulting from canal preparation. Int Endod J 39: 931 - 939.
Versluis A, Versluis-Tantbirojn D (2011) Filling cavities or restoring teeth? J Tenn Dent Assoc 91: 36 - 42, quiz 42 - 33.
Vire DE (1991) Failure of endodontically treated teeth: classification and evaluation. J Endod 17: 338 - 342.
Wilcox LR, Roskelley C, Sutton T (1997) The relationship of root canal enlargement to finger-spreader induced vertical root fracture. J Endod 23: 533 - 534.
Yared G (2008) Canal preparation using only one Ni-Ti rotary instrument: preliminary observations. Int Endod J 41: 339 - 344.
Yoldas O, Yilmaz S, Atakan G, Kuden C, Kasan Z (2012) Dentinal microcrack formation during root canal preparations by different NiTi rotary instruments and the self-adjusting file. J Endod 38: 232 - 235.
Zhi-Yue L, Yu-Xing Z (2003) Effects of post-core design and ferrule on fracture resistance of endodontically treated maxillary central incisors. J Prosthet Dent 89: 368 - 373.

根管治疗后的牙体修复：
制订治疗计划的思路

3

福阿德·巴德尔（Fouad Badr）
沃克-金·西奥格（Wook-Jin Seong）
乔奇·佩尔迪高（Jorge Perdigão）

摘　要

　　本章节旨在通过提供各种治疗思路，指导临床医师为根管治疗后患牙制订符合循证牙科学的治疗计划。值得注意的是，鉴于现有的部分文献缺乏临床相关性，其报道结果在实际运用于临床牙科学时仍面临局限性。

　　对牙体结构异常薄弱的活髓牙或死髓牙（包括剩余健康牙体组织很少，牙本质肩领不完整，以及邻面接触点少于 2 个）进行修复时，可能发生一些已知的临床并发症。在决定是否对患牙实施根管治疗前，患牙在整体牙列中预期行使的功能以及能否长期行使功能均应纳入考虑范畴。无论活髓牙还是死髓牙，一旦牙釉质和牙本质完整性遭到破坏，应考虑采用冠覆盖的修复方式。另外的章节将对各种不同桩核材料与其他修复手段展开讨论。

　　最后，作为临床医师，我们有责任告知患者尝试保存和修复患牙可能带来的风险效益以及所需付出的努力。

3.1　引言

　　牙齿存在于复杂的口腔环境中。人类的牙齿经历了各自不同的修复和/或创伤后，呈现出各式各样的形态。目前，牙科医师还不能通过基于干细胞的生物性牙修复与再生技术实现牙体修复。但作为临床医师，我们时常在工作中感觉自己不得不承担起"英雄牙医"的角色。在同一名患者口腔中发现多种牙体修复材料（比如金箔、硅酸盐水门汀、银汞合金、复合树脂、陶瓷等)的现象并不少见。有时,甚至能在同一颗牙上看到多种修复材料。无论在常规口腔检查还是对外伤或根尖周感染急诊患者进行临床评估时,医师都必须与患者在对患牙的处理意见上达成一致。对根尖周感染的患牙、因龋病或外伤导致大面积充填或严重破坏的患牙做出临床处理之前,医师必须首先从整体角度对全口牙列的临床状况进行评价,其次再检查患牙,并明确了解患者的临床症状、体征及其主诉。医师应根据患者的需求与偏好,科学结合患者本人的感受,实践循证牙科学原则。任何临床情况下,不管患牙是否接受过根管治疗,实践循证法都有利于为患牙制订治疗计划提供思路。

本章节将讨论临床医师在面对中重度破坏的患牙(伴或不伴牙髓来源的感染)时必须掌握的治疗思路。首先对患牙的牙髓活力进行判断,并对剩余健康牙体组织及其与牙周组织的关系进行评估,然后再决定患牙是否可以修复。如果患牙有修复的可能,且患者也愿意保留患牙,那么我们应进一步考虑患牙在整体牙列中预期行使的功能与可能承受的应力。为了使修复后的患牙彻底发挥预期功能,是否需要对患牙进行根管治疗或根管再治疗?是否有必要进行全冠或桩核修复?是否能通过牙本质肩领产生箍效应,抑或者患牙是否需要接受冠延长术或正畸牵引?本章节也将针对这些治疗方法带来的影响与后果展开讨论。最后,如果患者最终决定拔除患牙,本章节将回顾一些拔牙后不同的修复方案。

3.2 诊断

3.2.1 评估牙髓状态

在提供合理治疗方案之前,临床医师首先必须做出准确的诊断。通过详细采集临床和口腔病史,了解患者必要的背景信息后,医师必须重视患者现有的症状和体征,从而对患牙的牙髓状态做出判断。由于牙髓状态会随时间逐步发生改变,所以尽管实施了一系列临床检查,我们仍然很难对牙髓状态做出精确诊断。本章节将不对牙髓诊断的具体细节进行展开。通常,当牙髓状态为不可复性牙髓炎或牙髓坏死时,我们会对患牙采取根管治疗。但是,当患牙没有足够健康的牙体组织作为后续修复治疗的基础时,即使牙髓状态为深龋伴可复性牙髓炎或正常牙髓,我们也可对患牙选择性地进行根管治疗(Carrotte 2004)。

3.2.2 牙髓/牙周病变

无论是通过根尖孔或根管侧支,牙周组织和牙髓组织之间通常都存在紧密联系。牙髓病变可以导致根尖周病变,并且呈现类似于牙周病的影像学表现。综合患牙的牙髓状态、根尖周病损、是否存在隐裂纹或牙根纵裂这一系列信息进行精确分析,有助于临床医师做出正确诊断,并判断患牙病变是牙髓来源,还是牙周来源,抑或者牙髓牙周联合来源。

虽然通过临床检查可以判断牙髓状态,但即使是坏死牙髓也可能存在会被刺激的疼痛受体,从而导致检查出现假阳性(Dummer 等 1980)。有时,在进行牙髓活力测试时,邻近含金属的修复体可能会导致诊断错误(Stock 1995)。大部分情况下,如果检测显示牙髓有病变,常规根管治疗可以促进根尖周病损的愈合。局限于单个牙齿的牙周病变并不常见,牙周来源的患牙通常有更宽的牙周袋。

牙体发育异常、失败的根管治疗、不良冠方修复体带来的细菌感染也会导致根尖周病损(Ray 和 Trope 1985;Saunders 和 Saunders 1990,1994)。大面积龋坏引起的牙根穿孔、吸收,或根管机械预备过程中的医源性因素同样可能引发牙周牙髓联合病变(Seltzer 等 1970)。

3.2.3 牙吸收

牙髓是完整机体的一部分,当正常牙髓内的神经血供遭到破坏时,细菌就可能侵入并导致牙髓坏死(Andreasen 和 Kahler 2015),当然也会对牙周组织与周围骨组织造成潜在损伤。牙髓神经血供以及牙周膜的损伤可能导致牙吸收,这种吸收有时经适当治疗后可以停止(图3-1)。在牙吸收造成大量牙体组织破坏之前,临床医师可以通过根管治疗术(Heithersay 1999)或截冠术(Malmgren 等 2006)保留牙齿。但医师必须明白,牙吸收可能是创伤性的或特发性的(Rivera 和 Walton 1994),也可能伴发于牙根折裂。明确是哪种类型的牙吸收很重要,因为有些牙吸收需要进行根管治疗,而有些则不需要。牙体牙髓科医师必须对此做出适当的评估。

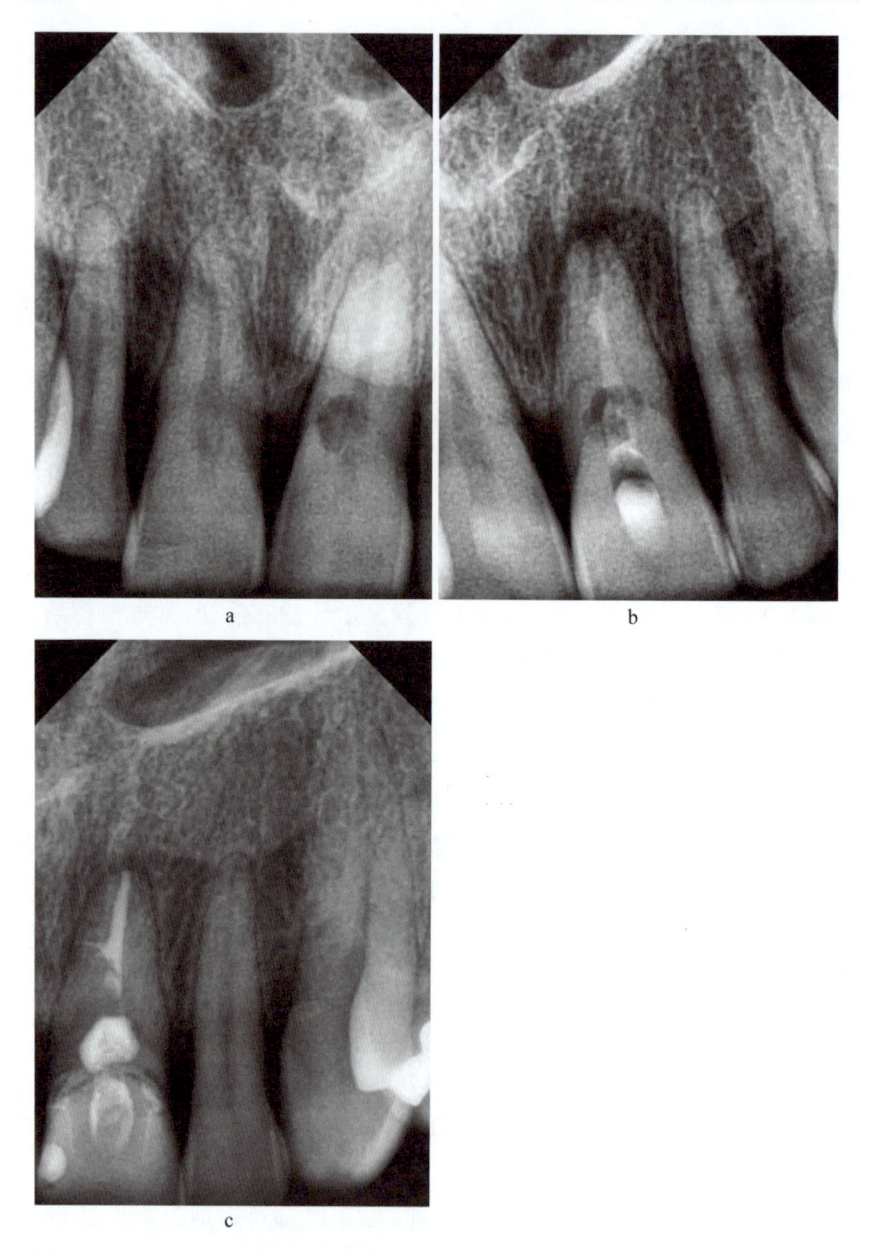

图 3-1　a. 患者主诉牙龈异常肿物。口内检查发现左上中切牙的唇颊侧黏膜局限性肿胀，牙周探诊在正常范围内，并且患者无症状。所有前牙叩痛不明显。患者自诉1年前有牙外伤史。左上中切牙根尖片显示根尖有阴影，伴随疑似内外穿通的炎症性吸收，牙髓测试无活力；b. 医师开始对患牙进行根管治疗，并使用氢氧化钙封药试图形成钙化；c. 根管治疗完成后，医师通过外科手术在患牙牙根颊侧，即牙根吸收导致根管与牙周膜间隙相通的地方放置了 ProRoot MTA（Dentsply Tulsa Dental Specialties）。随后在根管内黏结纤维桩，并制作临时冠。

3.2.4 牙周评估

评估牙周状态需要考虑很多因素。判断患牙预后时,患者年龄、最初骨丧失量、牙周探诊深度、临床附着丧失、松动度、牙根形态、根分叉病变以及患者吸烟与否,这些因素都需要被考虑在内。在一项回顾性研究中,米勒(Miller)等对 102 名患者(816 颗磨牙)进行了常规牙周治疗,并根据牙周预后因素对所有牙齿进行评分。他们发现所有被评估的因素中,吸烟是最大的危险因子(吸烟者发生牙齿丧失的可能性比不吸烟者增加了 246%),远超过牙周袋深度、松动度以及根分叉病变的影响。研究者同时提到,78.3% 的磨牙经治疗后不会被拔除,并可平均保留 24.2 年,这说明可以通过预防性的牙周支持治疗保持牙周健康(Miller 等 2014)。但这项研究的局限性在于没有评估根分叉病变的严重程度,只涉及了根分叉病变的存在与否。而维护口腔健康的专业人员都知道,根分叉病变越严重,患者保持口腔卫生的难度越大。同样,牙周袋超过 3 mm 也不利于维持口腔卫生,牙周手术则能通过减小牙周袋深度,更有利于维持口腔卫生。

另该研究中,针对预后评估中用于准确预测患牙使用寿命的常用临床参数,为了检测其有效性,研究者对 100 名接受了牙周治疗并处于牙周维护期的患者(2 509 颗牙齿)开展了历时 16 年的前瞻性研究。结果发现,最初探诊深度、最初根分叉病变、最初松动度、最初冠根比以及不戴殆垫情况下的口腔不良习惯均与牙齿缺失有关(McGuire 和 Nunn 1996)。固定局部义齿的基牙缺失率低于可摘局部义齿的基牙。有趣的是,研究者认为固定局部义齿基牙有更高的存留率可能与选择基牙的条件有关,因为只有非常健康的牙齿才会被选作固定义齿基牙。

许多学者均指出,牙周因素是导致拔牙最常见的原因,42.6% 被拔除的牙齿以及 59.4% 根管治疗后被拔除的患牙都是源于牙周因素(Fonzar 等 2009)。当美学形态不佳的牙齿发生根尖周炎或需要根管再治疗时,研究者更推荐拔除患牙并进行种植修复(Setzer 和 Kim 2014)。然而,就如上述讨论的,如果进行适当的牙周治疗,即使患牙有中度垂直型骨吸收或根分叉病变,也可取得较好的预后(Setzer 和 Kim 2014)。

任何牙齿的坚固程度取决于其最薄弱部分。如果牙齿的根基受到损害,整体预后也将不容乐观。除口腔急诊外,任何治疗开始前都应该先确保并维持牙周健康。正如我们在随后讨论中提到的,牙齿会受到来自各个方向的机械力。牙齿的牙周支持力越弱,施加在牙体牙周整体系统上的水平力量可能增加,修复体和牙周组织将承受更多应力。对于非完美但尚健康的牙周组织,临床医师必须考虑在修复过程中实现应力分布,这对减轻非正中运动时的咬合力具有重要意义。例如,在修复一个冠根比不佳但尚在接受范围内的尖牙时,医师应该考虑选择组牙功能𬌗而非尖牙保护𬌗。

3.3 牙体修复

根据流程图(图3-2)制订综合治疗计划前,有必要对包括患牙在内的整体口腔进行评估。临床医师必须评估整体牙周支持组织状况、咬合关系以及患者是否存在口腔不良习惯。在考虑整体治疗计划中𬌗平面的问题时,与𬌗平面不协调的伸长牙可能导致其与对𬌗牙之间没有足够的垂直空间。如果此时需要修复对𬌗牙,那么治疗计划中可能包括对伸长牙进行正畸压低或牙冠高度修整,并可能需要进行根管治疗(图3-3)。同时,对于已完成根管治疗的患牙,医师必须评估根管治疗的质量。正如第1章所述,根管治疗质量不佳仍是修复失败的一个主要原因。

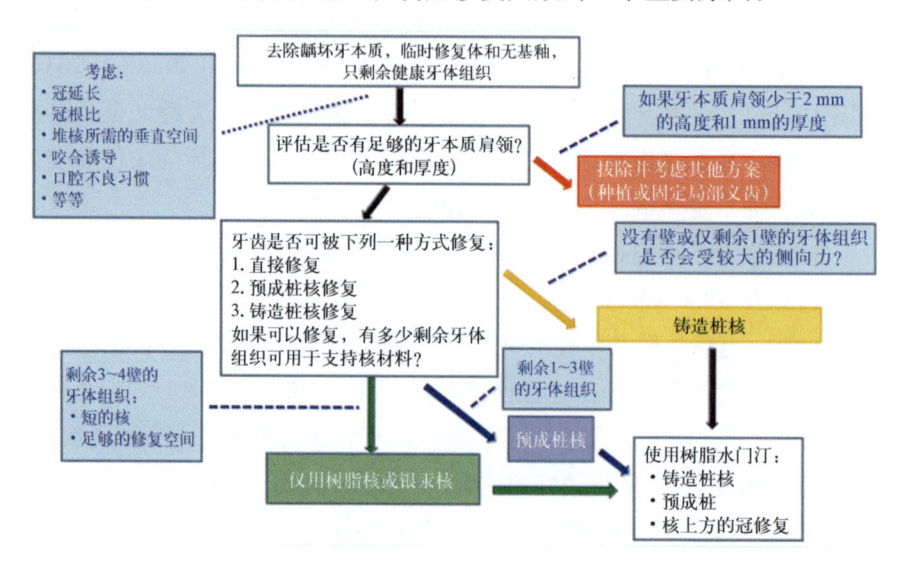

图3-2 贯穿第3章的治疗计划流程图

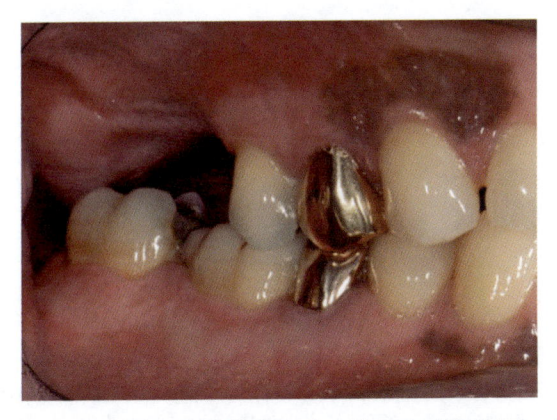

图3-3 这张照片显示右下第二磨牙(镜像)已向上萌出至对颌无牙区。右上第一磨牙拔除多年后,患者现在考虑修复右上第一磨牙。为使右下第二磨牙回到正常的殆平面上,可能需要进行多学科间合作治疗,包括正畸移动和/或牙冠高度修整和/或根管治疗。

固定局部义齿或可摘局部义齿基牙承受的应力与单冠基牙不同。最后,在决定是否需要对基牙进行冠延长时,基牙的冠根比、牙根锥度、根分叉位置等因素都必须纳入考虑范畴。

3.3.1 剩余牙体组织的评估

有些临床情况(比如牙根纵折或隐裂延伸至根尖到达牙周膜)可以考虑直接拔除患牙,尤其当患者不希望医师通过手术探查明确患牙可修复性的时候。而在另一些拔牙指征并不明确的情况下,临床医师需要将龋坏的牙本质和/或不良修复体去除后才能合理评估患牙的整体状态(图3-4)。也只有通过这样做,我们才能判断拟制作的修复体边缘是否会违反生物学原则(见图1-2),以及剩余健康牙体组织是否能够提供足够的支持力保证修复体使用寿命和功能。同时在这一阶段,我们还需评估患牙的冠根比及其在牙列中受到的咬合力大小,从而判断是否有必要实施冠延长术(图3-2)。

3.3.2 牙本质肩领

去除龋坏牙本质和不良修复体后,牙体四周都必须留有健康的牙体组织形成颈部的牙本质肩领,更多关于牙本质肩领的详细解释参考第1章。

如果即使对患牙进行辅助外科手术和/或正畸治疗(手术与正畸治疗的前提是不会严重影响牙齿预后),也仍然无法获得2 mm高度的牙本质

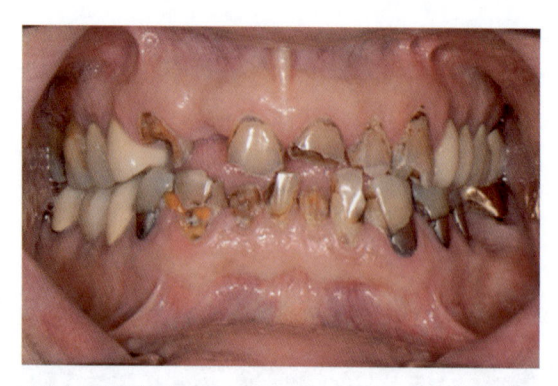

图 3-4 即使不去除龋坏牙本质和不良修复体，我们也可以明确患者有些牙齿已无法修复。无论是否进行根管治疗，通过冠延长术在健康牙体组织上获得足够的牙本质肩领都会破坏冠根比。考虑到牙根的锥度，任何形式的全冠牙体预备都会使剩余牙本质壁变得很薄。

肩领，那么就应该选择拔除患牙（图 3-4）。如果患牙在去除龋坏牙本质或不良修复体，经历外伤或根管治疗后已有大量牙体组织缺损，但仍有至少高 2 mm 和厚 1 mm 的牙本质肩领时，临床医师必须考虑在进行全冠修复牙备之前先恢复基本的牙体结构。有时，牙体组织破坏范围太大以至于接近髓腔，这种情况下有必要选择性地进行根管治疗和堆核，后者可以增强未来修复体的固位力和抗力性。

根据汉普顿（Hempton）和多米尼奇（Dominici）（2010）的研究，导致修复体脱落的力量大多发生在修复体下 1/3，因此修复体边缘的位置至关重要。临床医师必须避免将修复体边缘部分或全部放置在所堆的核上，警惕避免咬合产生的应力传导到恢复牙体基本结构的充填体上，或在有桩核修复的情况下传导到桩与牙根的交界面上。桩与牙根之间通常靠水门汀黏结，殆力作用下黏结剂疲劳可能会导致桩核脱落或基牙折裂。在一项体外研究中，皮洛（Pilo）等（2008）建议为了防止基牙折裂，限定牙本质肩领的最小厚度和高度相当重要。他们认为折裂通常发生于牙体组织而非核材料，且发生牙体折裂的概率与去除的牙本量直接相关。

3.3.3 牙本质和牙釉质完整性

值得一提的是，在预备根管和桩道时必须格外小心。过量预备会导致根管过分扩大以及不必要的牙本质去除。为防止牙体折裂，并在预备堆核的情况下对核材料提供适当的支持作用，必须保证至少有 1 mm 的根管牙本质厚度（Quzounian 和 Schilder 1991）。

正如前面章节所述,根管治疗后牙本质的机械性能会发生改变。然而,窝洞预备类型对牙尖变形(牙尖分离)的影响可能更显著。有一项研究指出,完整下颌磨牙牙尖变形幅度不超过 1 μm,近中邻𬌗面洞患牙的变形幅度小于 2 μm,近远中邻𬌗面洞患牙的变形幅度为 3~5 μm。根管治疗后,近中邻𬌗面洞组的牙尖变形幅度为 7.0~8.0 μm,近远中邻𬌗面洞组的幅度为 12.0~17.0 μm(Panitvisai 和 Messer 1995)。研究者提倡保护牙釉质的连续性,这将有助于保持牙齿的刚度;今后,临床医师必须重视保护牙尖,尤其对于根管治疗后的患牙,制备近远中邻𬌗面洞导致的牙尖变形幅度将比近中邻𬌗面洞增加 2~3 倍。

相比根管治疗后牙本质的机械性能,我们似乎更应关注最初造成患牙需要接受根管治疗的牙体形态破坏。患牙釉质的完整性可能比是否做过根管治疗更重要。接下来,我们将进一步探讨牙体完整性对患牙整体预后影响的相关报道。

回顾治疗计划流程图(图 3-2),在对牙齿承受的应力进行评估后,我们需要回答两个问题:① 是否有足够的剩余健康牙体组织支持堆核?② 剩余牙体组织是否足够坚固到可以抵抗牙颈部冠折?如果这两个问题的答案都是"否",那么需要考虑使用铸造桩核或预成桩核。如果这两个问题的答案都是"是",那么可以考虑仅使用(复合树脂或银汞)核修复(图 3-2 和图 3-5)。

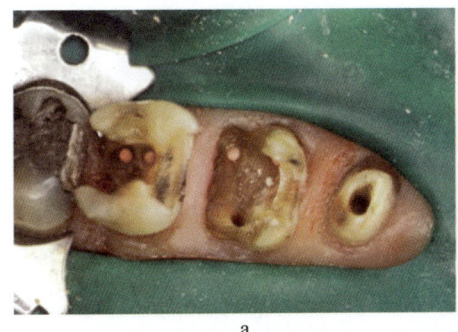

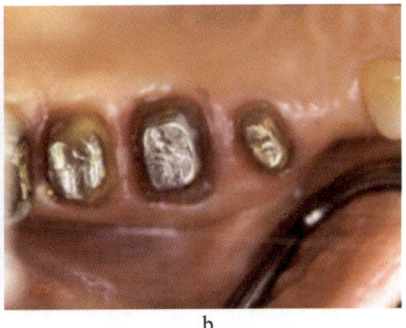

图 3-5 a. 去除龋坏牙本质和薄壁后,患者右上第二前磨牙的剩余牙体组织量已经不足以支持堆核,并且强度无法抵抗牙颈部的冠折。右上第一磨牙只剩余不到 3 个壁,因此需要通过打桩支持堆核。而右上第二磨牙有足够的剩余壁,可以支持堆核以及抵抗牙颈部冠折;b. 医师对右上第二前磨牙采用铸造桩核,在右上第一磨牙的腭根内放置预成金属桩,并在其上堆了银汞核。另外,采用银汞核重建右上第二磨牙缺失的牙体组织。

在一项为期3年的随机临床试验中，卡吉迪亚科（Cagidiaco）等（2008）根据根管治疗后，基牙预备前冠方牙本质的剩余量，将360颗前磨牙分成6组，每组60颗。再将每组60颗牙齿随机分为使用和不使用纤维桩的两个亚组。他们认为，当剩余牙体有4个完整壁时不需要使用（纤维）桩，但一旦有1个壁缺失，那么不使用桩的牙齿就会出现修复失败。在安放桩的牙齿中，只有1个壁残留，以及冠方没有壁并且有或没有2 mm牙本质肩领的牙齿修复失败率增加。法拉利（Ferrari）等的两项研究（2007，2012）同样指出，纤维桩的使用能在很大程度上降低根管治疗后前磨牙的修复失败率。冠方保留一侧牙体壁可以明显降低修复失败风险。

在冠方有3个或4个牙体壁保留的情况下，临床医师需在不同的核材料中进行选择。在一项疲劳研究中，科瓦里克（Kovarik）等（1992）测试了玻璃离子水门汀（glass ionomer cement，GIC）、复合树脂以及银汞作为冠下方核材料的抗疲劳性能。使用GIC核的冠在20 000次应力循环后全部破损。80%使用复合树脂核的冠在50 000次循环后破损。对于使用银汞核的冠，有30%在70 000次循环后遭到破损。盖图（Gateau）等（2001）报道指出，基于GIC的两种核材料相比银汞更易发生破损，提示GIC类材料的抗疲劳强度并不适用于桩核修复。有些医师曾采用银加强型GIC类材料（即金属陶瓷）堆核。正如康贝（Combe）等（1999）所述，尽管金属陶瓷GIC材料在耐压强度方面与某些树脂相似，但它在抗拉伸、抗弯曲以及各种模量方面是最弱的材料之一。金属陶瓷GIC材料并不适用于后牙堆核。

3.4 根管治疗后牙齿的预后

如果不考虑修复，根管消毒和根管充填都完善到位，那么根管治疗的效果是可预见的。对于术前不存在根尖周炎症的患牙而言，初次根管治疗的成功率在90%以上（Marquis等2006）。但若患牙术前已存在根尖周炎，那么成功率将降低至80%左右（Sjogren等1990；de Chevigny等2008）。

吉伦（Gillen）等（2011）在系统综述中指出，各方面治疗都会影响患牙的整体预后，包括牙周、根管以及修复治疗。若冠方修复体不密合，微生物将通过修复体边缘的缺陷处进入,那么患牙根尖周炎症维持愈合状态的概率就会降低。

3.4.1 前牙根管治疗后的存留率

人们通常认为根管治疗后未行冠修复的前牙相较于后牙更不易发生折断。但是,近期一项基于140万颗根管治疗后患牙的研究(Salehrabi和Rotstein 2004)表明,被拔除的前牙中83%未行冠修复,9.7%行冠桩修复,7.3%行冠而未行桩修复。2004年的这次大规模研究结果与索伦森和马丁诺夫在1984年报道的结果不同。1984年,索伦森和马丁诺夫的研究结果表明,根管治疗后的前牙若行冠修复,其预后与不行冠修复相比无明显改善。关于纤维桩对修复根管治疗后的前牙带来的积极影响请参阅第6章。

3.4.2 后牙根管治疗后的存留率

后牙根管治疗后若未行冠修复,其发生折裂的可能性大于活髓牙(Aquilino和Caplan 2002)。另一项研究表明,未行冠修复的患牙保存的平均周期为50个月,而行全冠修复的死髓牙保存的平均周期为安放修复体后87个月(Vire 1991)。一项回顾性队列研究显示,对于除开髓孔外无缺损的根管治疗后磨牙,可使用复合树脂充填体进行成功修复。有趣的是,复合树脂充填体的临床效果比银汞合金更好。修复后2年,复合树脂充填的修复成功率为90%,而银汞合金为77%。修复后5年,两种充填材料修复成功率均明显下降,复合树脂及银汞合金分别为38%和17%(Nagasiri和Chitmongkolsuk 2005)。类似地,一项3年的调查发现,根管治疗后的前磨牙若仅行桩修复,并直接使用复合树脂充填Ⅱ类洞,其成功率与全冠修复的前磨牙相当(Mannocci等2002)。

如第1章所述,银汞合金在有足够厚度的前提下可用于覆盖与牙齿缺失边缘嵴相邻的牙尖。为起到保护作用,建议银汞合金的厚度在功能尖处为4.0 mm,在非功能尖处为3.0 mm(Liberman等1987)。

为了从整体角度出发考虑患牙的可修复性,我们有必要评估牙齿未来将承受的应力。有科学证据表明,根管治疗后的牙齿在牙弓中的位置和功能会影响其存留率,这部分内容我们将在下一节中讨论。另外,第6

章还涵盖了纤维桩放置对根管治疗后的后牙使用寿命和预后的影响。

3.4.3 邻面接触点的重要性

患牙存在两个邻面接触点有助于提高其根管治疗后的存留率(Aquilino 和 Caplan 2002；Caplan 等 2002)。卡普兰(Caplan)等(2002)对 280 名患者(400 颗牙齿)的病历和 X 线照片进行了回顾性研究，认为根管治疗后的牙齿如果邻面接触点少于 2 个，其存留率低于 2 个邻面接触点均存在的患牙。为了强调这一点，一项基于 14 项临床研究的 meta 分析也印证了这个结果。以下因素有利于提高根管治疗后患牙的存留率，按影响程度从大到小依次排列：① 根管治疗后行全冠修复；② 同时有近远中邻面接触的牙；③ 不作为活动或固定修复基牙的牙；④ 牙齿类型，特别是非磨牙的牙(Balto 2011)。

另一项历时 4 年，包括 759 颗初次根管治疗和 858 颗根管再治疗牙齿的前瞻性研究表明，有 2 个邻面接触点的患牙缺失风险相较于邻面接触点少于 2 个的患牙低 50%。这项研究还指出，位于牙列末端的患牙缺失率相较于非末端牙增加近乎 96%(Ng 等 2011)。在一项 10 年的随访研究中，阿奎里诺(Aquilino)和卡普兰证实了第二磨牙的存留率明显低于其他任何类型的牙。根管治疗后第二磨牙的存留率较其他牙低至 5 倍以上，其原因可能是第二磨牙承受的𬌗力较大，而且根管治疗中直线通路建立受阻和视野受限也增加了第二磨牙的治疗难度(Aquilino 和 Caplan 2002)。

现已证实，根管治疗后牙齿在牙列中的位置，以及邻面接触点的存在或缺失对其存留率具有显著影响。这可能是因为位于远中或邻面接触点缺失的牙齿需承受更大的𬌗力与非轴向力。同时，若不考虑患者的咀嚼力，当对𬌗为常规全口义齿丙烯酸牙时，根管治疗后牙齿承受的压力比对𬌗为种植体单冠时更小。这种压力主要取决于对𬌗修复体的回弹性能，而非修复体材料本身。

3.4.4 固定局部义齿和可摘局部义齿

多项临床研究表明，相比活髓牙，由根管治疗后的牙齿作为基牙的固定局部义齿失败率更高(Reuter 和 Brose 1984；Karlsson 1986；Palmqvist 和 Swartz 1993；Sundh 和 Odman 1997)。20 多年前，索伦森和马丁诺夫

(1985)回顾了超过6 000名患者的病历记录,针对其中1 273颗接受过根管治疗并作为固定局部义齿或可摘局部义齿基牙的牙齿,他们得出结论:根管治疗后牙齿作为固定局部义齿和可摘局部义齿基牙时的失败率明显高于单冠。根管治疗后的牙齿作为固定局部义齿和可摘局部义齿基牙时的成功率分别为89.2%和77.4%。有趣的是,他们还发现放置桩会导致患牙单冠修复时的成功率明显降低,但对其作为固定局部义齿基牙时的成功率没有明显影响,对其作为可摘局部义齿基牙时的成功率有明显提高。不过该研究为回顾性研究,研究中有一些未被记录的因素,可能影响可摘局部义齿的功能和根管治疗后牙齿所受应力,包括支托和固位体的设计、游离端基托的适应性以及咬合关系。此外,研究未对远中游离端的跨度进行记录,也未对牙支持式可摘局部义齿和远中端游离可摘局部义齿进行区分。

更近期的一项临床研究比较了固定局部义齿和单冠修复20年的预后。研究者发现,至少有一颗基牙接受过根管治疗的三单位固定桥与活髓牙作为基牙的固定局部义齿相比,两者成功率无明显差异。单端固定和三单位以上的固定局部义齿失败率更高(De Backer等2007)。再次强调,在考虑将根管治疗后的牙齿作为修复体基牙时,我们必须首先关注对颌的修复体(如果有的话)、基牙的牙周情况、骨组织支持和基牙将承受的应力大小。有些情况下,临床医师的判断将起到重要作用。如一种情况是一个三单位后牙固定局部义齿的两个固位体均为根管治疗后基牙,其对颌为稳定的常规全口义齿;另一种情况是一个非末端经根管治疗后单冠修复的后牙,其对颌为种植体单冠,关于这两种情况哪一种对根管治疗后牙齿预后更有利,现有的文献尚未给出结论。

3.5 辅助外科手术

3.5.1 生物学宽度

当龋坏的牙本质、窝洞或现有的修复体范围大且接近牙根时,如果计划对患牙实施冠延长术,那么我们必须考虑生物学宽度(见图1-2)。侵犯生物学宽度可能会引起慢性炎症(Gunay等2000),甚至导致牙周组织破坏

(Cunliffe 和 Grey 2008)。加吉洛(Gargiulo)等(1961)发表了最早关于生物学宽度大小问题的研究之一，计算出龈牙结合部的平均深度为 2.04 mm，上皮附着的平均值为 0.97 mm，结缔组织附着的平均值为 1.07 mm。

关于修复体边缘的位置，有些研究者主张从冠边缘到牙槽嵴顶必须保持 3 mm 的生物学距离，避免冠边缘的菌斑堆积导致牙周附着丧失(Nevins 和 Skurow 1984)。另一项回顾性研究指出，如果最初磨牙修复体边缘到牙槽骨的距离小于 4 mm，那么其中 40%的磨牙将在冠修复 5 年后发生根分叉病变(Dibart 等 2003)。

尽管通常认为牙槽嵴顶到修复体边缘的距离不小于 3 mm 可有效避免牙周附着丧失的发生，临床医师仍必须时刻谨记每位患者的牙体解剖是存在细微差异的。瓦切克(Vacek)等(1994)验证了与加吉洛等先前研究类似的假说，并报道了生物学宽度的范围(表 3-1)。临床检查中，充分的牙周探诊和适当的 X 线片对判断患牙生物学宽度非常重要。

表 3-1 生物学宽度的范围(上皮附着＋结缔组织附着)

牙 位	测量值(mm)	范围(mm)
前 牙	1.75±0.56	0.75～3.29
前磨牙	1.97±0.67	0.78～4.33
磨 牙	2.08±0.55	0.84～3.29

通常，我们会对修复体是否会侵犯生物学宽度产生疑虑。不过，如果患者愿意，有一种较好的方法是在决定进行冠延长术之前，先采用长期临时修复体检测上皮附着在修复体边缘刺激下可能发生的变化。尤其需要注意临时修复体的边缘必须密合，并且进行适当抛光，以防止边缘渗漏和/或诱导炎症反应的菌斑堆积。

3.5.2 冠延长术

当剩余牙体组织少、正常牙本质无法提供足够固位力和抗力性时，临床医师可能需要通过外科手术来"创造"更多的健康牙体组织。冠延长手术过程中可能需要结合正畸牵引术(图 3-6)。这一章节我们不具体讨论正畸牵引术的细节，有兴趣的读者可以在其他相关口腔医学论著上找到

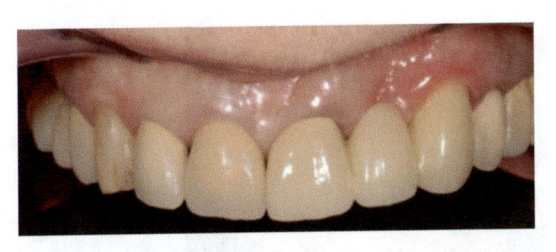

图 3-6 该临床病例中,患者的牙龈组织有明显炎症。固定局部义齿(9-X-11)的固位体边缘明显侵犯了上皮附着。若要施行冠延长术,临床医师必须在术中格外留意邻牙的龈缘水平,并可以考虑实施正畸牵引术结合冠延长术。

大量信息。通过冠延长术获得的健康牙体组织被后期修复体包绕,使殆力得以分散至牙周组织而不是桩-核-牙体组织界面。但由于牙齿的松动会导致殆力对修复体产生的水平分力增加,必须注意牙齿修复后的冠根比。牙周膜可以承担的轴向力是水平分力的 17 倍(Thayer 1980)。一些学者在对 10 颗天然中切牙进行桩冠修复时预备了 2 mm 牙本质肩领,并将其与 10 颗无牙本质肩领的对照牙进行比较,体外检测牙本质肩领对牙齿抗折强度的影响。研究者建议相较于牙本质肩领的存在与否,更应关注桩的长度。

我们不能仅仅为了使后期修复体可以包绕在健康的牙体组织周围提高抗折性,就决定采用冠延长术获得牙本质肩领。在整体治疗计划的制订过程中还有其他因素应被重视。

为保持修复体良好的稳定性,冠根比必须保持不超过 1∶1。考虑到牙周组织减少后仍要承受相同的负载,不合理的治疗计划可能导致牙齿松动度增加。此外,当牙根距离近时,很难在不破坏牙根的情况下移除牙间骨质。软组织不能向根向复位也会导致冠延长受限。

临床医师需谨记越向牙齿根方预备,牙本质壁就越薄,露髓或横向修复空间不足导致修复体外形突度过大的可能性就越高。医师必须尽量选择合适的终止线,特别对于下颌前牙(Borelli 等 2015)。

为了保持牙周健康和防止造成膜龈缺损,保持至少 2~3 mm 的附着龈宽度尤其重要(图 3-7)(Maynard 和 Wilson 1979)。

最后,临床医师需关注整个牙列和整体的治疗方案。对出于美学考虑进行治疗或者笑线较高的患者,嘴唇位置可能显露牙龈水平的不和谐并影响美学效果。在前牙被动萌出的情况下,如果临床牙冠较短,笑线较高,那

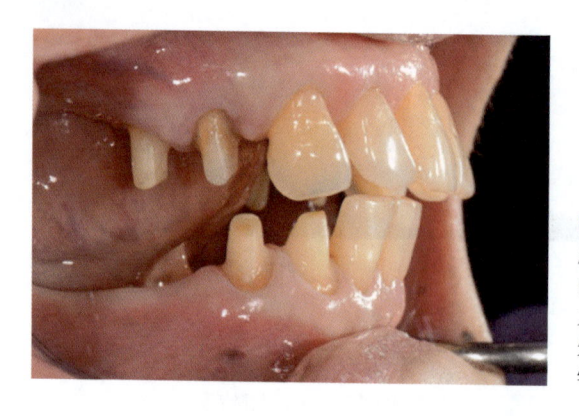

图 3-7 该患者的右侧上颌前磨牙经牙体预备后,尽管有足够的牙本质肩领,并且符合其他抗力和固位原则,但是附着龈的缺失明显,违反了牙体预备的生物学学则。

么有时会导致牙龈暴露过多。如果患者希望前牙区有更好的比例,那就可能有必要通过冠延长术暴露更多的解剖牙冠(Allen 1993;McGuire 1998)。在这些情况下,必须制作诊断蜡型为外科医师提供手术导板,从而合理确定新修复体的边缘位置。当龈下龋损并未向根方进展至牙根时,功能性和美学性的冠延长可以相结合。同时,需要特别关注邻间乳头可能出现丧失。医师必须决定是否需要对牙间牙槽骨进行切除手术,或是否手术应只限于唇侧。在因龈间隙增宽而导致美学效果不佳时,修复医师可能需要更好地调整修复体轮廓或增宽修复体接触区。当相邻牙间牙槽嵴顶和修复体接触点之间的距离大于 5 mm 时,相邻牙间会出现黑三角(Tarnow 等 1992)(图 3-8)。

3.6 缺失牙的修复方案选择

当一颗或几颗牙无法修复或预后不佳时,通常只能选择拔除患牙。在对缺失牙的修复方案进行讨论之前,临床医师必须先告知患者对患牙做出的诊断以及相关依据。

3.6.1 固定局部义齿

固定局部义齿许多年来都被认为是修复的金标准。它们相对制作较快,并且医师能对其预期的修复效果做出适当判断。不可否认的是,固定局部义齿的不足之处是需要对邻牙进行预备和难以清洁。不过,虽然修复体的桥体难以清洁,但更多时候是因为患者自身不愿对桥体下方进行

3 根管治疗后的牙体修复：制订治疗计划的思路　　57

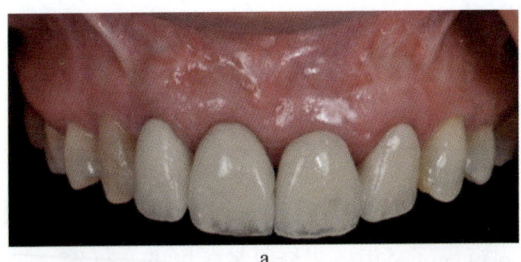

图3-8　a. 患者佩戴上颌右侧侧切牙、右侧中切牙（种植体）、左侧中切牙和左侧侧切牙的临时冠近6个月，使龈乳头逐渐长入龈间隙；b. 最终，医师仅对患者上颌左侧中切牙的唇侧施行了冠延长术，配合永久修复体合适的外形取得了令人满意的美学效果（感谢Remi Elkattah医师和Aram Torosian口腔技师提供该病例）。

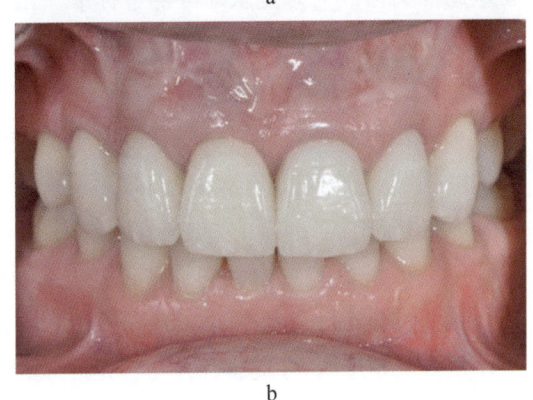

清洁，从而影响修复体的存留率，增加修复体边缘发生龋坏的风险。尽管已有一些桥体下方发生骨沉积的病例报道，但是由于缺乏牙周膜对牙槽骨的刺激作用，多数情况下桥体下方会发生骨丧失，导致修复科医师和口腔技工需要制作比正常形态更大的桥体或用粉红色瓷掩盖缺损。

　　一些研究者已报道了固定局部义齿的使用寿命。萨利纳斯（Salinas）等（2004）提出固定局部义齿15年的存留率是69%。另一些研究者认为20年存留率为50%～69%（Budtz-Jorgensen 1996）。固定局部义齿邻牙10年的存留率为92%（Aquilino等2001）。合适的修复方案必须符合循证牙科学，并满足患者的期望。今后，患者也可以选择其他治疗方式修复缺牙区。

3.6.2　可摘局部义齿

　　可摘局部义齿是一种相对廉价的缺失牙修复方式，并且具有修复软组织缺损的作用。遗憾的是，患者有时会有一种"满口异物"的感觉。根据临床情况的不同，可摘局部义齿也会对邻牙产生明显的扭力或应力，而且因为它有一部分是由下面的黏膜组织支持，所以在承重区下方可能会发生骨丧失。这种修复体 10 年的寿命是 50%（Budtz-Jorgensen 1996）。阿奎里诺等（2001）报道邻近缺牙区的牙齿 10 年存留率是 56%。

3.6.3　口腔骨内种植体

牙种植修复可以通过刺激牙槽骨帮助保持缺牙区的骨量，从而取代固定局部义齿成为修复缺牙区的金标准。虽然这种方式通常需要更长的治疗时间，涉及手术并且意味着初始成本增加，但是邻牙因不被累及而能保留更长时间，所以从远期角度看患者投入的成本明显减少。尽管种植修复不需要担心龋齿，但是种植体周围黏膜炎和种植体周围炎是随之产生的新问题。据威尔逊（Wilson）报道，在水门汀黏结型种植体植入 9 年后，即可出现由黏结剂引发的种植体周围炎（Wilson 2009）。另一方面，一些研究证实口腔骨内种植体 15～20 年的存留率在 95% 以上（Budtz-Jorgensen 1996；Salinas 等 2004）。

从修复角度看，牙周膜存在与否是导致种植牙和天然牙触觉敏感度明显不同的原因。牙齿的平均轴向位移 25～100 μm，而种植体是 3～5 μm（Schulte 1995；Kim 等 2005）。因此，牙种植修复体及其部件将承受更多应力，定期评估咬合对预防种植修复系统的折裂、崩瓷或技术性/机械性并发症至关重要。在一项 10 年回顾性研究中，维特内本（Wittneben）等（2014）评价了种植体支持固定义齿与单冠的机械性/技术性并发症发生率和修复失败率，并发现在 397 个固定种植修复体中，崩瓷是最常见的并发症（20.31%），其次是种植体固位螺丝松动（2.57%）和修复体脱落（2.06%）。

牙种植体具有保护余留牙的作用；某学者报道了种植体邻牙 10 年存留率为 99.5%（Priest 1999）。

最后，如果患者强烈要求，那么缺牙区也可以不修复。但这会不可避免地导致缺牙区发生骨丧失，并且影响邻牙的存留（Aquilino 等 2001）。

3.7　总结

简要地说，制订治疗计划的思路如下：

临床医师必须在评估患牙的同时评估整体口腔情况，这样才能制订出一个明确而综合的治疗计划。

1. 患牙目前的情况和预后如何?

(a) 牙周支持组织

(b) 根管治疗的质量

2. 以下操作之后有多少健康的牙体组织能保留?

(a) 去除龋坏组织

(b) 根管治疗

(c) 冠预备

3. 患牙未来将承受多大的应力?

(a) 作为单冠 vs.作为固定局部义齿/可摘局部义齿的基牙

(b) 承受非正中𬌗运动

(c) 咬合力(前牙 vs.后牙),夜磨牙/紧咬牙

4. 明确患牙剩余牙体组织和所受应力后,考虑存在多少垂直空间可用于堆核时,需要回答以下问题:

(1) 余留的健康牙体组织是否足以为修复体提供强有力的支持?(子问题:桩是否能增加核的固位?)

(2) 剩余牙体组织是否足以抵抗牙颈部出现的冠/核折裂(子问题:患牙的牙周袋深度?是否有可能并且有必要进行冠延长术?黏结桩是否会增强修复系统的强度?)

如果这两个问题的答案是"**是**",那么治疗方案是:

(a) 银汞或复合树脂核修复(剩余 4 个,3 个或 2 个牙体组织壁)(子问题:复合树脂核是否比银汞核更能降低牙尖劈裂的风险?)

(b) 预成桩(剩余 3 个或 2 个牙体组织壁)+堆核(子问题:如果是活髓牙,那么是否有必要选择进行根管治疗?即使有足够的牙体组织壁,增加纤维桩是否能改善患牙的预后?)

(c) 预成桩,如果上颌前牙进行过根管治疗并且需要冠修复。

如果这两个问题的答案是"**否**",那么治疗方案是:

(a) 预成桩(剩余 3 个,2 个或 1 个牙体组织壁)+堆核(子问题:如果是活髓牙,那么是否有必要选择进行根管治疗?)。

(b) 铸造桩核(剩余 1 个牙体组织壁,或只有牙本质肩领,或牙本质肩领高度与厚度不足)(子问题:如果是活髓牙,那么是否有必要选择进行根管治疗?)。

（c）冠延长术＋铸造桩核（子问题：如果是活髓牙，那么除了冠延长术，是否有必要选择进行根管治疗？）。

（d）拔牙，并用种植体或固定局部义齿进行修复。

（e）最后，从整个牙列角度考虑总体治疗计划，包括修复体使用寿命，其他可行的修复方案（种植体，固定局部义齿或可摘局部义齿），性价比和患者意愿等。

（唐子圣　译）

参考文献

Al-Hazaimah H, Gutteridge DL (2001) An in vitro study into the effect of the ferrule preparation on the fracture resistance of crowned teeth incorporating prefabricated post and composite core restoration. Int Endod J 34: 40 – 46.

Allen EP (1993) Surgical crown lengthening for function and esthetics. Dent Clin North Am 37: 163 – 179.

Andreasen FM, Kahler B (2015) Pulpal response after acute dental injury in the permanent dentition: clinical implication — a review. J Endod 41: 299 – 308.

Aquilino S, Caplan D (2002) Relationship between crown placement and the survival of endodontically treated teeth. J Prosthet Dent 87: 256 – 263.

Aquilino SA, Shugars DA, Bader JD, White BA (2001) Ten-year survival rates of teeth adjacent to treated and untreated posterior bounded edentulous spaces. J Prosthet Dent 85: 455 – 460.

Balto K (2011) Tooth survival after root canal treatment. Evid Based Dent 12: 10 – 11.

Borelli B, Sorrentino R, Goracci C, Amato M, Zarone F, Ferrari M (2015) Evaluating residual dentin thickness following various mandibular anterior tooth preparations for zirconia full-coverage single crowns: an in vitro analysis. Int J Periodontics Restorative Dent 35: 41 – 47.

Budtz-Jorgensen E (1996) Restoration of the partially edentulous mouth — a comparison of overdentures, removable partial dentures, fixed dental prosthesis and implant treatment. J Dent 24: 237 – 244.

Cagidiaco MC, Garcia-Godoy F, Vichi A, Grandini S, Goracci C, Ferrari M (2008) Placement of fiber prefabricated or custom made posts affects the 3-year survival of endodontically treated premolars. Am J Dent 21: 179 – 184.

Caplan DJ, Kolker J, Rivera EM, Walton RE (2002) Relationship between number of proximal contacts and survival of root canal treated teeth. Int Endod J 35: 193 – 199.

Carrotte P (2004) Endodontics: Part 2 Diagnosis and treatment planning. Br Dent J 197: 231 – 238.

Combe EC, Shaglouf AM, Watts DC, Wilson NH (1999) Mechanical properties of direct core build-up materials. Dent Mater 15: 158 – 165.

Cunliffe J, Grey N (2008) Crown lengthening surgery — indications and techniques. Dent Update 25: 29 – 35.

De Backer H, Van Maele G, Decock V, Van den Berghe L (2007) Long-term survival of complete crowns, fixed partial dentures, and cantilever fixed dental prostheses with posts and cores on root canal-treated teeth. Int J Prosthodont 20: 229 – 234.

de Chevigny C, Dao TT, Basrani BR, Marquis V, Farzaneh M, Abitbol S, Friedman S (2008)

Treatment outcome in endodontics: the Toronto study - phase 4: initial treatment. J Endod 34: 258 - 263.
Dibart S, Capri D, Kachouh I, Van Dyke T, Nun ME (2003) Crown lengthening in mandibular molars: a 5-year retrospective radiographic analysis. J Periodontol 74: 815 - 821.
Dummer PMH, Hicks R, Huws D (1980) Clinical signs and symptoms in pulp disease. Int Endod J 13: 27 - 35.
Ferrari M, Cagidiaco MC, Grandini S, De Sanctis M, Goracci C (2007) Post placement affects survival of endodontically treatment premolars. J Dent Res 86: 729 - 734.
Ferrari M, Vichi A, Fadda GM, Cagidiaco MC, Tay FR, Breschi L, Polimeni A, Goracci C (2012) A randomized controlled trial of endodontically treated and restored premolars. J Dent Res 91: 72S - 78S.
Fonzr F, Fonzar A, Buttolo P, Worthington HV, Esposito M (2009) The prognosis of root canal therapy: a 10-year retrospective cohort study on 411 patients with 1175 endodontically treated teeth. Eur J Oral Implantol 2: 201 - 208.
Gargiulo A, Wentz F, Orban B (1961) Dimensions and relations of the dentogingival junction in humans. J Periodontol 32: 261 - 267.
Gateau P, Sabek M, Dailey B (2001) In vitro fatigue resistance of glass ionomer cements used in post-and-core applications. J Prosthet Dent 86: 149 - 155.
Gillen BM, Looney SW, Gu LS, Loushine BA, Weller RN, Loushine RJ, Pashley DH, Tay FR (2011) Impact of the quality of coronal restoration versus the quality of root canal fillings on success of root canal treatment: a systematic review and meta-analysis. J Endod 37: 895 - 902.
Gunay H, Seeger A, Tschernitschek H, Geurtsen W (2000) Placement of the preparation line and periodontal health: a prospective 2-year clinical study. Int J Periodontics Restorative Dent 20: 171 - 181.
Heithersay GS (1999) Invasive cervical resorption following trauma. Aust Endod J 25: 79 - 85.
Hempton TJ, Dominici JT (2010) Contemporary crown-lengthening therapy: a review. J Am Dent Assoc 141: 647 - 655.
Karlsson S (1986) A clinical evaluation of fixed bridges, 10 years following insertion. J Oral Rehabil 13: 423 - 432.
Kim Y, Oh TJ, Misch CE, Want HL (2005) Occlusal considerations in implant therapy: clinical guidelines with biomechanical rationale. Clin Oral Implant Res 16: 26 - 35.
Kovarik RE, Breeding LC, Caughman WF (1992) Fatigue life of three core materials under simulated chewing conditions. J Prosthet Dent 68: 584 - 590.
Liberman R, Judes H, Cohen E, Eli I (1987) Restoration of posterior pulpless teeth: amalgam overlay versus cast gold inlay restoration. J Prosthet Dent 57: 540 - 543.
Malmgren B, Malmgren O, Andreasen JO (2006) Alveolar bone development after decoronation of ankylosed teeth. Endod Topics 14: 35 - 40.
Mannocci F, Bertelli E, Sherriff M, Watson TF, Ford TR (2002) Three-year clinical comparison of survival of endodontically treated teeth restored with either full cast coverage or with direct composite restorations. J Prosthet Dent 88: 297 - 301.
Marquis VL, Dao T, Farzaneh M, Abitbol S, Friedman S (2006) Treatment outcome in endodontics - the Toronto study. Phase III: Initial treatment. J Endod 32: 299 - 306.
Maynard JG Jr, Wilson RD (1979) Physiological dimensions of the periodontium significant to the restorative dentist. J Periodontol 50: 170 - 174.
McGuire MK (1998) Periodontal plastic surgery. Dent Clin North Am 42: 411 - 465.
McGuire MK, Nunn ME (1996) Prognosis versus actual outcome. III. The effectiveness of clinical parameters in accurately predicting tooth survival. J Periodontol 67: 666 - 674.
Miller PD Jr, McEntire ML, Marlow NM, Gellin RG (2014) An evidence-based scoring index to determine the periodontal prognosis on molars. J Periodontol 85: 214 - 225.
Nagasiri R, Chitmongkolsuk S (2005) Long-term survival of endodontically treated molars

without crown coverage: a retrospective cohort study. J Prosthet Dent 93: 164-170.

Nevins M, Skurow HM (1984) The intracrevicular restorative margin, the biologic width, and the maintenance of the gingival margin. Int J Periodontics Restorative Dent 4: 30-49.

Ng YL, Mann V, Gulabivala K (2011) A prospective study of the factors affecting outcomes of non-surgical root canal treatment: Part 2. Tooth survival. Int Endod J 44: 610-625.

Ouzounian ZS, Schilder H (1991) Remaining dentin thickness after endodontic cleaning and shaping before post space preparation. Oral Health 81: 13-15.

Palmqvist S, Swartz B (1993) Artificial crowns and fixed partial dentures 18 to 23 years after placement. Int J Prosthodont 6: 279-285.

Panitvisai P, Messer HH (1995) Cuspal deflection in molars in relation to endodontic and restorative procedures. J Endod 21: 57-61.

Pilo R, Shapenco E, Lewinstein I (2008) Residual dentin thickness in bifurcated maxillary first premolars after root canal and post space preparation with parallel-sided drills. J Prosthet Dent 99: 267-273.

Priest G (1999) Single-tooth implant and their role in preserving remaining teeth: a 10-year survival study. Int J Oral Maxillofac Implants 14: 181-188.

Ray HA, Trope M (1985) Periapical status of endodontically treated teeth in relation to the technical quality of the root filling and the coronal restoration. Int Endod J 28: 12-18.

Reuter JE, Brose MO (1984) Failures in full crown retained dental bridges. Br Dent J 157: 61-63.

Rivera ME, Walton RE (1994) Extensive idiopathic apical root resorption. A case report. Oral Surg Oral Med Oral Pathol 78: 673-677.

Salehrabi R, Rotstein I (2004) Endodontic treatment outcomes in a large patient population in the USA: an epidemiological study. J Endod 30: 846-850.

Salinas TJ, Block MS, Sadan A (2004) Fixed dental prosthesis or single-tooth implant restorations? Statistical considerations for sequencing and treatment. J Oral Maxillofac Surg 62: 2-16.

Saunders WP, Saunders EM (1990) Assessment of leakage in the restored pulp chamber of endodontically treated multi rooted teeth. Int Endod J 23: 28-33.

Saunders WP, Saunders EM (1994) Coronal leakage as a cause of failure in root canal therapy: a review. Endod Dent Traumatol 10: 105-108.

Schulte W (1995) Implants and the periodontium. Int Dent J 45: 16-26.

Seltzer S, Sinai I, August D (1970) Periodontal effects of root perforations before and during endodontic procedures. J Dent Res 49: 109-114.

Setzer FC, Kim S (2014) Comparison of long-term survival of implants and endodontically treated teeth. J Dent Res 93: 19-26.

Sjogren U, Hagglund B, Sundqvist G, Wing K (1990) Factors affecting the long-term results of endodontic treatment. J Endod 16: 498-504.

Sorensen JA, Martinoff JT (1984) Intracoronal reinforcement and coronal coverage: a study of endodontically treated teeth. J Prosthet Dent 51: 780-784.

Sorensen JA, Martinoff JT (1985) Endodontically treated teeth as abutments. J Prosthet Dent 53: 631-636.

Stock CJR (1995) Patient assessment. In: Stock CJR, Gulabivala K, Walker RT, Goodman JR (eds) Endodontics, 2nd edn. Mosby-Wolfe, London, pp. 43-46.

Sundh B, Odman P (1997) A study of fixed prosthodontics performed at a university clinic 18 years after insertion. Int J Prosthodont 10: 513-519.

Tarnow DP, Magner AW, Fletcher P (1992) The effect of the distance from the contact point to the crest of bone on the presence or absence of the inter proximal dental papilla. J Periodontol 63: 995-996.

Thayer H (1980) Overdentures and the periodontium. Dent Clin North Am 24: 369-377.

Vacek JS, Gher ME, Assad DA, Richardson AC, Giambarresi LI (1994) The dimensions of the human dentogingival junction. Int J Periodontics Restorative Dent 14: 154-165.

Vire DE (1991) Failure of endodontically treated teeth: classification and evaluation. J Endod 17: 338-342.

Wilson TG Jr (2009) The positive relationship between excess cement and peri-implant disease: a prospective clinical endoscopic study. J Periodontol 80: 1388-1392.

Wittneben JG, Buser D, Salvi GE, Burgin W, Hicklin S, Bragger U (2014) Complication and failure rates with implant-supported fixed dental prostheses and single crowns: a 10-year retro-spective study. Clin Implant Dent Relat Res 16: 356-364.

4 纤维增强牙科材料在根管治疗后牙齿修复中的应用

约翰娜·坦纳(Johanna Tanner)
安娜-玛丽亚·勒贝尔-罗诺夫(Anna-Maria Le Bell-Rönnlöf)

摘 要

纤维增强复合材料(fiber-reinforced composites，FRC)是一类不含金属的轻型牙科材料，具有各向异性的性质特征。它们相对成本较低，与牙齿颜色接近，并能与黏结剂、直接充填技术同时运用。现代的牙科纤维增强复合材料主要由玻璃纤维和二甲基丙烯酸酯树脂组成。为了获得最佳临床效果，临床医师有必要充分了解这些复合材料的性能表现。纤维增强复合材料中的纤维提供强度和刚度，基质聚合物将纤维结合在一起，在纤维加固部分的周围形成连续相。为了发挥最佳的机械性能，纤维必须与基质聚合物紧密黏附，并被聚合物充分浸润。另外一些因素也能影响纤维增强复合材料的机械性能、光学性能和黏结性能，包括纤维和基质聚合物的种类、数量、位置和纤维的方向。现代牙科纤维增强复合材料主要采用单向或多向连续的长纤维，以及不连续的短纤维，并在根管治疗(RCT)后牙齿修复方面存在一些优势。由于纤维增强复合材料具有接近天然牙本质的弹性模量、高抗拉强度，并且能应用于高性价比的椅旁技术中，使得这种材料非常适合用于修复根管治疗后牙体结构变得薄弱的牙齿。

4.1 关于牙科纤维增强复合材料的介绍

纤维增强复合材料是一种不含金属的轻型材料，具有良好的机械性能，比如较高的抗疲劳性和断裂韧度。现代纤维增强复合材料适用于对静动态强度与断裂韧度要求较高的领域,在工业上应用广泛,例如运动设备和船体制造。纤维增强复合材料第一次在牙科中的应用可以追溯到20世纪60年代,被报道用于增强义齿的丙烯酸树脂基托(Smith 1962;Schwickerath 1965)。20世纪90年代,操作性能方面的改进最终使纤维增强复合材料开始大规模应用于牙科材料中。

纤维增强复合材料最初主要用于加固可摘义齿的丙烯酸树脂基托(Ladizesky 等 1992;Vallittu 1997a;Cheng 和 Chow 1999),其加固效果比传统金属丝更好(Vallittu 1996)。随着加强纤维能与二甲基丙烯酸酯树脂和颗粒填料复合物成功结合,纤维增强复合材料可以进一步应用于固定义齿修复和其他牙科领域。有文献报道纤维增强复合材料可用于制作固定局部义齿(Freilich 等 1998a,b;Behr 等 2000;Meiers 和 Freilich 2000;Vallittu 和 Sevelius 2000;Ahlstrand 和 Finger 2002;Göhring 等 2002;Kolbeck 等 2002)、种植体上部结构(Freilich 等 2002;Meiers 和 Freilich 2006;Ballo 等 2009;Zhao 等 2009)、牙周夹板(Meiers 等 1998;Sewón 等 2000)、正畸保持器(Rantala 等 2003;Kirzioĝlu 和 Ertük 2004)。纤维增强复合材料在牙体修复方面的应用包括制作根管桩(Mannocci 等 1999a,b;Qualthrough 等 2003)、修复断裂瓷贴面(Valittu 2000;Özcan 等 2006)、加固充填复合物(Fernnis 等 2005;Garoushi 等 2013)。结合黏结技术,并采用特定的纤维方向和分布位置改变充填材料物理性能,可以使纤维增强复合材料实现创伤更小,保留更多牙体组织的修复技术。促进纤维增强复合材料应用的其他优点是材料的性价比高,而且对玻璃和二氧化硅纤维而言,纤维半透明的特点使材料具有良好的美观性。对纤维增强复合材料的应用进行风险评估,并正确选择符合适应证的患者,对确保材料应用成功具有重要意义。

4.2 纤维增强复合材料的结构和特点

纤维增强复合材料由嵌入聚合物基质的增强纤维组成。与通常用于牙科修复材料的颗粒填料相比,纤维增强复合材料中高长宽比的填料具有增强作用,它们以其长度比截面更长为特征,典型的是纤维或晶须。在纤维增强复合材料中,纤维提供强度和刚度,基质聚合物将纤维结合在一起,在纤维加固部分的周围形成连续相,一方面将负荷转移给纤维;另一方面保护纤维不被湿润的口腔环境侵蚀。为达到更好的机械性能,纤维必须与基质聚合物紧密黏附(Beech 和 Brown 1972),并被聚合物充分浸润(Vallittu 1995a)。高黏度的树脂系统很难浸润纤维,如丙烯酸树脂的义齿基托或颗粒填料复合物。如果因为树脂黏度太高或发生聚合收缩,导致纤维没有被完全浸润,那么材料就不能发挥最佳的机械性能(Vallitti 1998a)。因此制造商需要对纤维进行预浸润,从而确保树脂能充分浸润纤维。除了纤维与树脂界面间的黏附,纤维的延伸性和体积含量等其他一些参数,也会影响复合材料中纤维的加固作用。

纤维的类型、位置、方向很大程度上决定了复合材料的机械性能(Murphy 1998)。根据复合材料的设计要求,增强纤维可以是单向的,全部相互平行,也可以是多向的,朝着两个或多个方向。纤维浓度,也就是说纤维体积含量越高,复合材料的抗拉强度越大。但事实上,在复合材料结构的张力侧,放置相对少量的纤维就能起到足够的加固作用。相比全纤维,牙科应用中更多时候会选择部分纤维增强材料机械性能(Vallittu 和 Narva 1997;Vallittu 1997a)。在应力最集中的区域采用增强纤维,并在其上方覆盖另一层材料满足美学和卫生需求。因此,修复过程通常包含多个步骤,比如采用桩核修复根管治疗后的牙齿。各部分材料的强度、刚度以及它们之间的黏附都会影响整个修复体的性能。

4.2.1 纤维的长度和方向

当增强纤维的方向沿着应力方向时,能发挥最强的增强效果。但是,当应力与纤维长轴垂直时,纤维对聚合物没有任何增强效果。纤维增强复合材料的机械性能取决于纤维长轴的方向,这个性质称为各向异性。Krenchel 因子表示纤维长度和方向对纤维增强效果的影响(图 4-1)。通过改变纤维位置和方向,可以使纤维增强复合材料在受力方向上具有高强度,并发挥更好的增强效果。除了机械性能,纤维增强复合材料的光学性能、表面物理性能和聚合收缩性能都与纤维方向有关。

根据使用的纤维纵横比,可以将纤维增强复合材料分为不连续的短纤维增强复合材料和连续的长纤维增强复合材料。根管桩是连续长纤维复合增强材料的典型应用,而不连续的短纤维增强复合材料能被用来增

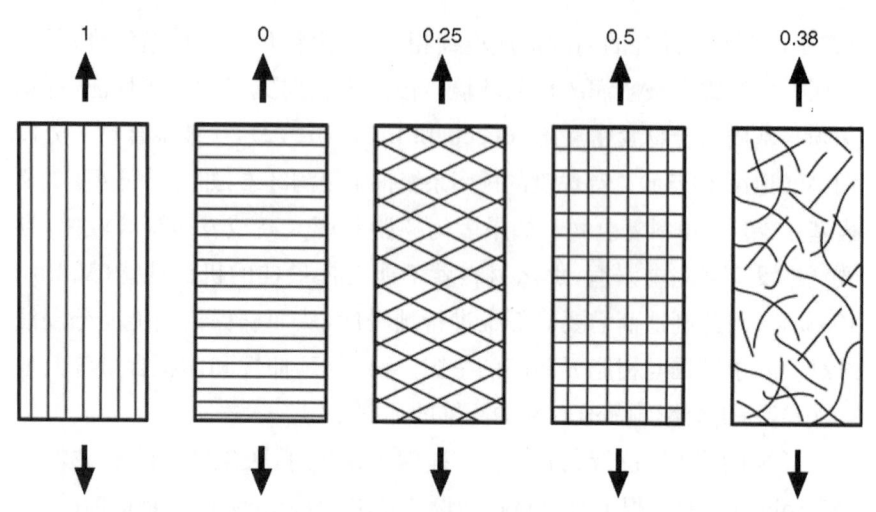

图4-1 Krenchel因子显示纤维方向对材料增强效果的影响
从左到右依次为：沿着受力方向的单向纤维，与受力方向呈90°的单向纤维，与受力方向分别呈45°的双向纤维，与受力方向分别呈0°和90°的双向纤维，不规则的短纤维。箭头方向代表受力方向。

强牙科充填复合材料（Garoushi等2013）。即使纤维体积含量一样，短、长纤维复合增强材料的机械性能也有所不同（Kamos 1993）。当连续单向纤维被纵横比较小的不连续纵向纤维代替时，复合材料最终的抗拉强度会减弱，但是材料依然保持各向异性（图4-1）。但如果短纤维杂乱排列，材料则会变成各向同性，同时抗拉强度显著下降。由于不连续纤维增强材料不具备单向连续纤维增强材料的高抗拉强度，所以两者的修复失败类型是不同的。不连续短纤维复合材料的失败原因，包括聚合物基质破裂、纤维剥脱、纤维断裂，而单向连续纤维增强复合材料最常见的失败原因主要是轴向拉力、水平向拉力和剪切力带来的破坏（Vallittu 2015）。纤维长度、纤维纵横比、纤维与基质聚合物之间的黏附，都是影响复合材料失败原因的因素。

4.2.2 纤维类型

为了使纤维发挥增强效果，其弯曲模量必须比基质聚合物更大。有些类型的纤维经测试后，被认为适用于增强牙科聚合物材料，最常见的是玻璃、碳/石墨和聚乙烯纤维。

现今，玻璃纤维是最适用于临床牙科学的纤维，其优点包括高抗拉强度、低延展性、良好的抗压与抗冲击性，以及低成本。玻璃纤维的透明外观也非常适用于对美学要求较高的牙科领域，比如制作前牙根管桩。不过，玻璃纤维成功背后最重要的因素无疑是其表面化学性能，通过硅烷偶联剂能使玻璃纤维与牙科聚合物发生黏附。玻璃纤维在应力下均匀拉伸至断裂极限，在达到断裂极限之前去除负荷，纤维会恢复原先的长度。这一特性结合高机械强度，使得玻璃纤维可以储存和释放大量能量（Murphy 1998）。根据玻璃的化学组成，玻璃纤维被分为 A（碱性的）、C（抗化学腐蚀的）、D（绝缘的）、E（导电的）、R（耐久的）、S（高强度的）这几种类型，它们的机械性和耐化学腐蚀性不同。在增强复合材料中最常用的玻璃纤维是 E 玻璃（99% 由玻璃纤维构成）（Vallittu 1998b），其组成中含有硼硅酸铝钙。随着牙科纤维增强复合材料技术发展，对纤维体积含量和聚合物基质性能的不断改进，使单向 E 玻璃纤维的弯曲强度更高（达 1 150 Mpa）（Lassila 等 2002；Alander 等 2004），几乎接近铸造钴铬合金（1 200 MPa）（Vallittu 1997b）。

　　碳纤维或碳/石墨纤维被广泛应用于增强复合材料中，并有良好的性能表现。碳纤维比铁更强，比铝更轻，比钛更硬（Murphy 1998）。碳纤维的机械性能随着化学组成改变而不同，但通常碳/石墨纤维在拉力和压力下都能展现出很高的强度。碳/石墨纤维第一次在牙科中的应用是在 20 世纪 70 年代，被用于增强聚甲基丙烯酸甲酯（polymethyl methacrylate，PMMA）（Schreiber 1971），使 PMMA 的弯曲强度提高近 100%。限制碳/石墨纤维牙科应用的主要缺点是纤维呈黑色，并在制造和操作方面存在困难。碳/石墨纤维在牙科中最主要用于制作根管预成桩（Isidor 等 1996；Purton 和 Payne 1996；Torbjörner 等 1996；Fredriksson 等 1998）。

　　超高分子量（ultrahigh molecular weight，UHMW）聚乙烯纤维是现有最强的增强纤维，由排成直线的聚合物链构成，具有低弹性模量、低密度以及良好的抗冲击强度（Murphy 1998）。这种纤维的颜色呈白色，所以适用于牙科。一些研究者检测了聚乙烯纤维对牙科聚合物材料的增强效果（Ladizesky 等 1990；Gutteridge 1992）。尽管超高分子量聚乙烯纤维具有优良的弯曲强度，但其临床应用仍受到限制，主要是因为该纤维与牙科树脂间的黏结存在困难。虽然有研究试图采用等离子喷涂等方法，改善超高分子量聚乙烯纤维的黏结性能，但效果并不理想（Ladizesky 等

1990)。另外，超高分子量聚乙烯纤维对蛋白质和口腔细菌具有高亲和力，会导致蛋白质和细菌黏附其表面，限制了该纤维作为牙科材料的应用（Tanner 等 2003，2005）。

4.2.3 黏结性能

与其他复合材料一样，纤维增强材料由不止一种材料组成。在纤维增强复合材料中，树脂基质、纤维和无机物填料都可以作为黏结底物。如果纤维暴露在表面，其他牙科修复复合材料或黏结剂与纤维增强复合材料之间的黏结主要取决于纤维自身的黏结性能。玻璃和硅纤维能通过硅烷化与牙科树脂发生黏结，由此决定了复合材料结构的黏结强度（Vallittu 1993）。硅烷偶联剂通过与玻璃表面形成氢键，并与牙科树脂的甲基丙烯酸酯基团形成共价键，从而促进两者之间的黏结（Matinlinna 等 2004）。

与纤维增强复合材料的其他主要部分，即聚合物基质的黏结主要取决于牙科聚合物采用的树脂系统类型。现代牙科树脂系统主要基于二甲基丙烯酸酯。纤维增强复合材料基质一般采用环氧树脂与二甲基丙烯酸酯，而大多数牙科纤维增强复合材料选择的树脂系统以双酚-A-二甲基丙烯酸缩水甘油酯（bisphenol-A diglycidyl methacrylate，bis-GMA）、三缩四乙二醇二甲基丙烯酸酯（triethylene glycol dimethacrylate，TEGDMA）、二甲基丙烯酸氨基甲酸酯（urethane dimethacrylate，UDMA）为主。这些热固性多功能树脂形成高度交联的聚合物网络，减弱了纤维增强复合材料与其他牙科聚合物之间的黏结。例如，纤维增强复合材料桩中的环氧树脂基质与树脂黏结剂之间主要是通过机械黏结（Purton 和 Payne 1996）。一些制造商试图通过在纤维增强复合材料桩表面增加锯齿形来克服黏结效果不佳这一问题。

另一种提高材料黏结性能的方法是通过加入低度交联的聚合物链，改变纤维增强复合材料树脂基质的化学组成。这种多相基质聚合物，同时包含了热塑性和热固性聚合物链，被称为半互穿聚合物网络（semi-interpenetrating polymer network，semi-IPN）（Sperling 1994）。已有研究报道了采用热固性与热塑性树脂混合物浸润玻璃纤维的方法（Vallittu 1995b；Lastumäki 等 2003）。将 PMMA 线性聚合物加入基质中，不仅能增加纤维复合增强材料的韧性（Lassila 等 2004），还能提高其表面黏结性能。非交联热塑性聚合链（PMMA）能使黏结树脂单体扩散到之前已经聚合的基质中（Mannocci 等 2005）。一些研究者指出，半互穿聚合物网络结构有助于提高复合材料的黏结性能（Kallio 等 2003；Lastumäki 等 2003）。采用半互穿聚合物网络的纤维增强复合材料可用于制作根管桩和大块充填复合物（见 4.3.1 和 4.3.2）。

4.2.4 纤维增强复合材料的水解稳定性

口腔中的纤维增强复合材料结构暴露在温度和 pH 不断变化的潮湿环境中。这对所有牙科材料都是一种挑战，包括纤维增强复合材料。尽管纤维增强复合材料有一定的抗腐蚀性，但聚合物基质、玻璃纤维和两者间的界面仍能在水腐蚀性介质，比如口腔中发生降解。纤维增强复合材料吸收水分后，由于基质聚合物的膨胀和塑化作用，以及纤维/基质界面发生水解，导致材料的机械性能下降（Jancar 和 Dibenedetto 1993）。由玻璃纤维和半互穿聚合物网络基质组成的纤维增强复合材料在水中存放 30 天后，强度和弹性模量会降低大约 15%（Vallittu 2000）。对于高吸水性的聚合物而言，这一现象将更明显。例如，高吸水性的聚酰胺基质能降低复合材料 50% 的强度（Lastumaki 等 2001）。短时间储存（如 1 个月）所导致的材料弯曲性能下降是可逆的，纤维增强复合材料能通过脱水恢复最初的弯曲性能（Lassila 等 2002）。而在较长期的老化过程中，材料强度和刚度的减弱主要发生在第 1 个月，之后会进入缓慢下降的稳定水平，最终在长时间里总体弯曲性能下降 20%～25%（如 10 年）（Vallittu 2007）。

高度聚合、高质量的纤维增强复合材料很少由于吸水作用发生永久性的改变。水、酸、碱在聚合物基质中弥散缓慢。纤维增强复合材料修复体的制造主要采用多相设计，由表面复合物保护多纤维的底层结构。但是，如果水或者唾液直接与纤维接触，材料的降解速度会加剧。在完成修复进行调磨抛光或复合材料产生裂缝时，纤维可能暴露。连接纤维和基质聚合物的聚硅氧烷网容易发生水解，当聚硅氧烷网暴露时，形成一个薄弱界面层，并能通过毛细管作用促进材料水解，同时降低纤维增强复合材料的机械性能。

热循环可以导致由纤维增强复合材料制作的根管桩机械强度降低

10%～20%。有些报道中,材料机械性能的下降幅度甚至可达40%～65%(Torbjörner 等 1996；Lassila 等 2004)。结果上的明显差异可能由检测方法不同造成。另一个重要原因是检测选用的纤维增强复合材料质量不同。纤维增强复合材料预成桩的空隙能促进水分吸收,可能造成材料强度降低(Lassila 等 2004)。空隙中的氧会阻止自由基在接近空隙的聚合物表面发生聚合,导致水渗透增加(Valittu 1997a)。图 4-2 分别展现了致密的和基质中含空隙的纤维增强复合材料。

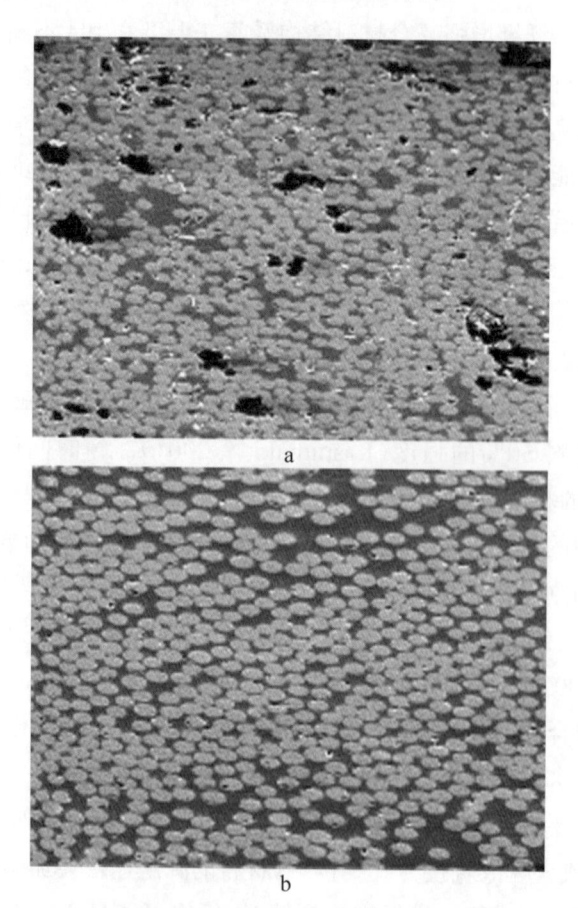

图 4-2　2种不同的纤维增强复合材料根管桩在扫描电子显微镜下的横截面图
a. 材料的聚合物基质中有空隙；b. 材料中致密的聚合物基质充分浸润纤维(图片来源 Elsevier,Rightslink®,编号 3580140154695)。

纤维自身在水环境中也是容易腐蚀降解的(Ehrenstein 等 1990)。玻璃纤维表面的化学组成影响其耐腐蚀性(Vallittu 1998b)。含钙高的玻璃更易被酸腐蚀。通过改变纤维表面化学成分，可以提高其抗酸性，比如添加氧化硼。然而，研究者认为这些碱金属离子、钙和氧化硼，在潮湿环境中会从玻璃纤维中析出，造成纤维表面降解（Vallittu 2014）。

4.3 纤维增强复合材料在根管治疗后牙齿修复中的应用

4.3.1 单向纤维增强复合材料

纤维增强复合材料在牙科中常用于制作根管桩。近几十年来，越来越多的医师采用纤维增强树脂桩将核、冠与牙根固定（Qualthrough 等 2003；Mannocci 等 2005）。单向纤维增强复合材料既可用于制作预先完全聚合固化的预成桩，也可用于制作在根管内聚合形成的个性化桩。

继 20 世纪 90 年代第一代预成碳或石墨纤维桩（Composipost，C-post）出现后，各种玻璃纤维和石英纤维逐步代替碳/石墨纤维，在临床上用于制作预成纤维增强树脂桩（Dallari 等 2006；Schmitter 等 2007）。第一批临床研究显示，运用碳纤维桩的牙齿存留率较高（Ferrari 等 2000；Hedlund 等 2003）。但之后，随访时间更长的研究也揭示了一些关于碳纤维桩的不足之处（Segerström 等 2006）。随着对桩的美学与弯曲性能要求提高，加速了玻璃纤维桩的发展。短期随访研究显示，玻璃纤维桩充分展现了良好的临床效果（Grandini 等 2005）。尽管近 15 年以来，已有不少临床研究报道了预成纤维增强树脂桩的各项性能，但设计合理，同时随访时间更长的随机临床试验仍然很少。

4.3.1.1 预成纤维增强树脂桩

预成纤维增强树脂桩是指在最终聚合的聚合物基质中含有大量连续单向增强纤维，由此形成符合预定直径的固体桩。预成纤维增强树脂桩采用的纤维是碳/石墨纤维或玻璃纤维（E 玻璃、S 玻璃、石英/二氧化硅），而基质通常是环氧聚合物，或具有高转化率和高度交联结构的环氧树脂与二甲基丙烯酸酯树脂混合物（图 4-3）。纤维为一般具有弹性的基质提供刚度和强度。根据制造商的不同，预成纤维增强树脂桩的纤维体积含量范围在 40%～65%（Torbjörner 和 Fransson 2004；Zicari 等 2013）。

相比传统的金属桩，预成纤维增强树脂桩有许多优点。合适的弹性

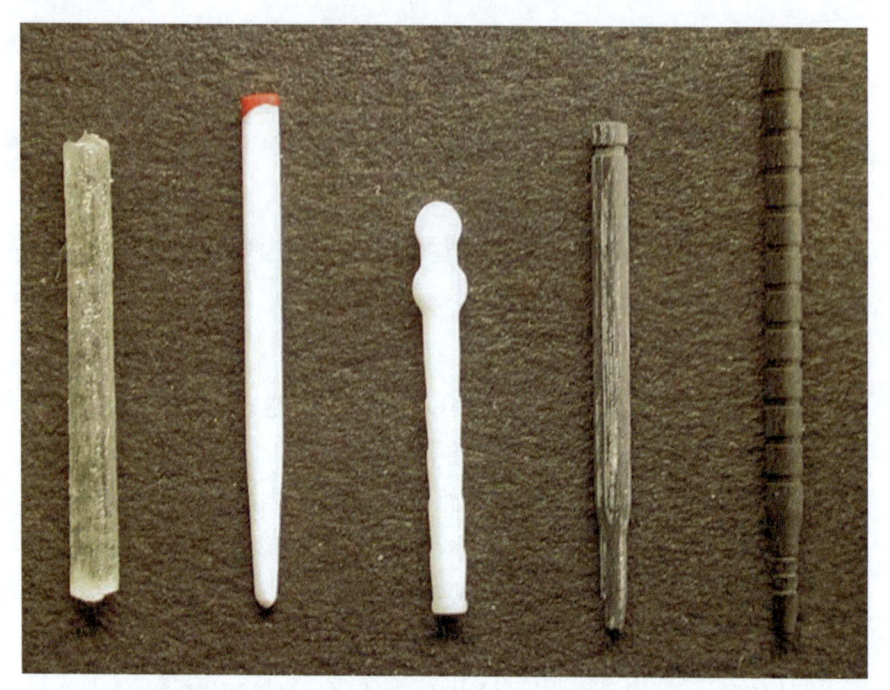

图 4-3 不同类型预成纤维增强树脂桩的照片
从左起依次为：everStick，SnowPost，ParaPost Fiber White，C-post，锯齿状 C-post。

模量是玻璃纤维增强树脂桩最主要的优点之一，能有效减少根折及其他导致修复失败的因素发生（Fokkinga 等 2004）。预成纤维增强树脂桩的优点还包括在口腔中易于操作、方便取出、美学效果佳，尤其是预成玻璃纤维增强树脂桩。

玻璃纤维增强树脂桩的优点在一些研究中已有所阐述（详见第 6 章）。尽管预成纤维增强树脂桩具备许多良好的性能，但也存在不足之处。纤维桩预成的形状很难与根管解剖形态相符。因此，在放置预成纤维桩的时候，冠方存在较大的空隙需由树脂黏结剂填补，并且可能导致根方牙本质不必要的过度去除（图 4-4a、4-5a）。此外，预成纤维增强树脂桩核系统的冠方刚度较弱，不足以抵抗由咬合力在冠部及牙颈部产生的较大应力（Pegoretti 等 2002）。因此，这样的桩核系统承受负荷的能力有限，修复后的牙齿无法抵抗颈部修复体边缘受到的较大应力。这将导致修复体受拉力侧的黏结剂脱落，边缘出现缺损，最终形成继发龋（Schmitter 等 2011），并且这一问题在牙本质肩领缺失时更易发生（图 4-4）（Creugers 等 2005）。

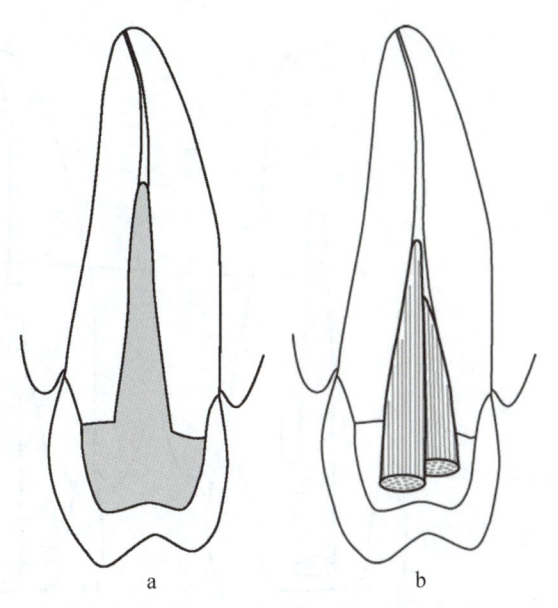

图 4-4 个性化纤维增强树脂桩的修复原理示意图
a. 传统定制的金属铸造桩核是根据根管解剖形态,由根方向冠方逐渐增粗的;b. 如今,类似的结构可以采用现代纤维增强复合材料直接在口内形成。

预成纤维增强树脂桩通过黏结剂和复合树脂水门汀,与根管内牙本质结合。然而,纤维桩高度交联的聚合物基质具有高转化率,不易发生反应,因此很难与树脂水门汀以及树脂核产生黏结(Kallio 等 2001)。一些纤维增强树脂桩基质中的环氧树脂主要依靠机械力与复合树脂水门汀以及树脂核黏结(Purton 和 Payne 1996;Torbjörner 和 Fransson 2004)。为了克服黏结不良的问题,一些制造商在纤维增强树脂桩表面增加了特殊结构,如锯齿状突出(Love 和 Purton 1996;Al-Harbi 和 Nathanson 2003),从而加强树脂水门汀与树脂核的机械固位。但由于纤维增强树脂桩具有各向异性,这样做不但不利于黏结,还可能反而会降低纤维桩的黏结性能与弯曲强度(Soares 等 2012;Zicari 等 2013)。此外,制造商也尝试过其他化学与机械性的表面处理,改善预成纤维增强树脂桩的黏结性能(Mannocci 等 1999a,b;Lastumäki 等 2002;Kallio 等 2003;Sahafi 等 2003),包括喷砂、硅烷化和树脂浸润。

4.3.1.2 个性化纤维增强树脂桩

为克服预成纤维增强树脂桩的缺点,研究者发展了新技术进一步改

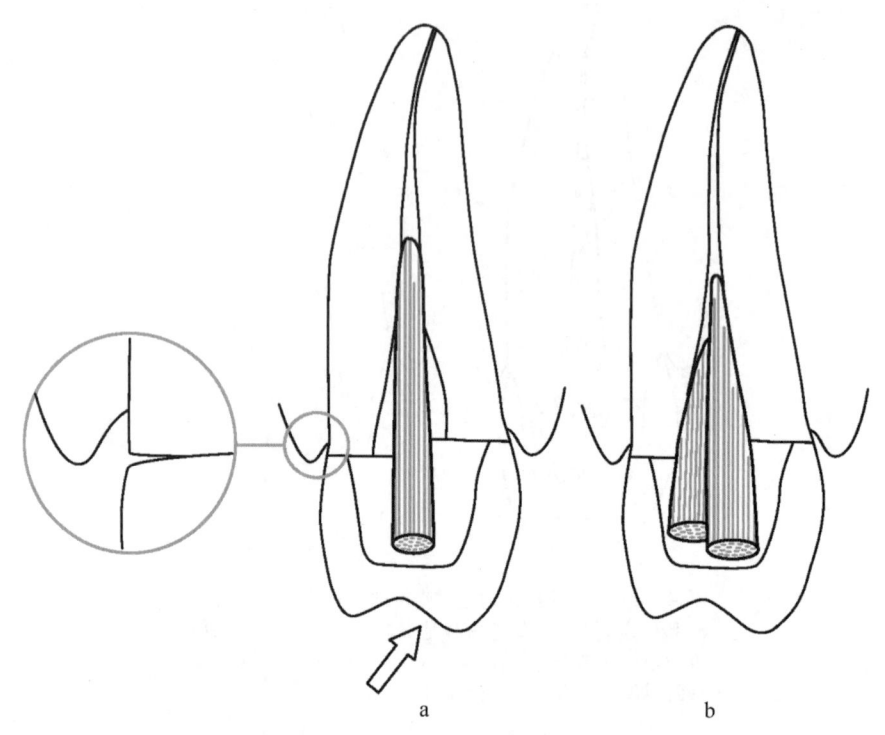

图 4-5　对缺少牙本质肩领的根管治疗后牙齿进行直接修复的模式图
a. 采用结构刚度不足的预成纤维增强树脂桩,可能导致修复体在咬合力作用下受力侧黏结失败;b. 采用个性化纤维增强树脂桩,可以通过增加纤维体积含量,增加修复体冠方关键区的刚度。

进根管治疗后牙齿的桩修复。不同的研究小组使用不同材料,对个性化纤维增强树脂桩系统的发展进行了评估。有一项研究采用冷等离子体处理后的聚乙烯编织纤维制作个性化纤维桩(Terry 等 2001)。据报道,个性化纤维增强树脂桩与预成桩相比,抗负荷和抗折能力更强(Corsalini 等 2007)。研究者曾在一例病例报道中提到,在半透明的纤维桩表面覆盖一层光固化树脂放入根管内,可以获得更符合根管形态的桩,即所谓的根管解剖型桩(Grandini 等 2003)。

研究报道显示,个性化玻璃纤维增强树脂桩与预成桩相比,黏结强度和抗疲劳强度显著提高(Qualthrough 和 Mannocci 2003；Lassila 等 2004；Le Bell 等 2004,2005；Bitter 等 2007)。这些个性化纤维增强树脂桩含有半互穿网络聚合物基质,由包含玻璃纤维和光固化树脂基质的非聚合纤维-树脂预浸料构成(图 4-3)。个性化或定制纤维增强树脂桩

4　纤维增强牙科材料在根管治疗后牙齿修复中的应用　　77

的目的是在根管横截面上,使纤维桩与根管壁之间无空隙,并通过制备符合根管解剖形态的桩,尽可能减少牙体预备量(图4-6b)。这样,更多的增强纤维可能放置在拉伸应力更高的根管上方,增强修复体的抗力性(Bitter 等 2007;Le Bell‒Rönnlöf 等 2011)。增加根管上方的纤维数量可以提高桩系统的负荷承受力。采用这种技术的纤维增强树脂桩类似于传统铸造桩核。桩由根方向冠方逐渐增粗,符合现代冠方扩大根管预备所获得的根管解剖形态,从而使根管治疗后原本牙体就较薄弱的牙齿可以保留更多牙本质(图4-6、图4-7)。

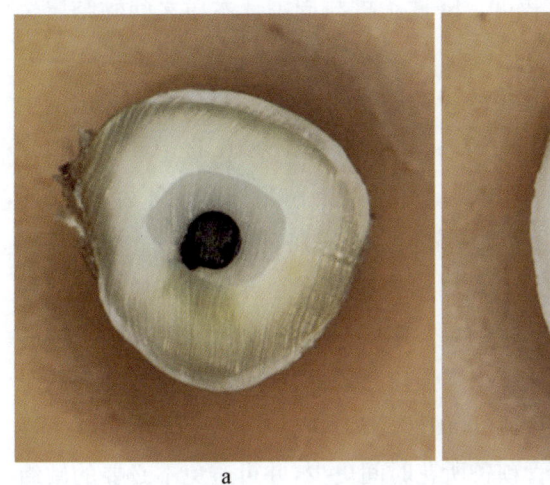

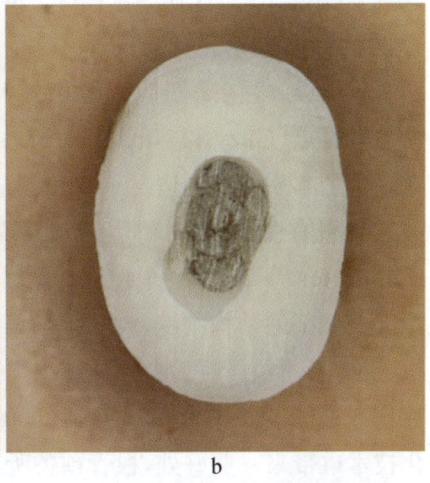

图4-6　a.采用预成碳/石墨纤维桩修复根管治疗后的前磨牙;b.采用个性化玻璃纤维桩修复根管治疗后的前磨牙。图中的牙齿在龈缘水平横截。对于冠方扩大的根管,个性化纤维桩可以充满根管管腔,更有效地发挥加固作用。

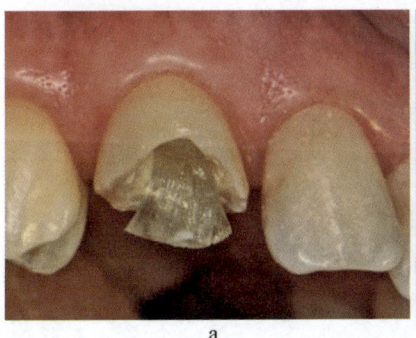

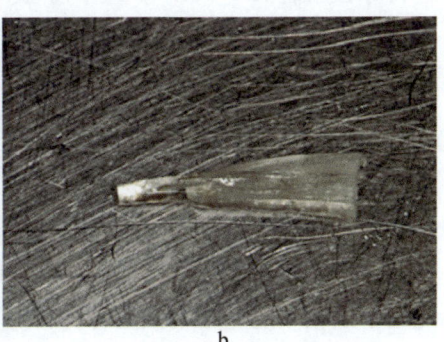

图4-7　a.采用个性化纤维增强树脂根管桩修复上颌尖牙的临床照片;b.纤维增强树脂桩插入根管前显示具有冠方扩大的解剖形态。

个性化技术的另一个是优点在于提高黏结性能。个性化纤维增强树脂桩的纤维之间由半互穿网络聚合物基质组成,最大程度上克服了桩和水门汀之间难以黏结的问题。椅旁技术中,抑氧层也可用以促进黏结。当树脂或树脂基复合材料,比如个性化根管桩,在空气中聚合时表面会形成一层非聚合层,称为抑氧层(Vallittu 1997b)。树脂水门汀可以与抑氧层发生黏结,并形成持久的结合。据报道,个性化纤维增强树脂桩与树脂水门汀之间的结合良好(Le Bell 等 2004,2005;Mannocci 等 2005;Bitter 等 2007)。当桩的尺寸与根管口尺寸非常接近时,黏结剂的厚度可以减少(图 4-5),这在一定程度上降低了桩与周围牙本质之间黏结层聚合收缩产生的应力。

将纤维放置在靠近应力集中的牙本质壁处,可以更好地模拟牙齿的生物力学特点(Guzy 和 Nicholls 1979;Torbjörner 2000;Hatta 等 2011)。在缺少牙本质肩领的情况下采用预成纤维增强树脂桩修复牙齿,常见的失败类型有黏结失败和边缘微渗漏,尤其是在牙齿承受拉力的一侧(Schmitter 等 2011)。个性化纤维增强树脂桩修复方法旨在通过增加牙颈部关键区的结构刚度和抗力性,减少修复黏结失败(见图 4-4)。另有报道称,采用短而粗的个性化纤维增强树脂桩修复牙齿,相比细而长的个性化纤维桩,可以承受更大负荷(Hatta 等 2011)。从操作角度而言,个性化技术也带来一些好处,根管预备所花时间更少,并可避免不必要的硬组织切除。

个性化纤维增强树脂桩聚合物基质的转化率足以使纤维桩在根管内进行原位聚合(Le Bell 等 2003)。此外,从抗折性和防止微渗漏方面而言,个性化纤维增强树脂桩与树脂水门汀在根管内直接同时聚合的方法可能优于纤维桩预先聚合(Hatta 等 2011;Makarewicz 等 2013)。

4.3.2 短而不连续的纤维增强复合材料在根管治疗后牙齿修复中的应用

许多研究已开始关注纤维对复合充填材料的加强作用(Krause 等 1999;Petersen 2005)。由于充填材料直接用于填充牙齿预备后的洞型,应用于该领域的纤维增强复合材料需要具备一些特殊性能。有些研究尝试采用纤维加强复合充填材料,却因纤维长度不足而失败。在充填材料中加入增强纤维导致充填体表面抛光性能不佳,也会造成修复失败。为了保持充填材料的适用性,纤维必须短而不连续,但事实上纤维长度仍应高于一定的临界阈值,以便能显著改善充填材料的机械性能与聚合收缩性能(Vallittu 2015)。优质的纤维长度应超过纤维直径的 50 倍(临界纤维长度)(Kardos 1993)。通过计算现代牙科纤维增强复合材料的长径比($1/d-$),临界纤维长度确定在 750~900 μm(Vallittu 1998a,b)。

目前,通常将纤维增强复合材料作为牙科充填体的一部分起到增强作用,这部分中的纤维相对较长,使充填体具备一定的强度和硬度。在纤维增强复合材料层的表面,再覆盖常规含颗粒填料的树脂复合物,从而获得较好的美学效果和抛光性能。含短纤维增强复合材料的填料能为充填体提供良好的机械强度与抗折性,对表面含颗粒填料的树脂层起支持作用,并能作为防裂层防止裂纹扩展。体外试验表明,由下方纤维增强复合材料与上方常规充填树脂组成的双层结构,可以提高充填体的抗折性能(Fennis 等 2005;Garoushi 等 2005,2006)。短纤维复合树脂核也可以对根管治疗后磨牙的复合树脂冠修复起到明显增强作用(Lammi 等 2011)。

当根管治疗后牙齿冠方有足够的牙本质时,尤其是磨牙,可以考虑不用安放桩。短纤维复合材料可以很好地用于修复冠方缺失的牙本质。图 4-8 表示采用短纤维复合材料修复中度缺损的根管治疗后磨牙。短纤维增强复合材料与窝洞壁以及上层复合树脂结合良好,可以将咬合力均匀地传递到牙齿上。而且,光照可以穿透纤维,增加树脂的聚合深度,从而实现更简便的大块充填技术。填充施加的力量可以使原本方向随机的纤维长轴与洞壁垂直。如前所述,纤维增强复合材料在沿纤维长轴方向上的聚合收缩最小(Tezvergil 等 2006)。为了控制聚合收缩带来的影响,最佳纤维长度为 1~3 mm(Garoushi 等 2007)。富含纤维的充填层也可以防止充填体上的裂纹扩展。相比仅含颗粒填料的复合材料,采用短纤维复合树脂核修复的牙齿在体外表现出更好的抗折性能(Lammi 等 2011)。关于短纤维增强复合材料在根管治疗后牙齿修复中的应用已积累了一些初步临床数据。一项随访 1 年的临床研究报告指出,短纤维增强复合材料非常适合在临床上用来修复大面积冠方缺损的活髓牙和死髓牙(Garoushi 等 2012)。为了更好地评价短纤维增强复合材料在根管治疗后牙齿修复中的应用价值,我们还需要进行更长期的随访与临床对照研究(图 4-8、图 4-9)。

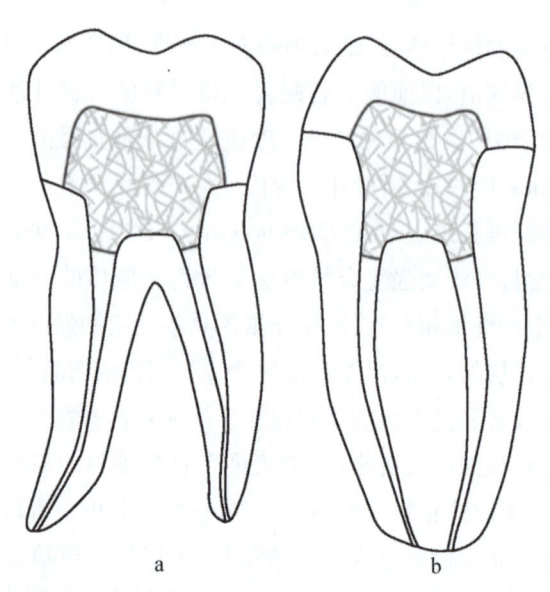

图4-8 采用短纤维复合充填材料与含颗粒增强复合材料的高嵌体修复根管治疗后中度缺损的磨牙模式图
a.颊舌面;b.近中面。

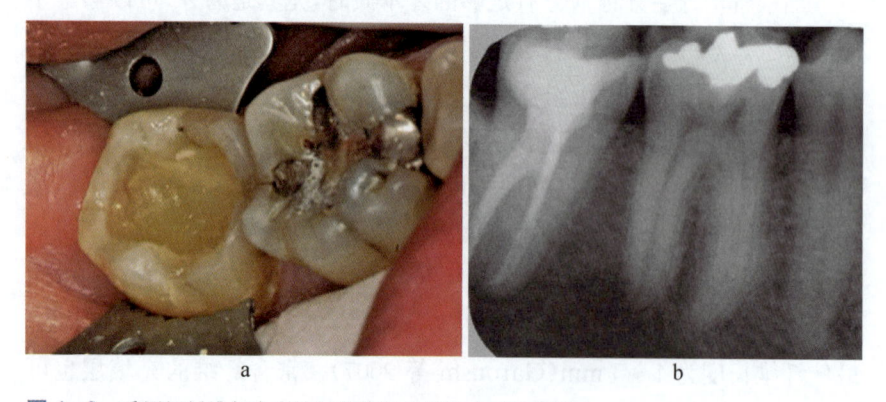

图4-9 采用短纤维复合充填材料修复根管治疗后的磨牙
a.临床照片;b.X线片。

结 论

纤维增强复合材料是一组具有各向异性的牙科材料。相对较低的成本,以及与牙齿接近的颜色,使纤维增强复合材料能与黏结剂、直接充填技术一同使用。纤维增强复合材料在根管治疗后牙体修复方面具有一些优势。弹性模量接近天然牙本质,抗拉强度高,在性价比高的椅旁技术中具有实用性，这些优点都使纤维增强复合材料非常适合修复根管治疗后牙体缺损的患牙。为了获得最佳的临床修复效果，医生必须充分了解影响这些复合材料性能的因素。

（唐子圣　译）

参考文献

Ahlstrand WM, Finger WJ (2002) Direct and indirect fiber-reinforced fixed partial dentures: case reports. Quintessence Int 33: 359-365.

Alander P, Lassila LVJ, Tezvergil A, Vallittu PK (2004) Acoustic emission analysis of fiber-reinforced composite in flexural testing. Dent Mater 20: 305-312.

Al-Harbi F, Nathanson D (2003) In vitro assessment of retention of four esthetic dowels to resin core foundation and teeth. J Prosthet Dent 90: 547-555.

Ballo AM, Akca EA, Ozen T, Lassila LVJ, Vallittu PK, Närhi TO (2009) Bone tissue responses to glass fiber-reinforced composite implants — a histomorphometric study. Clin Oral Impl Res 20: 608-615.

Beech D, Brown D (1972) The role of the filler-matrix interface in composite restorative materials based on polymethylmethacrylate. Br Dent J 133: 297-300.

Behr M, Rosentritt M, Lang R, Handel G (2000) Flexural properties of fiber reinforced composite using a vacuum/pressure or a manual adaptation manufacturing process. J Dent 28: 509-514.

Bitter K, Noetzel J, Neumann K, Kielbassa AM (2007) Effect of silanization on bond strengths of fiber posts to various resin cements. Quintessence Int 38: 121-128.

Cheng YY, Chow TW (1999) Fabrication of complete denture bases reinforced with polyethylene woven fabric. J Prosthodont 8: 268-272.

Corsalini M, Genovese K, Lamberti L, Pappalettere C, Carella M, Carossa S (2007) A laboratory comparison on individual Targis/Vectris posts with standard fiberglass posts. Int J Prosthodont 20: 190-192.

Creugers NHJ, Mentnik A, Fokkinga WA, Kreulen CM (2005) 5-year follow-up of a prospective clinical study on various types of core restorations. Int J Prosthodont 18: 34-39.

Dallari A, Rovatti L, Dallari B, Mason PN, Suh BI (2006) Translucent quartz-fiber post luted in vivo with self-curing composite cement: case report and microscopic examination at a two-year clinical follow-up. J Adhes Dent 8: 189-195.

Ehrenstein G, Schmiemann A, Bledzki A, Spaude R (1990) Corrosion phenomena in glass-fiber-reinforced thermosetting resins. In: Cheremisinoff N (ed) Handbook of ceramics and composites. Marcel Dekker, New York, pp. 231-268.

Fennis WM, Tezvergil A, Kuijs RH, Lassila LV, Kreulen CM, Creugers NH, Vallittu PK (2005) In vitro fracture resistance of fiber reinforced cusp-replacing composite restorations. Dent Mater 21: 565-572.

Ferrari M, Vichi A, Mannocci F, Mason PN (2000) Retrospective study of the clinical performance of fiber posts. Am J Dent 13: 9B-13B.

Fokkinga WA, Kreulen CM, Vallittu PK, Creugers NHJ (2004) A structured analysis of in vitro failure loads and failure modes of fiber, metal and ceramic post-and-core systems. Int J Prosthodont 17: 476-482.

Fredriksson M, Astbäck J, Pamenius M, Arvidson K (1998) A retrospective study of 236 patients with teeth restored by carbon fiber-reinforced epoxy resin posts. J Prosthet Dent 80: 151-157.

Freilich MA, Karmarker AC, Burstone CJ, Goldberg AJ (1998a) Development and clinical application of a light-polymerized fiber-reinforced composite. J Prosthet Dent 80: 311-318.

Freilich MA, Duncan JP, Meiers JC, Goldberg AJ (1998b) Preimpregnated fiber-reinforced pros-theses. Part I. Basic rationale and complete coverage and intra-coronal fixed partial denture design. Quintessence Int 29: 689-696.

Freilich MA, Duncan JP, Alarcon EK, Eckrote KA, Goldberg AJ (2002) The design and fabrication of fiber-reinforced implant prostheses. J Prosthet Dent 88: 449-454.

Garoushi S, Lassila LVJ, Tezvergil A, Vallittu PK (2005) Load bearing capacity of fibre-reinforced and particulate filler composite resin combination. J Dent 34: 179-184.

Garoushi S, Lassila LVJ, Tezvergil A, Vallittu PK (2006) Fiber-reinforced composite substructure: load bearing capacity of an onlay restoration and flexural properties of the material. J Contemp Dent Pract 7: 1-8.

Garoushi S, Vallittu PK, Lassila LVJ (2007) Fracture resistance of short random oriented glass fiber reinforced composite premolar crown. Acta Biomater 3: 779-784.

Garoushi S, Tanner J, Vallittu PK, Lassila L (2012) Preliminary clinical evaluation of short fiber-reinforced composite resin in posterior teeth: 12-months report. Open Dent J 6: 41-45.

Garoushi S, Säilynoja E, Vallittu PK, Lassila LVJ (2013) Physical properties and depth of cure of a new short fiber reinforced composite. Dent Mater 29: 835-841.

Grandini S, Sapio S, Simonetti M (2003) Use of anatomic post and core for reconstructing an endodontically treated tooth: a case report. J Adhes Dent 5: 243-247.

Grandini S, Goracci C, Tay FR, Grandini R, Ferrari M (2005) Clinical evaluation of the use of fiber posts and direct resin restorations for endodontically treated teeth. Int J Prosthodont 18: 399-404.

Gutteridge D (1992) Reinforcement of poly(methyl methacrylate) with ultra-high-modulus-polyethylene fibers. J Dent 20: 50-54.

Guzy GE, Nicholls JI (1979) In vitro comparison of intact endodontically treated teeth with and without endo-post reinforcement. J Prosthet Dent 42: 39-44.

Göhring TN, Schmidlin PR, Lutzt F (2002) Two-year clinical and SEM evaluation of glass-fiber-reinforced inlay fixed partial dentures. Am J Dent 15: 35-40.

Hatta M, Shinya A, Vallittu PK, Shinya A, Lassila LV (2011) High volume individual fibre post versus low volume fibre post: the fracture load of the restored tooth. J Dent 39: 65-71.

Hedlund SO, Johansson NG, Sjögren G (2003) A retrospective study of pre-fabricated carbon fibre root canal posts. J Oral Rehabil 30: 1036-1040.

Isidor F, Odman P, Brøndum K (1996) Intermittent loading of teeth restored using prefabricated carbon fiber posts. Int J Prosthodont 9: 131-136.

Jancar J, Dibenedetto AT (1993) Fibre reinforced thermoplastic composites for dentistry. Part I Hydrolytic stability of the interface. J Mater Sci Mater Med 4: 555-561.

Kallio TT, Lastumäki TM, Vallittu PK (2001) Bonding of restorative and veneering composite resin to some polymeric composites. Dent Mater 17: 80-86.

Kallio TT, Lastumäki TM, Vallittu PK (2003) Effect of resin application time on bond strength of polymer substrate repaired with particulate filler composite. J Mater Sci Mater Med 14: 999-1004.

Kardos JL (1993) Short-fiber-reinforced polymeric composites, structure - property relations. In: Lee SM (ed) Handbook of composites. Wiley-VCH, Palo Alto, p 593.

Kirzioğlu Z, Ertük MS (2004) Success of reinforced fiber material space maintainer. J Dent Child (Chic) 71: 158-162.

Kolbeck C, Rosenritt M, Behr M, Lang R, Handel G (2002) In vitro examination of the fracture strength of 3 different fiber- reinforced composite and 1 all-ceramic posterior inlay fixed partial denture systems. J Prosthodont 11: 248-253.

Krause WR, Park SH, Straup RA (1999) Mechanical properties of BIS-GMA resin short glass fiber composites. J Biomed Mater Res 23: 1195-1211.

Ladizesky NH, Chow TW, Ward IM (1990) The effect of highly drawn polyethylene fibres on the mechanical properties of denture base resins. Clin Mater 6: 209-225.

Ladizesky NH, Ho CF, Chow TW (1992) Reinforcement of complete denture bases with continuous high performance polyethylene fibers. J Prosthet Dent 68: 934-939.

Lammi M, Tanner J, Le Bell-Rönnlöf A, Lassila L, Vallittu P (2011) Restoration of endodontically treated molars using fiber reinforced composite substructure. J Dent Res 90 (Spec Iss A): Abst 2517.

Lassila LVJ, Nohrström T, Vallittu PK (2002) The influence of short-term water storage on the flexural properties of unidirectional glass fiber-reinforced composites. Biomaterials 23: 2221-2229.

Lastumäki T, Lassila L, Vallittu PK (2001) Flexural properties of bulk fiber-reinforced composite DC-Tell used in fixed partial dentures. Int J Prosthodont 14: 22-26.

Lastumäki TM, Kallio TT, Vallittu PK (2002) The bond strength of light-curing composite resin to finally polymerized and aged glass fiber-reinforced composite substrate. Biomaterials 23: 4533-4539.

Lastumäki TM, Lassila LV, Vallittu PK (2003) The semi-interpenetrating polymer network matrix of fiber-reinforced composite and its effect on the surface adhesive properties. J Mater Sci Mater Med 14: 803-809.

Le Bell AM, Tanner J, Lassila LV, Kangasniemi I, Vallittu PK (2003) Depth of light-initiated polymerization of glass fiber-reinforced composite in a simulated root canal. Int J Prosthodont 16: 403-408.

Le Bell AM, Tanner J, Lassila LVJ, Kangasniemi I, Vallittu PK (2004) Bonding of composite resin luting cement to fiber-reinforced composite root canal post. J Adhes Dent 6: 319-325.

Le Bell AM, Lassila LV, Kangasniemi I, Vallittu PK (2005) Bonding of fibre-reinforced composite post to root canal dentin. J Dent 33: 533-539.

Le Bell-Rönnlöf AM, Lassila LV, Kangasniemi I, Vallittu PK (2011) Load-bearing capacity of human incisor restored with various fiber-reinforced composite posts. Dent Mater 27: e107-e115.

Lassila LV, Tanner J, Le Bell AM, Narva K, Vallittu PK (2004) Flexural properties of fiber reinforced root canal posts. Dent Mater 20: 29-36.

Love RM, Purton DG (1996) The effect of serrations on carbon fiber posts-retention within the root canal, core retention, and post rigidity. Int J Prosthodont 9: 484-488.

Makarewicz D, Le Bell-Rönnlöf AM, Lassila LV, Vallittu PK (2013) Effect of cementation technique of individually formed fiber-reinforced composite post on bond strength and microleak-age. Open Dent J 7: 68-75.

Mannocci F, Innocenti M, Ferrari M, Watson TF (1999a) Confocal and scanning electron microscopic study of teeth restored with fiber posts, metal posts, and composite resins. J Endod 25: 789-794.

Mannocci F, Ferrari M, Watson TF (1999b) Intermittent loading of teeth restored using quartz fiber, carbon-quartz fiber and zirconium dioxide ceramic root canal posts. J Adhes Dent 1: 153-158.

Mannocci F, Sheriff M, Watson TF, Vallittu PK (2005) Penetration of bonding resins into fibre-reinforced posts: a confocal microscopic study. Int Endod J 38: 46-51.

Matinlinna JP, Lassila LV, Özcan M, Yli-Urpo A, Vallittu PK (2004) An introduction to silanes and their clinical applications in dentistry. Int J Prosthodont 17: 155-164.

Meiers JC, Duncan JP, Freilich MA, Goldberg AJ (1998) Preimpregnated fiber-reinforced prostheses. Part II. Direct applications: splints and fixed partial dentures. Quintessence Int 29: 761-768.

Meiers JC, Freilich MA (2000) Conservative anterior tooth replacement using fiber-reinforced composite. Oper Dent 25: 239-243.

Meiers JC, Freilich MA (2006) Use of a prefabricated fiber-reinforced composite resin framework to provide a provisional fixed partial denture over an integrating implant: a clinical report. J Prosthet Dent 95: 14-18.

Murphy J (1998) Reinforced plastics handbook, 2nd edn. Elsevier Advanced Technology, Oxford, UK.

Özcan M, van der Sleen JM, Kurunmäki H, Vallittu PK (2006) Comparison of repair methods for ceramic-fused-to-metal crowns. J Prosthodont 15: 283-288.

Pegoretti A, Fambri L, Zappini G, Bianchetti M (2002) Finite element analysis of a glass fibre-reinforced composite endodontic post. Biomaterials 23: 2667-2682.

Petersen RC (2005) Discontinuous fiber-reinforced composites above critical length. J Dent Res 84: 365-370.

Purton DG, Payne JA (1996) Comparison of carbon fiber and stainless steel root canal posts. Quintessence Int 27: 93-97.

Qualthrough AJ, Chandler NP, Purton DG (2003) A comparison of the retention of tooth colored posts. Quintessence Int 34: 199-201.

Qualthrough AJ, Mannocci F (2003) Tooth-colored post systems: a review. Oper Dent 28: 86-91.

Rantala LI, Lastumäki TM, Peltomäki T, Vallittu PK (2003) Fatigue resistance of orthodontic appliance reinforced with glass fiber weave. J Oral Rehabil 30: 501-506.

SahafiA, Peutzfeldt A, Asmussen E, Gotfredsen K (2003) Bond strength of resin cement to dentin and to surface-treated posts of titanium alloy, glass fiber, and zirconia. J Adhes Dent 5: 153-162.

Schmitter M, Rammelsberg P, Gabbert O, Ohlmann B (2007) Infl uence of clinical baseline findings on the survival of 2 post systems: a randomized clinical trial. Int J Prosthodont 20: 173-178.

Schmitter M, Hamadi K, Rammelsberg P (2011) Survival of two post systems — Five year results of a randomized clinical trial. Quintessence Int 42: 843-850.

Schreiber CK (1971) Polymethylmethacrylate reinforced with carbon fibers. Br Dent J 130: 29-30.

Schwickerath H (1965) Glasfaser und Kunststoffverstärkung. Zahnarztl Welt Zahnarztl Rundsch ZWR Zahnarztl Reform 66: 364-367.

Segerström S, Astbäck J, Ekstrand KD (2006) A retrospective long term study of teeth restored with prefabricated carbon fiber reinforced epoxy resin posts. Swed Dent J 30: 1-8.

Sewón LA, Ampula L, Vallittu PK (2000) Rehabilitation of a periodontal patient with rapidly progressing marginal alveolar bone loss. A case report. J Clin Periodontol 27: 615-619.

Smith DC (1962) Recent developments and prospects in dental polymers. J Prosthet Dent 12: 1066-1078.

Soares CJ, Pereira JC, Valdivia ADCM, Novais VR, Meneses MS (2012) Influence of resin cement and post configuration on bond strength to root dentin. Int Endod J 45: 136-145.

Sperling LH (1994) Interpenetrating polymer networks: an overview. In: Klempner D, Sperling LH, Utracki LA (eds) Interpenetrating polymer networks, 1st edn. American Chemical Society, Washington, pp. 3-39, 356.

Tanner J, Carlén A, Söderling E, Vallittu PK (2003) Adsorption of parotid saliva proteins and adhesion of *Streptococcus mutans* ATCC 21752 to dental fiber-reinforced composites. J Biomed Mater Res B Appl Biomater 15: 391-398.

Tanner J, Robinson C, Söderling E, Vallittu P (2005) Early plaque formation on fibre-reinforced composites *in vivo*. Clin Oral Investig 9: 154-160.

Terry DA, Triolo PT, Swift EJ (2001) Fabrication of direct fiber-reinforced posts: a structural design concept. J Esthet Restor Dent 13: 228-240.

Tezvergil A, Lassila LV, Vallittu PK (2006) The effect of fiber orientation on the polymerization shrinkage strain of fiber-reinforced composites. Dent Mater 22: 610 - 616.

Torbjörner A (2000) Post and cores. In: Karlsson S, Nilner K, Dahl B (eds) A textbook of fixed prosthodontics: The Scandinavian approach. Förlagshuset Gothia AB, Stockholm, pp. 173 - 186.

Torbjörner A, Fransson B (2004) A literature review on the prosthetic treatment of structurally compromised teeth. Int J Prosthodont 17: 369 - 376.

Torbjörner A, Karlsson S, Syverud M, Hensten-Pettersson A (1996) Carbon fiber reinforced root canal posts. Mechanical and cytotoxic properties. Eur J Oral Sci 104: 605 - 611.

Vallittu PK (1993) Comparison of two different silane compounds used for improving adhesion between fibers and acrylic denture base material. J Oral Rehabil 20: 533 - 539.

Vallittu PK (1995a) The effect of void space and polymerization time on transverse strength of acrylic-glass fiber composite. J Oral Rehabil 22: 257 - 261.

Vallittu PK (1995b) Impregnation of glass fibers with polymethylmethacrylate using powder-coating method. Appl Compos Mater 2: 51 - 58.

Vallittu PK (1996) Comparison of the in vitro fatigue resistance of an acrylic resin removable partial denture reinforced with continuous glass fibers or metal wires. J Prosthodont 5: 115 - 121.

Vallittu PK (1997a) Glass fiber reinforcement in repaired acrylic resin removable dentures: preliminary results of a clinical study. Quintessence Int 28: 39 - 44.

Vallittu PK (1997b) Oxygen inhibition of autopolymerization of polymethylmethacrylate-glass fiber composite. J Mater Sci Mater Med 8: 489 - 492.

Vallittu PK (1997c) Transverse strength, ductility, and qualitative elemental analysis of cobalt-chromium alloy after various durations of induction melting. J Prosthodont 6: 55 - 60.

Vallittu PK (1998a) Some aspects of the tensile strength of unidirectional glass fibre-polymethyl methacrylate composite used in dentures. J Oral Rehabil 25: 100 - 105.

Vallittu PK (1998b) Compositional and weave pattern analyses of glass fibers in dental polymer fiber composites. J Prosthodont 7: 170 - 176.

Valittu PK (2000) Effect of 180-week water storage on the flexural properties of E-glass and silica fiber acrylic resin composite. Int J Prosthodont 13: 334 - 339.

Vallittu PK (2007) Effect of 10 years of in vitro aging on the flexural properties of fiber-reinforced resin composites. Int J Prosthodont 20: 43 - 45.

Vallittu PK (2015) High-aspect ratio fillers: Fiber-reinforced composites and their anisotropic properties. Dent Mater 31: 1 - 7.

Vallittu PK (2014) Glass fibers in fiber-reinforced composites. In: Matinlinna J (ed) Handbook of oral biomaterials, Pan Stanford Publishing Pte Ltd, Singapore, pp. 255 - 279.

Vallittu PK, Narva K (1997) Impact strength of a modified continuous glass fiber-polymethylmethacrylate. Int J Prosthodont 10: 142 - 148.

Vallittu PK, Sevelius C (2000) Resin-bonded, glass fiber-reinforced composite fixed partial dentures: a clinical study. J Prosthet Dent 84: 413 - 418.

Vallittu PK, Ruyter IE, Ekstrand K (1998) Effect of water storage the flexural properties of E-glass and silica fiber acrylic resin composite. Int J Prosthodont 11: 340 - 350.

Zhao DS, Moritz N, Laurila P, Mattila R, Lassila LVJ, Strandberg N, Mäntylä B, Vallittu PK, Aro HT (2009) Development of a biomechanically optimized multi-component fiber-reinforced composite implant for load-sharing conditions. Med Eng Phys 31: 461 - 491.

Zicari F, Coutinho E, Scotti R, Van Meerbeek B, Naert I (2013) Mechanical properties and micro-morphology of fiber posts. Dent Mater 29: e45 - e52.

纤维加强型树脂桩修复根管治疗后牙齿的生物力学原则

5

卡洛斯·何塞·苏亚雷斯(Carlos José Soares)
安西尼斯·凡尔路易斯(Antheunis Versluis)
达拉尼·坦比罗恩(Daranee Tantbirojn)
惠昂-凯奥尔·金(Hyeon-Cheol Kim)
克里斯尼科夫·维瑞西莫(Crisnicaw Veríssimo)
保罗·塞萨尔(Paulo César)
弗雷塔斯·桑托斯-菲子霍(Freitas Santos-Filho)

摘 要

桩的使用影响根管治疗后牙齿的生物力学效应。本章节讨论根管治疗后前牙和后牙用纤维加强型树脂桩修复时的生物力学特征,以及桩系统、桩长度、黏结步骤、肩台设计和冠修复时对之的影响。本章节探讨根管治疗后缺损严重的牙齿在用玻璃纤维桩修复时的组织学特性,以及髓腔固位冠修复的黏结特性。

根管治疗后的牙齿由于龋坏、髓腔通路以及力学、化学和物理特性的改变而变得结构脆弱(Theodosopoulou and Chochlidakis 2009；Tang et al. 2010)。通常这样的牙齿需要桩来行冠修复。与金属桩相比,纤维加强型的树脂桩被认为更适用于根管治疗后牙齿(Soares et al. 2012)。纤维桩最大的优点是其弹性模量与牙本质弹性模量相似,这样咬合力通过牙根的时候可以更加均匀分布(Santos-Filho et al. 2014a, b；Verissimo et al. 2014)。用纤维加强型的树脂桩修复根管治疗后牙齿的压力/张力分布取决于几种因素。作者在本章节探讨用纤维加强型的树脂桩修复根管治疗后牙齿的生物力学原则。

5.1 桩系统的力学特性和桩-牙本质相互作用对修复后牙齿的压力/张力

传统上,铸造金属桩核和预成金属桩用于临床并获得相对的成功

(Theodosopoulou and Chochlidakis 2009；Tang et al. 2010)。但是，铸造金属桩核弹性模量并与高发的根折相关。为了寻求与牙根牙本质相似弹性和力学特性的材料，非金属桩得以发展。在这些非金属桩中，目前使用的有碳纤维加强型的环氧树脂桩，石英或玻璃纤维加强型的环氧树脂桩或甲基丙烯酸树脂桩，氧化锆桩和纤维加强型的聚乙烯桩。实验室和临床研究表明在用于根管治疗后牙齿的修复时，纤维加强型的树脂桩("纤维桩")可以很好地取代金属桩(Goracci and Ferrari 2011；Soares et al. 2012)。

纤维桩成功率高的原因很大程度是由其刚度特性决定的。纤维桩由环氧树脂聚合物基体和嵌入其内的纤维组成。这些成分的整合使得纤维桩的刚度行为与牙本质相近(弹性模量 18 GPa)并保持了牙齿的天然弹性。纤维桩和牙本质相似的弹性模量减少了应力集中，使得应力分布接近健康牙齿(图 5-1a，图 5-1c)。与根部牙本质相比，铸造桩核弹性模量高很多，其形成的更加坚硬的修复体产生高的应力集中(图 5-1b)。这种高的应力集中很容易导致牙根的垂直折裂(Lertchirakarn et al. 2003)。有研究显示玻璃纤维桩的低弹性模量降低了黏结失败的风险，而这是由于桩-黏结剂界面较低的应力所致(Santos et al. 2010；Goracci and Ferrari 2011)。玻璃纤维桩修复的牙齿根折风险较低的原因是因为树脂核和桩之间更易发生失败。而且，不像玻璃纤维桩那样，铸造桩核不与牙本质结合，这使得修复的牙齿中容易产生高的应力(图 5-1c)。

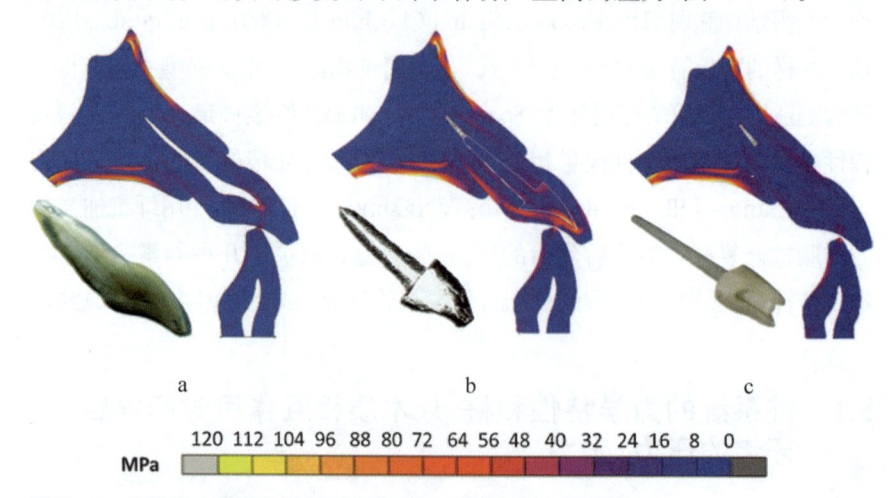

图 5-1 根管治疗后牙齿使用不同桩系统二维有限元应力分析
a. 健康牙齿；b. 金属铸造桩核；c. 玻璃纤维桩。

5 纤维加强型树脂桩修复根管治疗后牙齿的生物力学原则

在桩选择方面另一个需要考虑的因素是放置桩时应力产生的数量。金属螺纹桩的每个螺纹都会在根部牙本质产生高度的应力集中,图5-2中扫描电镜发现其所致的张力可以在牙本质产生裂纹(Santos Filho et al. 2013)。

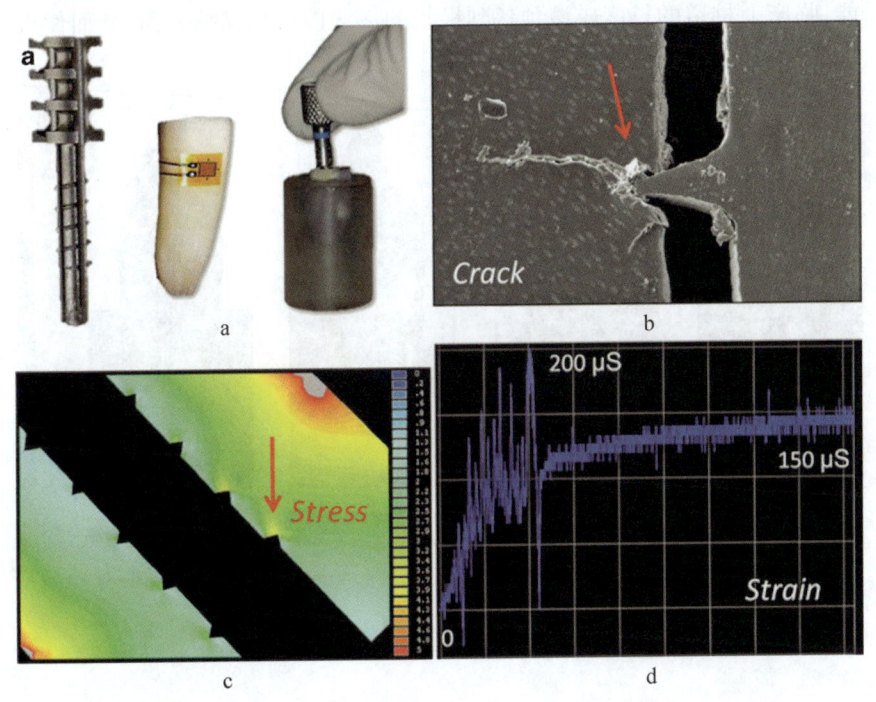

图5-2 金属螺纹桩(Radix-Anker)的应变分析
a. 手工置入螺纹桩诱发应变;b. 扫描电镜显示螺纹桩产生的裂纹;c. 桩的螺纹处产生 Von Mises 应力;d. 螺纹桩产生的外部牙根张力(图摘自 Santos Filho et al. 2013)。

5.2 桩的长度对根管治疗后牙齿的力学特性分析

根管治疗后牙齿的修复受肩领的数量、桩的直径和桩的材质等几种因素的影响。这些因素改变了牙齿的应力分布,进而影响了牙齿的抗折能力。短的铸造桩核的生物力学性能很差,其失败率也非常高(Santos-Filho et al. 2014b)。有研究表明桩的长度至少要与冠的长度相等或为剩余根长的2/3。然而由于铸造桩核的固位依靠摩擦力,所以这种观点也有所改变。临床上桩的长度受根管弯曲程度以及根管堵塞程度的影响。与铸造桩核相比,玻璃纤维桩因其能与牙本质结合的优势,其长度受限较小(Santos-Filho et al. 2008)。

有限元分析显示,玻璃纤维桩修复根管治疗后牙齿的应力分布受桩的长度影响不大(图5-3)(Santos-Filho et al. 2014b)。然而,只要有可能,临床上桩道的长度应该预备到根长的2/3以增加黏结表面,从而使玻璃纤维桩和根管之间有更好的固位。

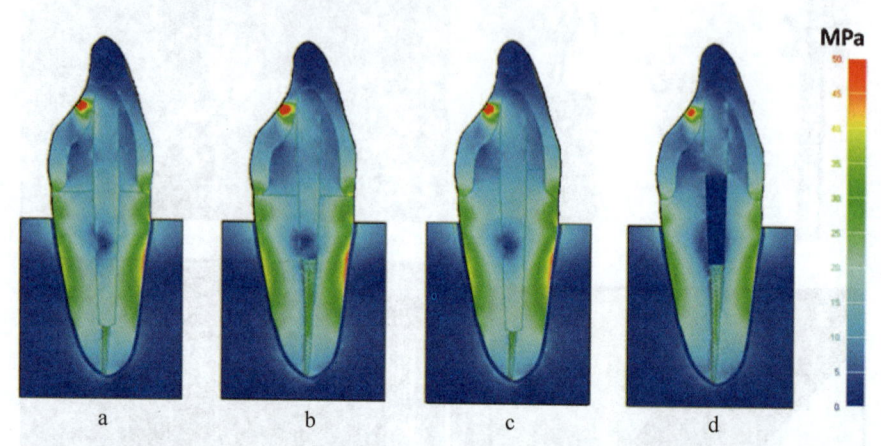

图5-3 不同桩系统和桩长度修复根管治疗后牙齿的三维有限元应力分析
a. 没有肩领桩长12 mm;b. 没有肩领桩长7 mm;c. 有2 mm肩领桩长12 mm;d. 有2 mm肩领桩长7 mm。

5.3 前牙和后牙纤维桩的生物力学性能

前牙和后牙在口腔中功能各异,这就决定了其载荷条件和解剖特点。有研究说前牙(切牙和尖牙)桩的失败率是后牙(磨牙和前磨牙)的3倍(Naumann et al. 2005)。这可能是由于前牙比后牙更容易受到水平向的力(Naumann et al. 2005)。玻璃纤维桩在前后牙的成功率都比较高,但是其在切牙和前磨牙的抗折能力比尖牙和磨牙要低(Castro et al. 2012)。铸造桩核失败率很高。玻璃纤维桩在根管治疗后磨牙剩余牙体结构较少时修复效果也很好(Santana et al. 2011)。

5.4 解剖型纤维桩修复根管治疗后的薄弱牙齿

根管治疗后的牙齿由于龋病破坏以及髓腔通路和/或根管过度预备

5 纤维加强型树脂桩修复根管治疗后牙齿的生物力学原则

被扩大后明显变弱(Silva et al. 2011)。由于这些严重薄弱的牙齿易于折裂和疲劳使得其修复具有挑战性。与预备后根管相匹配的纤维桩还尚未可得。铸造金属桩核一直在使用,但是扩大的根管形态容易形成宽大,有锥度且没有固位效果的桩。而且,如前所述,高弹性模量的金属容易引起高度应力集中(图5-4)。标准形态的纤维桩需要配合大量的黏结剂以填满扩大的根管。这些黏结剂所在的位置是潜在的薄弱区,进而影响预后(Silva et al. 2011)。

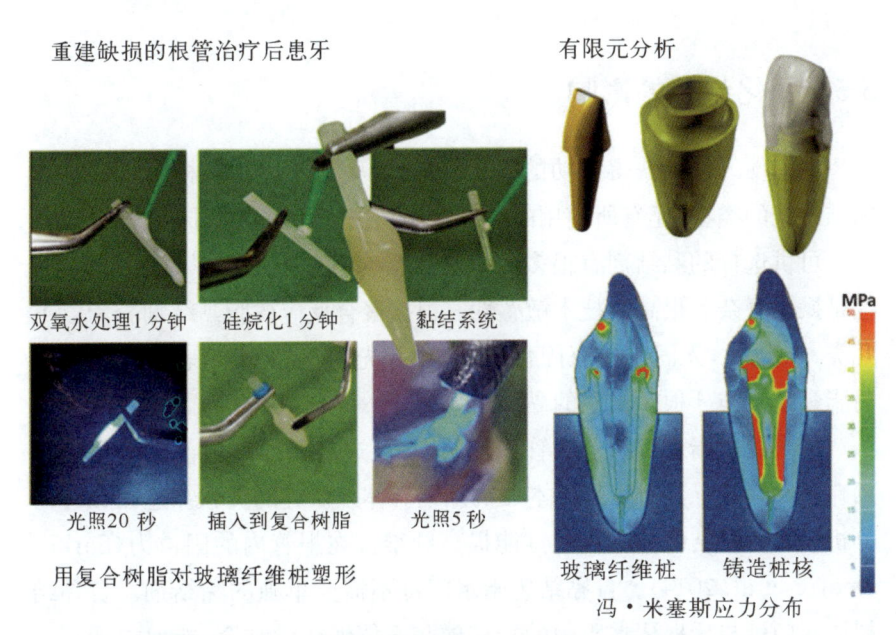

图5-4 用纤维桩和复合树脂在黏结前复原脆弱的根管治疗后患牙

一种简单可用的方法是用复合树脂对纤维桩进行塑形(图5-4)。桩的表面用24%的过氧化氢处理3分钟,然后用硅烷和黏结系统处理后黏结(de Sousa Menezes et al. 2011)。临床医师可以用诊室内漂白所用的35%的过氧化氢来处理,处理时间减至1分钟(Menezes et al. 2014)。桩的表面处理后,根管壁隔离水溶胶。然后加入复合树脂形成一个与扩大根管匹配的有解剖外形的桩。未固化的复合树脂置于纤维桩周围并插入根管内。固化前必须取出桩并再次插入根管以确保在没有卡住的情况下有较好的匹配能力,复合树脂光照5秒。彻底的复合树脂光固位在根管外面完成(20秒)。塑形后树脂表面用37%的磷酸处理,然后用气-水冲洗20秒。随后使用黏结系统并光照固化。固化前解剖型的纤维桩应该能够再次插入根管并能很好地适应根管形状。

解剖型的桩减少了光固化黏结剂的使用并能与根管壁贴合。因为复合树脂与牙本质的弹性模量相似,这样在解剖型的树脂桩与牙本质表面有均匀的应力分布,接近健康牙齿(Santos et al. 2010；Silva et al. 2011；Santos-Filho et al. 2014a)。与其他方法相比,树脂塑形的解剖型桩的抗折能力最高。

5.5 固化步骤的影响

要想使纤维桩获得成功的固化,黏结步骤必不可少。树脂水门汀和黏结系统的类型,还有所使用的根管封闭剂决定了固化的步骤。

可供选择的黏结剂有很多。树脂黏结剂有很好的力学和黏结特性,但是操作复杂有很高的技术敏感性。根据聚合反应树脂黏结剂分为以下几类:自固化,光固化或双固化(自固化和光固化)。文献表明双固化的树脂黏结剂与牙根牙本质的黏结效果最好。

传统的树脂水门汀受根管深度的影响,这是因为根尖部牙本质小管稀疏从而降低了其对根部牙本质的黏结。体外研究的文献综述和meta-分析表明自黏结的树脂水门汀能提高纤维桩在根管内的固位力(Sarkis-Onofre et al. 2014)。自黏结树脂水门汀不需要单独的黏结剂。自黏结树脂水门汀与牙根牙本质中的羟基磷灰石能够化学结合,能促进牙本质轻度脱矿并渗入其内。因此,这些水门汀有化学固位和微机械固位。近来的研究表明这些水门汀的黏结强度比传统的树脂水门汀要高,并且受根管深度的影响较小。

如果修复体固定的话,黏结步骤决定着纤维桩的成功率。黏结步骤的影响因素在本书的其他章节进行讨论。本章节所强调的独特技术是在水门汀混合和光固化反应之间的时间延长。这种延迟能提高双固化树脂水门汀与牙本质的结合并且不影响其力学特性(Khoroushi et al. 2012；Faria-e-Silva et al. 2014)。立即光照能快速增加水门汀的黏性,从而阻止酸性单体与牙齿结构的反应并减弱结合能力。双固化树脂水门汀的延迟光照能降低聚合收缩应力。无论何种树脂水门汀体系,5分钟延迟光

5 纤维加强型树脂桩修复根管治疗后牙齿的生物力学原则

照能提高树脂水门汀的力学特性,并能降低因收缩产生的应力(图 5-5)(Faria-e-Silva et al. 2014；Pereira et al. 2015)。

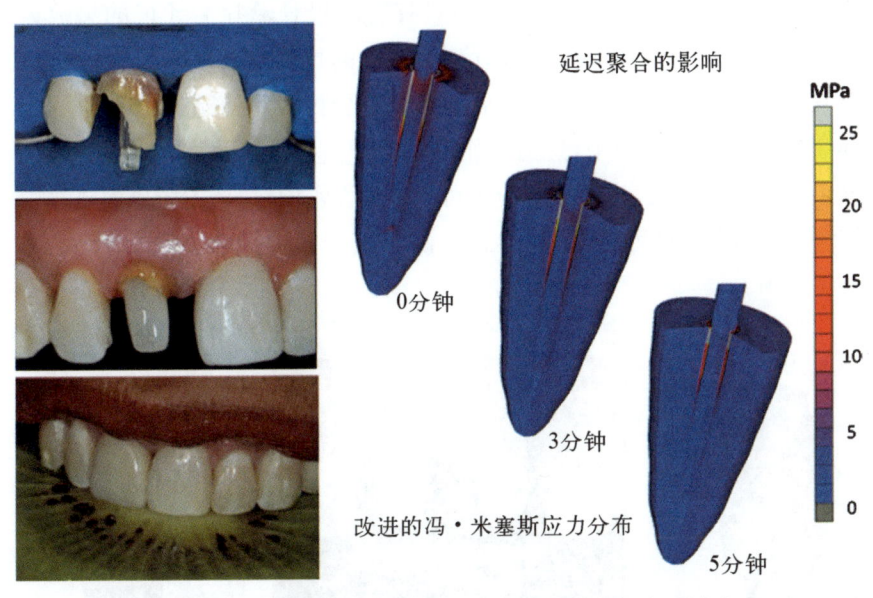

图 5-5 黏结步骤和 0,3,5 延迟聚合对树脂水门汀收缩应力的影响(图来自 Pereira et al. 2015)

　　纤维桩可以和冠部的重建一起进行。然而,根管封闭剂的类型可以影响根部牙本质和桩的黏结强度。如果黏结过程在牙髓治疗后进行,临床医师需要注意丁香油类封闭剂的影响。作为酚类化合物,丁香油能抑制树脂基质材料的聚合反应。丁香油中的羟基能与树脂聚合收缩中形成的自由基发生反应,从而降低这些材料的转化程度并降低结合强度。当使用氢氧化钙基质封闭剂的时候,不管黏结步骤是在根管充填后立即进行还是 7 天后进行,纤维桩的结合强度都不会降低(Menezes et al. 2008)。在使用氢氧化钙基质的牙髓封闭剂时,可以在完成牙髓治疗后立即进行桩的黏结。然而这个主题与第 6、第 7、第 9 章所探讨的内容仍有争议。

5.6 肩领设计对牙髓治疗后修复牙齿生物力学行为的影响

　　剩余冠部牙本质的高度称为肩领(见第 1 章),它可以支持余留牙冠部结构抵抗咬合力和插入桩时导致的侧方力。不论选择什么样的桩系统,肩领的存在可以改善牙根的应力分布,提高根管治疗后牙齿的抗折能力(图 5-6)。但是,桩系统却对有肩领根管治疗后牙齿的失败模式有影响。对失败模式的理解对避免严重的折裂方式非常重要。没有肩领的铸造金属桩核失败率非常高。应力分析显示铸造桩核在根的内部产生很高的应力集中,这为初始的垂直根折创造了条件(Sterzenbach et al. 2012)。而且,这种高的应力可以导致在水门汀-牙本质界面或水门汀-桩界面产生微间隙,从而导致细菌定植和根尖周病变(Sterzenbach et al. 2012)。

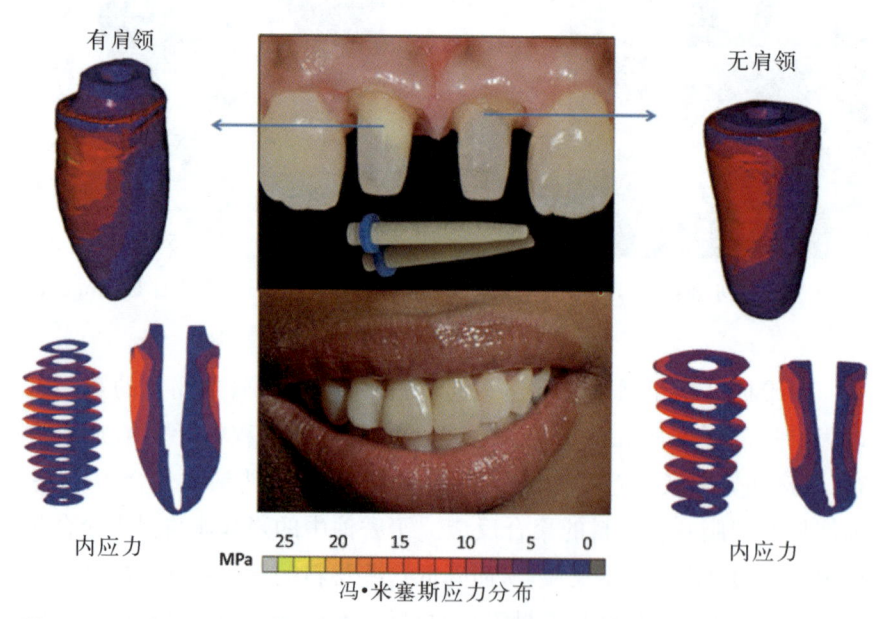

图 5-6 有肩领和无肩领纤维桩修复患牙的三维有限元分析(图摘自 PhD Thesis of Andrea D. Valdivia, Federal University of Uberlândia)

通过体外实验和有限元分析,有学者发现 2 mm 大小的肩领能对根管治疗后牙齿产生最好的应力分布。文献综述证实在冠的边缘能有 1.5~2 mm 大小的冠部结构延伸会有比较好的预后(Juloski et al. 2012)。如果临床上不能获得完整的肩领,不完全肩领仍然比没有肩领好。保留牙齿结构如同选择合适的修复材料一样重要能够产生最佳的生物力学行为。

5.7 冠修复对纤维桩修复后牙齿的生物力学行为的影响

根管治疗后牙齿重建的最后一步是冠部的修复。修复的选择主要受剩余牙齿结构的影响。选择范围从复合树脂修复到复合树脂全冠，陶瓷全冠和金属冠。

对于根管治疗后牙齿的Ⅲ类修复，如果不用纤维桩直接用复合树脂贴面修复将会增高根折发生率（Valdivia et al. 2012）。全瓷冠对低弹性模量的核材料和纤维桩有好的保护作用，这是因为高弹性模量的冠能够把高载荷扩展到更大的区域。所以全瓷冠能在核、桩和牙齿结构出现问题前先出现失败（da Silva et al. 2010）。

5.8 纤维桩修复之外：根管治疗后牙齿嵌体冠整体黏结修复

根管治疗后牙齿的通常通过核、桩或无桩和冠来修复。随着牙科黏结材料的出现，桩和核的使用不再明显（Biacchi et al. 2013）。桩、核和冠的黏结通常一起进行。然而每个黏结界面都有结合失败的风险，因此每个界面的黏结都是修复预后的关键因素。对某些根管治疗后的牙齿，嵌体冠也许是更好的修复选择。嵌体冠是一种整体的黏结修复方式，包括冠部和凸入髓腔和根管内的部分（图 5-7）。凸入髓室和冠方根管的部分提供了固位功能（Bindl and Mormann 1999；Gohring and Peters 2003）。

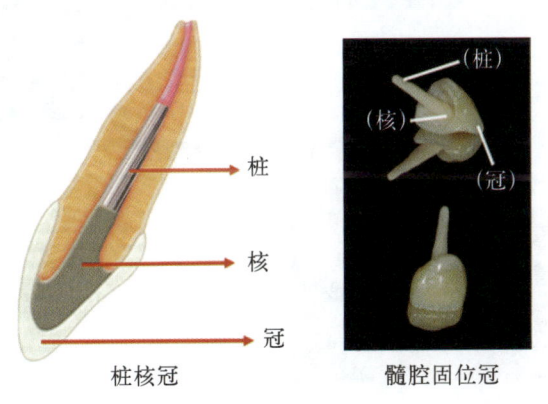

图 5-7 传统桩核冠和嵌体冠的比较

通过消除或减少黏结界面的数目,嵌体冠减少了黏结降解对修复的影响。临床上,嵌体冠的修复步骤并不复杂,更加实用,而且比桩核冠的修复步骤简单(Dejak and Mlotkowski 2013)。

嵌体冠的失败概率与传统冠相似。牙本质和黏结嵌体冠的水门汀中应力值比传统冠中的要低。有限元分析显示嵌体冠的失败可能性比纤维桩低(Dejak and Mlotkowski 2013)。威布尔分析表明与传统冠相比嵌体冠失败的概率降低很多。临床研究也证实嵌体冠的寿命比较长(Biacchi et al. 2013)。

嵌体冠修复的优点体现在功能、美学、生物力学、费用及较少的临床时间方面(图 5-8 和图 5-9)(Lin et al. 2010)。嵌体冠适用于大面积的冠缺损,这是因为其用大面积髓腔固位而不是根管桩固位(Pissis 1995;Zarow et al. 2009)。嵌体冠简单有效的观念与生物整体修复的理念相一致。这种类型的修复重建尚未普及,但应该会很快开展起来(Biacchi and Basting 2012;Fages and Bennasar 2013)。

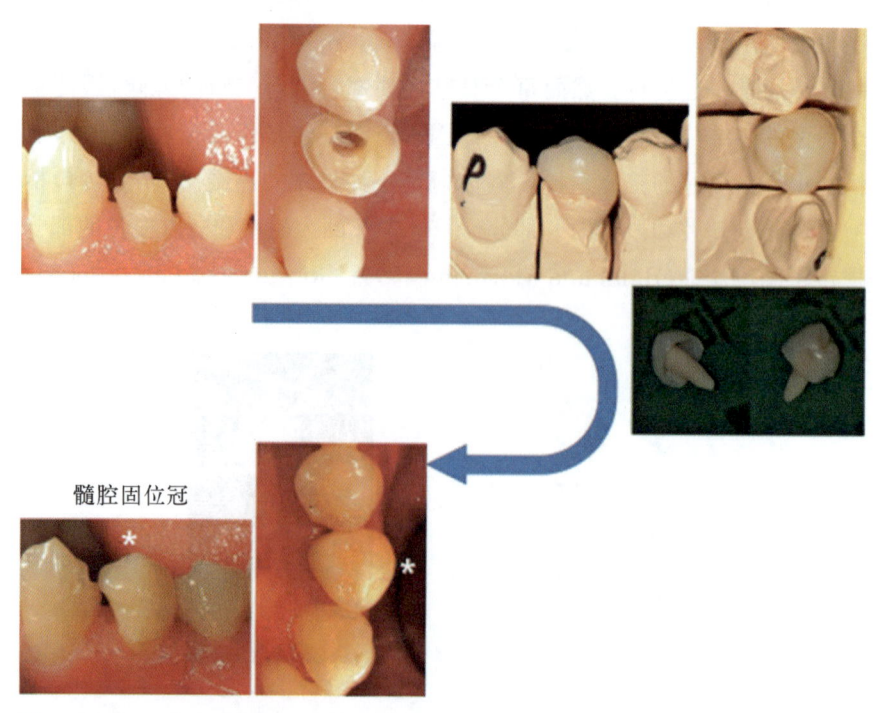

图 5-8　使用 Tescera(Bisco DentalProducts)修复下颌第一前磨牙的嵌体冠病例(*)

髓腔固位冠

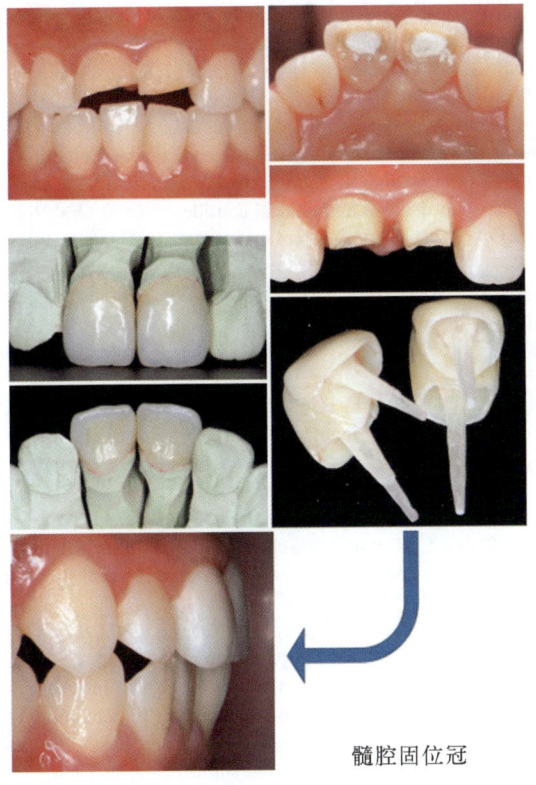

图 5-9 矫正牙长轴的上颌中切牙的嵌体冠病例

（朱来宽 译）

参考文献

Biacchi GR，Basting RT（2012）Comparison of fracture strength of endocrowns and glass fiber post-retained conventional crowns. Oper Dent 37：130-136.

Biacchi GR，Mello B，Basting RT（2013）The endocrown：an alternative approach for restoring extensively damaged molars. J Esthet Restor Dent 25：383-390.

Bindl A，Mormann WH（1999）Clinical evaluation of adhesively placed cerec endo-crowns after 2 years-preliminary results. J Adhes Dent 1：255-265.

Castro CG，Santana FR，Roscoe MG，et al.，Soares CJ（2012）Fracture resistance and mode of failure of various types of root filled teeth. Int Endod J 45：840-847.

da Silva NR，Raposo LH，Versluis A，et al.，Soares CJ（2010）The effect of post, core, crown type，and ferrule presence on the biomechanical behavior of endodontically treated bovine anterior teeth. J Prosthet Dent 104：306-317.

de Sousa Menezes M，Queiroz EC，Soares PV，et al.，Martins LR（2011）Fiber post etching with hydrogen peroxide：effect of concentration and application time. J Endod 37：398-402.

Dejak B, Mlotkowski A (2013) 3d-finite element analysis of molars restored with endocrowns and posts during masticatory simulation. Dent Mater 29: e309-e317.

Fages M, Bennasar B (2013) The endocrown: a different type of all-ceramic reconstruction for molars. J Can Dent Assoc 79: d140.

Faria-e-Silva AL, Peixoto AC, Borges MG, Menezes Mde S, Moraes RR (2014) Immediate and delayed photoactivation of self-adhesive resin cements and retention of glass-fiber posts. Braz Oral Res 28(1) Ferracane JL, Stansbury JW, Burke FJ (2011) Self-adhesive resin cements — chemistry, properties and clinical considerations. J Oral Rehabil 38: 295-314.

Gohring TN, Peters OA (2003) Restoration of endodontically treated teeth without posts. Am J Dent 16: 313-317.

Goracci C, Ferrari M (2011) Current perspectives on post systems: a literature review. Aust Dent J 56(Suppl 1): 77-83.

Juloski J, Radovic I, Goracci C, et al., Ferrari M (2012) Ferrule effect: a literature review. J Endod 38: 11-19.

Khoroushi M, Karvandi TM, Sadeghi R (2012) Effect of prewarming and/or delayed light activation on resin-modified glass ionomer bond strength to tooth structures. Oper Dent 37: 54-62.

Lertchirakarn V, Palamara JE, Messer HH (2003) Patterns of vertical root fracture: factors affecting stress distribution in the root canal. J Endod 29: 523-528.

Lin CL, Chang YH, Chang CY, et al., Huang SF (2010) Finite element and weibull analyses to estimate failure risks in the ceramic endocrown and classical crown for endodontically treated maxillary premolar. Eur J Oral Sci 118: 87-93.

Menezes MS, Faria-e-Silva AL, Silva FP, et al., Martins LR (2014) Etching a fiber post surface with high-concentration bleaching agents. Oper Dent 39: E16-E21.

Menezes MS, Queiroz EC, Campos RE, et al., Soares CJ (2008) Influence of endodontic sealer cement on fibre glass post bond strength to root dentine. Int Endod J 41: 476-484.

Naumann M, Blankenstein F, Dietrich T (2005) Survival of glass fibre reinforced composite post restorations after 2 years-an observational clinical study. J Dent 33: 305-312.

Pereira RD, Valdivia AD, Bicalho AA, et al., Soares CJ (2015) Effect of photo-activation timing on mechanical properties of resin cements and bond strength of fiber glass posts to root dentin. Oper Dent (in press)

Pissis P (1995) Fabrication of a metal-free ceramic restoration utilizing the monobloc technique. Pract Periodontics Aesthet Dent 7: 83-94.

Santana FR, Castro CG, Simamoto-Junior PC, et al., Soares CJ (2011) Influence of post system and remaining coronal tooth tissue on biomechanical behavior of root filled molar teeth. Int Endod J 44: 386-394.

Santos AF, Meira JB, Tanaka CB, et al., Versluis A (2010) Can fiber posts increase root stresses and reduce fracture? J Dent Res 89: 587-591.

Santos Filho PC, Soares PV, Reis BR, et al., Soares CJ (2013) Effects of threaded post placement on strain and stress distribution of endodontically treated teeth. Braz Oral Res 27: 305-310.

Santos-Filho PC, Castro CG, Silva GR, et al., Soares CJ (2008) Effects of post system and length on the strain and fracture resistance of root filled bovine teeth. Int Endod J 41: 493-501.

Santos-Filho PC, Verissimo C, Raposo LH, et al., Marcondes Martins LR (2014a) Influence of ferrule, post system, and length on stress distribution of weakened root-filled teeth. J Endod 40: 1874-1878.

Santos-Filho PC, Verissimo C, Soares PV, et al., Soares CJ (2014b) Influence of ferrule, post system, and length on biomechanical behavior of endodontically treated anterior teeth. J Endod 40: 119-123.

Sarkis-Onofre R, Skupien JA, Cenci MS, et al., Pereira-Cenci T (2014) The role of resin cement on bond strength of glass-fiber posts luted into root canals: a systematic review and meta-analysis of in vitro studies. Oper Dent 39: E31-E44.

Silva GR, Santos-Filho PC, Simamoto-Junior PC, et al., Soares CJ (2011) Effect of post type and restorative techniques on the strain and fracture resistance of flared incisor roots. Braz Dent J 22: 230-237.

Soares CJ, Valdivia AD, da Silva GR, et al., Menezes Mde S (2012) Longitudinal clinical evaluation of post systems: a literature review. Braz Dent J 23: 135-740.

Sterzenbach G, Franke A, Naumann M (2012) Rigid versus flexible dentine-like endodontic posts - clinical testing of a biomechanical concept: seven-year results of a randomized controlled clinical pilot trial on endodontically treated abutment teeth with severe hard tissue loss. J Endod 38: 1557-1563.

Tang W, Wu Y, Smales RJ (2010) Identifying and reducing risks for potential fractures in endodontically treated teeth. J Endod 36: 609-617.

Theodosopoulou JN, Chochlidakis KM (2009) A systematic review of dowel (post) and core materials and systems. J Prosthodont 18: 464-472.

Valdivia AD, Raposo LH, Simamoto-Junior PC, et al., Soares CJ (2012) The effect of fiber post presence and restorative technique on the biomechanical behavior of endodontically treated maxillary incisors: an in vitro study. J Prosthet Dent 108: 147-157.

Verissimo C, Simamoto Junior PC, Soares CJ, et al., Santos-Filho PC (2014) Effect of the crown, post, and remaining coronal dentin on the biomechanical behavior of endodontically treated maxillary central incisors. J Prosthet Dent 111: 234-246.

Zarow M, Devoto W, Saracinelli M (2009) Reconstruction of endodontically treated posterior teeth - with or without post? Guidelines for the dental practitioner. Eur J Esthet Dent 4: 312-327.

纤维加强型树脂桩(纤维桩)   6

乔奇·佩尔迪高(Jorge Perdigão)

摘 要

根管治疗后牙齿的修复争议了好多年。过去认为使用桩只是为了冠部修复固位。最近的研究表明纤维加强型树脂桩(或纤维桩)与黏结技术合用时可以巩固牙根。

纤维桩与牙本质的弹性模量相似,这使得其与根部牙本质力学兼容。临床研究显示纤维桩与硬的桩相比折裂的发生率低。临床治疗的成功依靠根管治疗的质量和冠部的修复两个方面,医师面临的挑战是如何使纤维桩和根管壁紧密密封,使纤维桩在根管壁上固位良好。

本章节探讨预成桩的种类、根管内使用的观点、优缺点以及与临床应用相关的考量。

6.1 前言

向根部延伸以获得安全的冠部修复观念存在已久。1871年,医生哈里斯(Harris)和奥斯汀(Austen)写到"当使用木质或金属轴的时候人工冠可以牢固地固定在牙根上,当使用这种轴的时候首选金或白金,因为银或贱金属容易被口腔中唾液氧化。"根管钉或桩是为了保护脆弱的根管治疗后牙齿出现根折,这种根折在内部应力集中的时候容易出现(Gutmann 1992)。

布莱克(Black)(1895)报道人无髓牙的牙本质抗碎强度比正常牙低。无髓牙矿化组织中水分比活髓组织中少了9%(Helfer et al. 1972)。詹姆森(Jameson)等(1993)报道含水和再水化的牙本质断裂张力和断裂能比脱水牙本质要高。无髓牙脆性增强与牙本质小管脱水相关(Huang et al. 1992)。

与后牙相比,前牙更容易脱水(Helfer 等 1972),这可以解释为什么前牙的失败率比后牙高(Mancebo 等 2010)。如第 2 章所述,作为无髓牙的牙本质水分减少的结果,可以认为根管治疗后牙齿比根管治疗前更容易折裂。然而,一般的观念是牙根牙本质的去除是牙齿变弱的重要因素(Schwartz and Robbins 2004)。目前认为与活髓牙相比,通路预备所致的牙齿完整结构的缺失是根管治疗后牙齿折裂发生的主要原因(Schwartz and Robbins 2004)。与只有通路预备没有桩道预备的牙相比,桩道预备能使根管治疗后牙齿变脆(Trope 等 1985)。窝洞预备时牙齿结构丢失的量与负荷所致的变形有直接关系(Tidmarsh,1976)。如第 2 章所述,根管通路预备去除了大量的冠部牙本质,使得牙齿在相对低负荷下也容易出现折裂。根管治疗后牙齿的抗折能力随着剩余牙本质的减少而减少,修复后牙齿的强度与剩余牙本质的量直接相关(Trabert et al. 1978;Mattison 1982;Sorenson and Martinoff 1984)。

牙根牙本质的改变也是影响修复后牙齿行为的一个因素。例如,根尖部的牙本质小管数量比冠部少(图 6-1)。随着牙齿增龄性变化以及牙

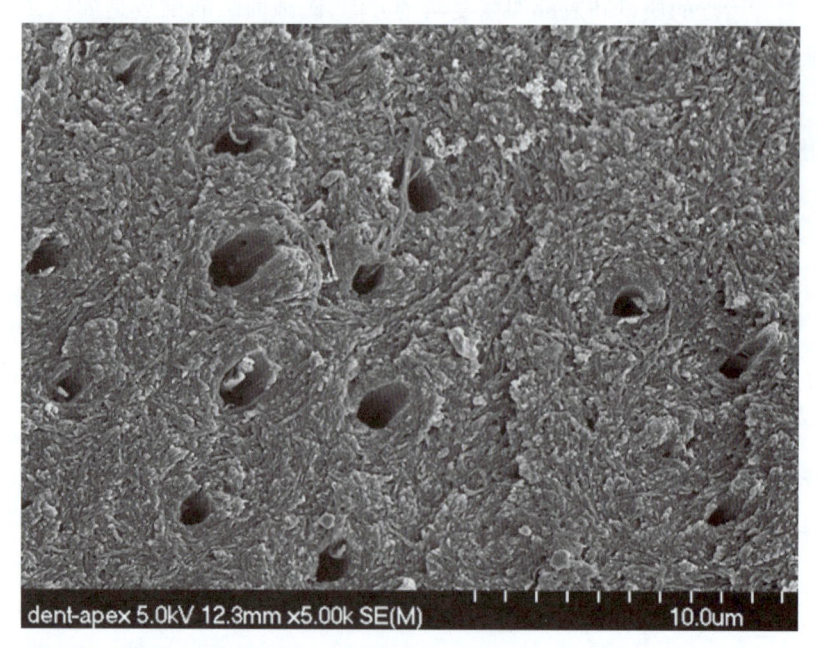

图 6-1　人磨牙根尖部 1/3 的扫描电镜图片。原始放大倍数 = ×5 000

6 纤维加强型树脂桩(纤维桩)

本质小管内管周牙本质的沉积,有机物和组织液的存在空间减少,这都使得与活髓牙相比其弹性减少。透明牙本质,有时称为硬化层(Nalbandian et al. 1960; Kinney et al. 2005),随着增龄化在根本形成(图 6-2)。正常和透明牙本质的结构和力学特性差异已有相关报道(Balooch et al. 2001; Kinney et al. 2005)。透明牙本质中的矿物质浓度明显比较高,使得牙本质小管管腔闭塞(图 6-3)。透明牙本质的弹性性能没有改变。然而,透明牙本质在失败前不会弯曲,这在正常牙本质中没有发现。透明牙本质的断裂韧性降低了 20%。随着增龄牙本质出现的变化如表 6-1 所示。

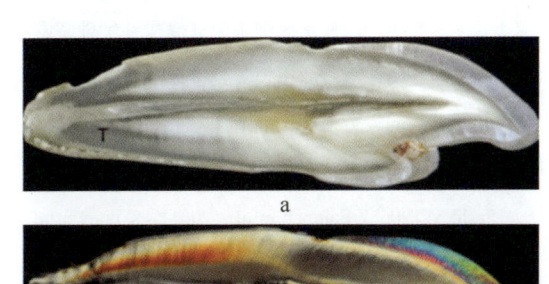

图 6-2 a.下颌尖牙的纵向切片,透明牙本质在根尖 1/3 形成;b.同一部位在偏振模式下的图示。

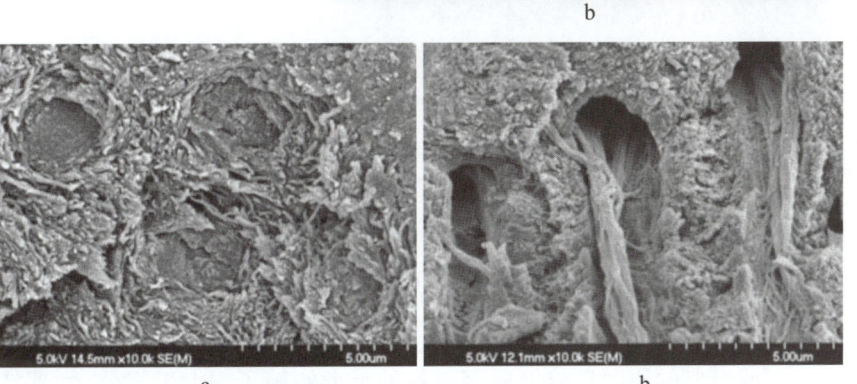

图 6-3 断裂牙本质的扫描电镜图
a.透明牙本质小管因矿物质沉积而消失;b.正常牙本质可以看到专有的牙本质小管。原始放大倍数 = ×10 000。

表 6-1 牙本质基质的增龄性变化

透明牙本质中矿物质浓度比正常牙本质高
管周基质的增加可以堵塞牙本质小管

(续表)

与正常牙本质不一样,透明牙本质在断裂前几乎不弯曲
随着年龄的增长牙本质的挠曲强度和张力强度明显减弱
透明牙本质的断裂韧性大约降低了 20%
增龄性变化增加了牙本质破坏启动及破坏延展的概率
增龄性变化降低了牙本质的渗透性
老龄牙本质的含水量较年轻牙本质低
增龄牙本质的硬度和弹性模量较年轻牙本质高
增龄牙本质中的成牙本质细胞和牙髓成纤维细胞密度降低
根尖 1/3 透明牙本质的积聚导致了牙本质小管直径的改变以及小管中矿物质的沉积
年轻牙本质的疲劳强度比老龄牙本质的高
与正常牙本质相比,硬化和老龄牙本质中杂合层变薄,树脂突变短,侧支变少

Pashley(1996),Balooch et al.(2001),Kinney et al.(2005),Prati et al.(1999),Murray et al.(2002),Jameson et al.(1993),Arola and Reprogel(2005),Kahler et al.(2003)

6.2 预成纤维桩的总则

能够修复根管治疗后牙齿的牙医增加了患者原本要拔除的患牙的保存机会。所以根管治疗后的牙齿都需要最后的修复治理才算是完整的,而且可以认为是成功的。根管治疗后牙齿恰当修复的失败可以导致牙髓治疗的失败(Safavi et al. 1987)。

根管内金属桩使根管治疗后牙齿的抗折能力翻倍。在纤维加强型树脂桩(纤维桩)和氧化锆桩出现很久以前,就认为很有必要使用销子预防根管治疗后牙齿的牙根折断。

一些经典的原则目前仍适用于各种类型的销子。由于成分、物理特性和独特黏结技术的不同,一些观念不能直接适用于纤维桩。桩主动或被动保持于根管内。主动的桩在插入时进入到牙本质壁中,被动的桩不进入牙本质壁中,而依靠黏结材料来固位(Smith et al. 1998)。因此,被动桩比主动桩固位力弱。主动桩在放置时产生更多的应力,这很可能是牙根出现断裂的薄弱点。为了避免根折,被动有锥度的桩开始使用起来(Gutmann 1992;Morgano 1996)。当使用被动桩时其固位力主要依赖于桩与根管壁的匹配程度以及黏结剂(Schmage et al. 2005)。铸造桩水门汀的厚度在 24～31 μm,预成桩水门汀的厚度在 30～50 μm,这可以最大程度的降低桩的失败率(Johnson and Sakumura 1978)。

根管治疗后患牙的寿命受多种因素影响,包括桩的设计、长度和厚度、肩领的影响、黏结和剩余牙体组织的影响(Lassila et al. 2004；Ferrari et al. 2012；Juloski et al. 2012)。以前的临床医师和研究人员认为桩应该是很硬的(Torbjörner et al. 1996)。硬的桩可以在抵抗载荷时不变形。然而,当应力传递至硬度低的部分,比如牙本质,可以导致机械性的失败(Torbjörner et al. 1996)。其他一些因素也可以影响根管治疗后牙齿的载荷能力,如牙齿的形态、修复的技术,还有最重要的一点,剩余的牙体组织是影响根管治疗后牙齿力学抗力的最基本的一些变量(Trope et al. 1985；Gutmann 1992；Sornkul and Stannard 1992；Fernandes and Dessai 2001)。

除了宽的直径(或厚度),高弹性模量(高硬度)的桩材料与桩-牙本质界面的高应力值相关。一直认为桩与牙本质的弹性模量(硬度)应该相似,这样可以使作用力沿着桩的长度平均分布,以避免应力集中并减少根折发生的概率。目前纤维桩似乎能满足这种要求,因为其弹性模量与牙本质相似(Zicari et al. 2013a)。与其他类型的桩相比,纤维桩的弹性模量与牙本质更加接近(Asmussen et al. 1999)。

纤维桩可以使应力沿着黏结剂-牙本质界面和剩余的牙体组织均匀分布。与此相反,铸造桩合金的弹性模量非常高。

6.3 桩的设计

6.3.1 桩的长度

如第 1 章所讨论的那样,阿布拉莫维茨(Abramovitz)等(2001)证实 3 mm 的牙胶体外根尖封闭的效果不可预知；所以应至少保留 5 mm 的牙胶(图 6-4)。当桩的长度占根长 2/3 时,平均长度的根和较短的根根尖封闭受到影响。当桩与冠长一致时,平均长度或长的根可能有足够的封闭效果。对于较短的根,即使桩的长度最短与冠的长度相等,其根尖封闭也会受到影响。

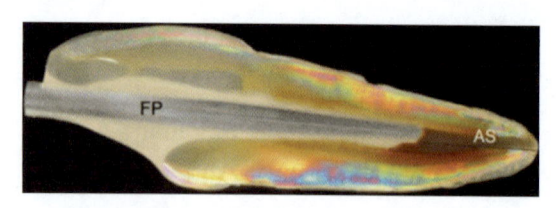

图 6-4 根管治疗后的上颌尖牙用自黏结水门汀黏结纤维桩(FP)的极化图像。牙胶尖的根尖封闭(AS)长度为 5 mm。

目前桩长度的大多数原则适用于当只有预成金属桩或铸造钉可选择的时候。索伦森和马丁诺夫(1984)报道,在下颌磨牙当桩的长度至少与冠的长度相等的时候成功率在 97%。古达克(Goodacre)和斯波尼克(Spolnik)(1995)推荐桩的长度为根长的 3/4。桩的长度至少为根长的 3/4 的时候可以提供最大的刚性和最小的牙根变形(弯曲)。这些桩的效果比只有根长 1/4 或 1/2 的桩要好(Leary et al. 1987)。

当从拔除的上颌侧切牙中进行桩移除实验的时候,占根长 3/4 或更长的桩移除所需要的拉力比只有根长一半或与冠长相等的桩多 20%～30%(Johnson and Sakumura 1978)。近来的一项体外研究,在破坏严重没有肩领的患牙,桩道预备 6 mm 或 3 mm 深,不能或者不能最大程度与根管壁匹配(Büttel et al. 2009)。纤维桩的深度为 6 mm 的实验组(匹配或最大程度不匹配)所承受的最大载荷力比 3 mm 的实验组要明显高很多。骨水平上方桩长度减少与桩尖部的应力增加相关(Al-Omiri et al. 2011)。

根管治疗后牙齿的抗折能力受桩长度的影响。

6.3.2 桩的厚度

关于铸造金属钉厚度的经典观念希灵堡(Shillingburg)等已做详述(1982)。作者写道"钉一定不要太大,这会破坏宝贵的牙齿结构、牙齿的结构完整性以及天然强度"。通过测试 50 个不同类型的恒牙(除外第三磨牙),作者认为下颌切牙桩的直径为 0.7 mm,上颌切牙为 1.7 mm。此外,在牙骨质-牙釉质联合处钉的直径不能大于牙根直径的 1/3。

根管治疗的过程中牙齿内部结构的去除伴随着相应的应力增加,尤其在牙颈部(Hunter et al. 1989)。桩的锥度与根管的匹配度,也称为形态一致性,一直被认为预成钛桩系统的一个重要因素(Schmage et al. 2005),纤维桩的固位看起来不受桩匹配程度的影响(Perdigão et al. 2007;Büttel et al. 2009)。最低程度的桩道预备实质上不会使牙齿变弱(Hunter et al. 1989),桩直径的增宽与应力的增加有关系(Al-Omiri et al. 2011)。

牙齿长度的增加能增加抗折能力(Trabert et al. 1978),桩道的过度预备插入金属桩后不会加固牙齿,但是降低了牙齿的抗折能力(Trabert et al. 1978;Mattison 1982)。根管治疗后牙齿的折裂强度不会因插入金属桩而增强(Trope et al. 1985;Goodacre and Spolnik 1994)。而且,通路开放结构完整的根管治疗后牙齿在插入金属桩时不会明显加固(Guzy and Nicholls 1979)。

纤维桩直径的增加可以增加其抗折最大载荷(Zicari et al. 2013a),但是随着桩直径的增加弯曲强度和弯曲模量却降低了。小直径的纤维桩不会导致牙根牙本质的过度去除,过度去除牙本质会降低抗折载荷导致修复体的失败。从临床角度来讲,在不同临床环境下选择合适纤维桩时纤维桩的弯曲强度能够平衡折裂载荷(Zicari et al. 2013a)。

当桩和牙本质有相似的弹性模量(硬度)的时候,如纤维桩,较小直径的桩可以有较好的应力分布(Al-Omiri et al. 2011)。

6.3.3 桩的形态

桩的形态多种多样(图6-5)——平行有凹凸表面、光滑表面、串珠形,锥度有凹凸表面、光滑表面、串珠形(Smith et al. 1998)。凹凸光滑的桩是预成金属桩被动固位效果最好的一种。把有锥度的桩道改为平行的桩道可以弱化牙齿(Lang et al. 2006)。虽然以前的研究提示使用平行的桩可以增加固位强度(Cohen et al. 1992;Morgano 1996;Teixeira et al. 2006),没有聚合的圆柱形的桩可以弱化根尖部的区域导致根折(Morgano 1996)。

推荐使用顶部有锥度的平行桩。

6.4 纤维桩的构成

牙科领域引入的第一个纤维桩,碳纤维加强型树脂桩(或碳纤维桩

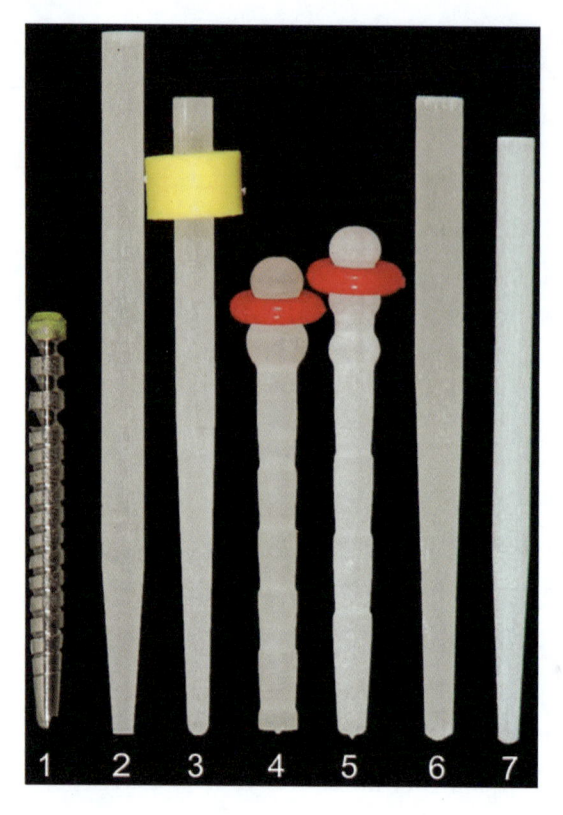

图6-5 目前使用的预成桩
1. Tenax（Coltene）；2. GC Fiber Post（GC Co.）；3. RelyX Fiber Post（3M ESPE）；4. Parapost Fiber Lux（Coltene）；5. Parapost Taper Lux（Coltene）；6. White Post（FGM）；7. Rebilda Post（VOCO GmbH）。

Duret et al. 1990)，是一个里程碑式的转折点，改变了根管治疗后牙齿修复的一些原则。最初的时候，碳纤维桩由环氧树脂基质（64%重量比）被直径 8 μm 单向的碳/石墨纤维加强后构成（Torbjörner et al. 1996）。然而，碳纤维是黑的，所以缺乏美容效果。碳纤维桩是替代铸造桩和预成金属桩或氧化锆桩的第一选择。至少在短期内的一些病例中，纤维桩固位的冠所展示的特性比其他预成桩好（King and Setchell 1990）。

目前美国市场上使用的一种纤维桩是 CF 碳纤维桩（J. Morita，USA）（图6-6a）。纤维的直径是 7.25 μm（图6-6b）。由玻璃或二氧化硅纤维制成的白的透明的桩，因其美观性已经用来替代了不美观的碳纤维桩（Lassila et al. 2004）。玻璃纤维的弹性模量（低硬度）较碳纤维的低（Lassila et al. 2004）。图6-7 显示了碳纤维桩（图6-7a）与目前使用的玻璃纤维桩的表面形态差异（图6-7b）。目前的纤维桩是透明的，由高体积百分比连续拉伸单向的坚强型玻璃纤维嵌入聚合物基质中制成，这

6 纤维加强型树脂桩(纤维桩)

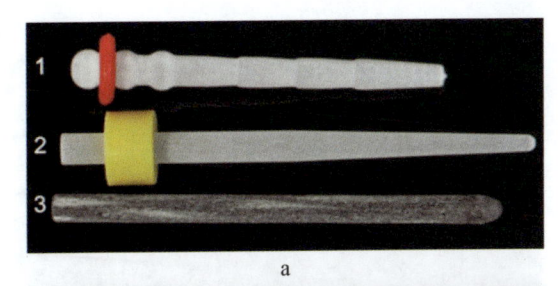

图 6-6 a. 不同的纤维桩。① 5# Parapost Taper Lux (Coltene);② 2# RelyX Fiber Post (3M ESPE);③ L2#，CF Carbon Fiber Post size L2 (J. Morita USA)。b. 扫描电镜所示的碳纤维(CF Carbon Fiber Post, J. Morita USA)。原始放大倍数=×10 000。

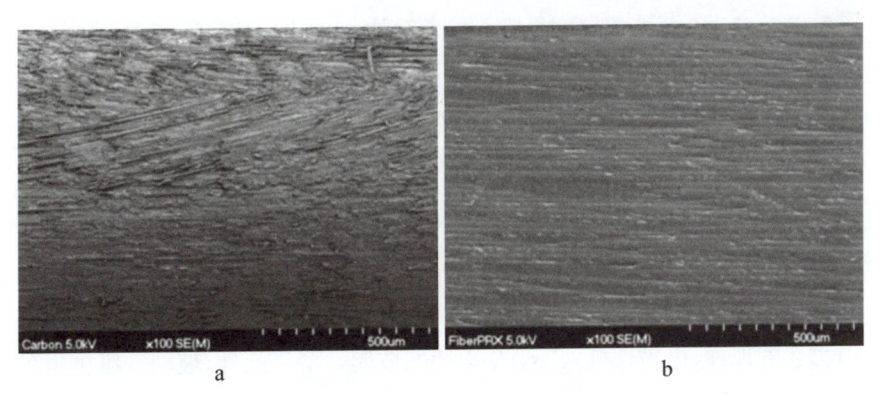

图 6-7 a. 扫描电镜所示的碳纤维桩侧面(CF Carbon Fiber Post，J. Morita USA)。原始放大倍数=×100；b. 扫描电镜所示玻璃纤维桩的侧面(RelyX Fiber Post，3M ESPE)。原始放大倍数=×100。

种聚合物使纤维保持在一起(图 6-8)。纤维-基质的比例范围从 40%～65%(Zicari et al. 2013a)。这种基质通常包含环氧树脂和/或甲基丙烯酸酯树脂高度变换高度交联的结构,可以使填料和阻射剂很好的加入其中(Zicari et al. 2013a)。一些桩系统也含有高分子重量的 PMMA 链。

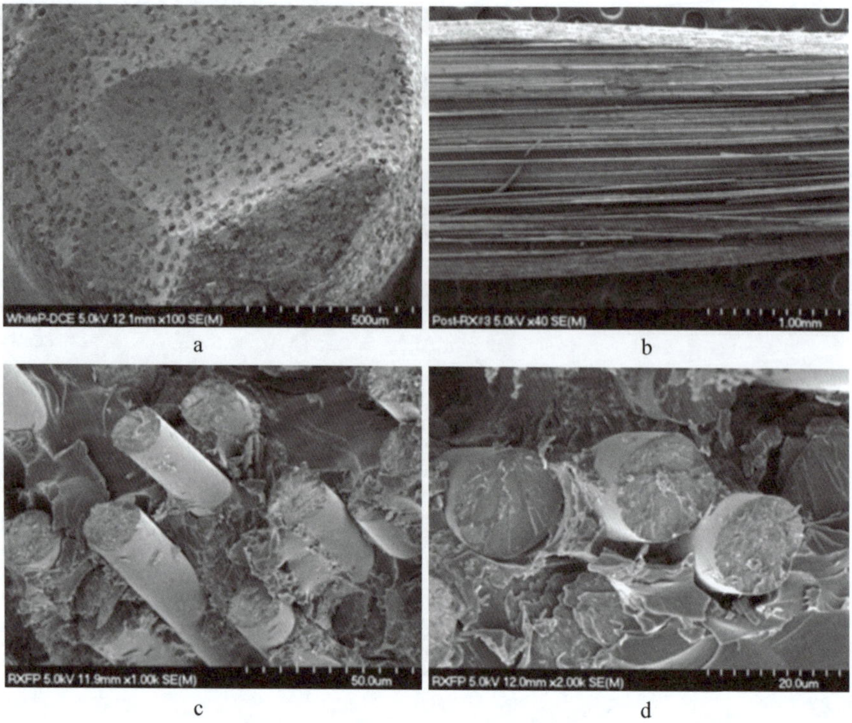

图 6-8　a. 扫描电镜所示玻璃纤维桩的冠方横断面(White Post DC‑E，FGM)，原始放大倍数 = ×100；b. 扫描电镜所示玻璃纤维桩的纵断面(RelyX Fiber Post，3M ESPE)。原始放大倍数 = ×40；c. 扫描电镜所示用金刚石车针切断的玻璃纤维桩断面(RelyX Fiber Post，3M ESPE)。原始放大倍数 = ×1 000；d. 扫描电镜所示用金刚石车针切断的玻璃纤维桩断面(RelyX Fiber Post，3M ESPE)。原始放大倍数 = ×2 000。

基质可以使纤维成分有高的机械强度并在纤维间分布应力(Lee and Peppas 1993)。纤维成分可以抵抗弯曲，而树脂基质可以抵抗压应力并与黏结水门汀中的功能性单体相互作用(Grandini et al. 2005)。如第 4 章描述的那样，电玻璃(E-glass)是常用的玻璃类型。此外，玻璃纤维桩也可以由石英纤维制成。石英是纯的二氧化硅晶体形式(Lassila et al. 2004)。

众所周知，环氧树脂的吸水性(Antoon et al. 1981)可以导致其降解(Lee and Peppas 1993)。有学者(1995)发现碳纤维加强型材料吸水降解后，横向拉伸强度有17%的降低。吸水性明显降低碳纤维桩弯曲模量和强度。疲劳试验发现无论是干燥还是含水饱和的桩，其弯曲模量和强度都明显降低。失败主要发生在纤维-基质界面和基质内的微裂部位。在水中存放和热循环后纤维和基质的黏结降低，也会出现基质裂隙(Torbjörner et al. 1996)。

玻璃纤维桩在热循环后降低了10%的弯曲模量。热循环后强度和断裂载荷降低了大约18%（Lassila et al. 2004）。在水中存放30天后纤维桩的力学性能出现降低，这种降低是由水所致的聚合物塑化导致的。由于纤维和树脂基质的弹性模量不同，纤维和基质界面容易出现应力。维利图（Vallittu）（2000）报道纤维-基质界面的质量影响了纤维加强型树脂材料（FRC）的力学特性。这两种材料如果没有充分的黏结，纤维就像基质内的空泡，从而弱化了纤维树脂复合物。

6.5 为什么是纤维桩？

以前的一些研究集中在基质-纤维比例（每平方毫米纤维所占的量）对纤维桩弯曲特性的影响。齐卡里（Zicari）等（2013）研究了不同纤维桩的结构特点，包括纤维密度、纤维直径、纤维-基质比例和纤维的分布。他们发现这些参数与弯曲强度之间没有关联。格兰迪尼（Grandini）等（2005）报道纤维桩的结构特性与耐疲劳程度无关，这些特性包括纤维直径、纤维密度和每平方毫米纤维所占的量。塞菲尔德（Seefeld）等（2007）发现纤维-基质的比例与纤维桩的弯曲强度有明显的线性关系。这些研究有点相互矛盾。

当比较相似参数的纤维桩弯曲强度的时候，某些特殊的桩比其他的明显要好很多。它们其中的一些是由于氧化锆填料的强度影响（Zicari et al. 2013a），这些填料在目前所使用的一些纤维桩中有分布。当用方向散射区域放射扫描电镜观察桩-水门汀界面的时候（佩尔迪高，未发表的观察结果）（图6-9），这些特殊纤维桩（图6-9b）基质中看到的填料颗粒与齐卡里（Zicari）等（2013a）所提到的一致。

6.5.1 纤维桩和金属桩的比较

很多体外研究表明与金属桩相比，纤维桩因其弹性模量与牙本质更接近而具备一些优势（Lassila et al. 2004；Zicari et al. 2013a,b）。然而，材料的模量只是影响应力发展的一个参数。

纤维桩比金属桩产生的应力低（Pegoretti et al. 2002；Santos et al.

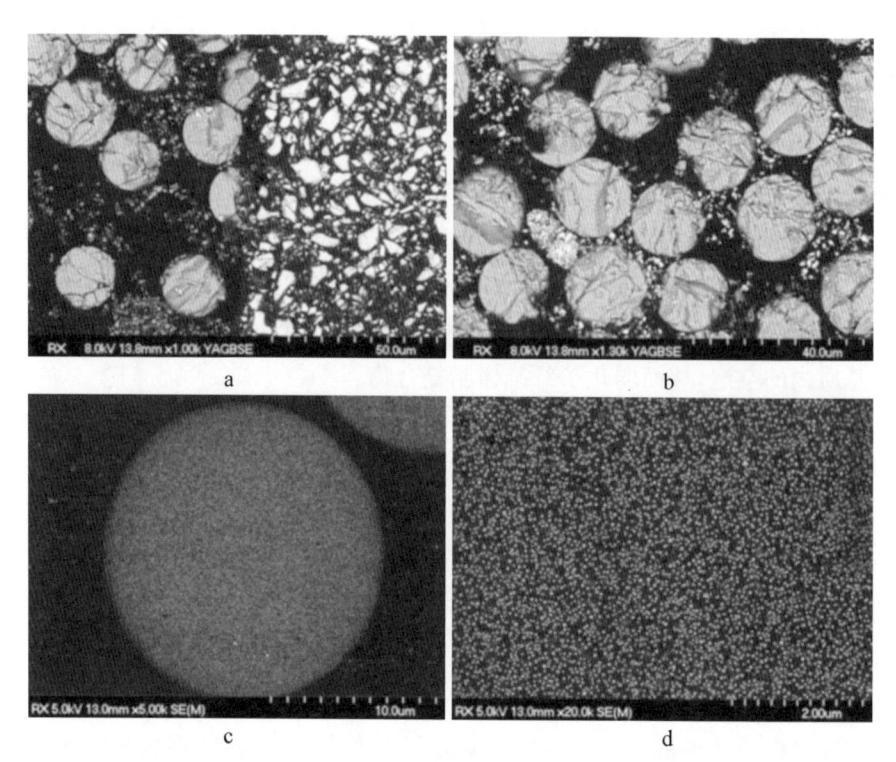

图6-9 a.扫描电镜所示 RelyX Fiber Post (3M ESPE)和自黏结水门汀的界面,原始放大倍数=×1 000;b.扫描电镜所示 RelyX Fiber Post (3M ESPE)。原始放大倍数=×1 300;c.扫描电镜所示 RelyX Fiber Post (3M ESPE)中单个的玻璃纤维。原始放大倍数=×5 000;d. c 中单个纤维的高放大倍数。原始放大倍数=×20 000。

2010)。而且,用纤维桩修复的根管治疗后牙齿折裂的可能性也较低(Santos et al. 2010)。1984~2003年的文献综述比较了失败模式与预成和传统的铸造金属桩,预成纤维桩的失败模式更有利(Fokkinga et al. 2004)。

通过有限元分析(FEA)计算了在受到外部载荷时的力学反应(Pegoretti et al. 2002)。其产生的应力与铸造金属桩和碳纤维桩产生的应力进行了比较,同时比较了天然牙的反应。铸造金属桩核在桩-牙本质界面产生了最大的应力集中。另一方面,纤维桩由于其弹性在颈部区域形成了高的应力。而纤维桩的刚度与牙本质相似,其所产生的最低应力在牙根内部。因此除了在颈缘产生应力集中外,纤维桩产生的应力区域与天然牙十分相似(Pegoretti et al. 2002)。

铸造金属桩10年后的成功率比较高(Gómez-Polo et al. 2010)。与纤维桩相比,铸造金属桩的抗折能力最强,但用其修复宽大的根管的时候可能产生不可修复的折断。纤维桩和塑形后的桩所发生的折断因提高了可修复断裂的发生概率从而提供了足够的抗折能力(Aggarwal et al. 2012)。近来的一项 meta 分析(Zhou and Wang 2013)也推断铸造桩的抗折能力也比纤维桩高。然而,**金属桩**修复的牙齿会发生灾难性的失败,比如在牙根的中 1/3 所发生的斜或水平的折断或者牙根的垂直折断。纤维桩所发生的折断可以修复,比如在牙根颈 1/3 发生的折断或在核部发生的折断(Zhou and Wang 2013)。

铸造金属桩和纤维桩都可以用来修复脆弱的牙齿。铸造桩黏结到牙齿结构上后能明显补偿根管治疗后牙齿肩领缺损所致的影响(Dorriz et al. 2009)。当颈 1/3 的根管因过度加宽而使牙根变脆弱的时候,与铸造金属桩相比,即使在所修复牙齿的预后有疑问时,颈部较宽的纤维桩仍是临床上最佳的选择。**纤维桩**所致的断裂是可以修复的(Wandscher et al. 2014)。

6.5.2 纤维桩和氧化锆桩的比较

Asmussen 等(1999)比较了碳纤维桩、氧化锆桩和钛桩。氧化锆桩的硬度是碳纤维桩的 5 倍。作者认为氧化锆桩因为没有延展性而非常脆。碳纤维桩拥有弹性极限,"该极限比强度值低,体现了一定程度的弹性行为"。

有学者(2002)比较了不同预成桩(钛、石英纤维、玻璃纤维和氧化锆桩)对根管治疗后牙齿冠修复后抗折强度和断裂模式的影响。桩用酸蚀-冲洗黏结和双固化树脂水门汀进行黏结。所有患牙用树脂核修复;金属冠用玻璃离子水门汀黏结。与其他 3 种桩相比,石英纤维桩修复的患牙所承受的破坏载荷明显比较高。纤维桩修复的患牙断裂可以被修复。氧化锆桩会导致灾难性的根折,而与钛桩和氧化锆桩相比,纤维桩修复的牙齿不易于折断(Akkayan and Gülmez 2002)。

伴有冠部缺损根管治疗后的上颌前牙用不同的桩核系统修复后,发现氧化锆桩伴树脂核修复后的牙齿的存活率和断裂强度,以及在人工口腔中的疲劳程度都是明显比较低的,因此作者不推荐在临床中使用氧化锆桩(Butz et al. 2001)。氧化锆桩的存活率明显比纤维桩低(Mannocci et al. 1999)。在该项研究中，用纤维桩树脂核和全瓷冠修复的患牙能最大程度的降低根折的风险。在湿性环境下间歇加载的实验中，纤维桩组只有1例断裂出现，而氧化锆组有6例断裂出现（1例冠折，5例根折+桩折）(Mannocci et al. 1999)。

纤维桩能降低根管治疗后牙齿的根折风险。

6.6　纤维桩的表面处理

增加纤维桩表面黏结特性的化学-机械表面处理方法有几种——氢氟酸、高锰酸钾、乙醇钠、喷砂和过氧化氢。所有这些方法都可以使处理过的纤维桩表面与复合树脂黏结剂之间形成互相渗透的网络(Monticelli et al. 2006)。树脂黏结材料渗透到纤维间的空隙可以增加表面粗糙度。实际上，氢氟酸、高锰酸钾、乙醇钠和喷砂都可以增加表面粗糙度氢氟酸、高锰酸钾、乙醇钠、喷砂(Mazzitelli et al. 2008)。

虽然不同的研究结果在一些病例中互相矛盾，作为一种有前途的方法，过氧化氢浸入可以增强纤维桩的黏结效果。有作者（2008）研究了过氧化氢和二氯甲烷对纤维桩和复合树脂之间抗剪切强度的影响。纤维桩的表面用10%过氧化氢处理20分钟能明显增强平均的抗剪切强度，这是由于过氧化氢能溶解纤维桩内的环氧树脂基质。纤维桩的表面用二氯甲烷处理5秒不能增强抗剪切强度。用30%过氧化氢或二氯甲烷处理5分钟或10分钟后能增强纤维桩和树脂核之间的黏结。在另一项研究中，24%和50%的过氧化氢在任何一种处理时间（1分钟、5分钟和10分钟）下都能增加树脂和纤维桩之间的平均黏结强度。没有处理的桩表面比较光滑，纤维没有暴露。过氧化氢能增加表面粗糙度并暴露个体纤维(de Sousa Menezes et al. 2011)。

马泽特利(Mazzitelli)等（2012）研究了2种自黏结树脂水门汀和5种纤维桩表面处理剂，包括硅烷、10%过氧化氢和硅酸盐喷砂。一种纤维桩，在所有的表面处理方法处理后平均推出黏结强度都相似。一种自黏结水门汀，只有硅烷化处理能提高推出黏结强度。有学者（2012）报道用硅酸盐喷砂处理组的平均推出黏结强度明显比硅烷处理组或无处理组高。

6 纤维加强型树脂桩(纤维桩)

在实验室中我们不能证实过氧化氢能改变纤维桩表面(图 6-10)。第 5 章和第 9 章会详细探讨纤维桩表面的处理。

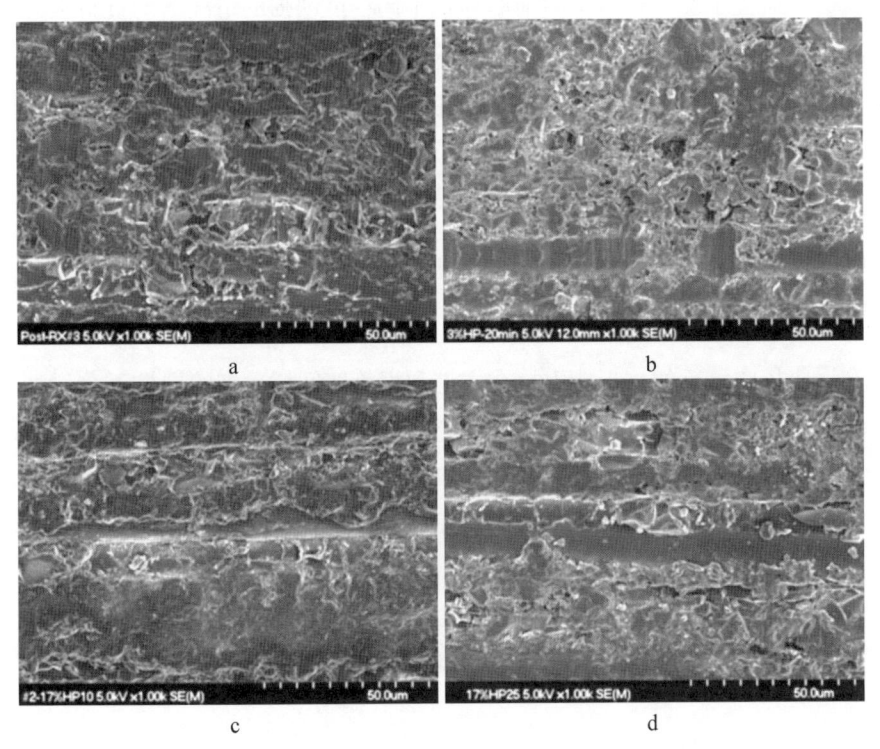

图 6-10 RelyX Fiber Post（3M ESPE)表面的扫描电镜图。原始放大倍数 = ×1 000 a. 未处理;b. 用 3%过氧化氢处理 20 分钟;c. 用 17%过氧化氢处理 10 分钟;d. 用 17%过氧化氢处理 25 分钟。

6.7 常见的观点

6.7.1 桩能加固残留的牙齿结构

桩的主要目的是保持用作保持最后义齿的核。过去 40 年内的一些作者认为,当金属桩使用传统的酸-碱水门汀黏结的时候,不能加固根管治疗后的牙齿。然而,当预成的金属桩用树脂类的水门汀黏结到根管内的时候,与使用磷酸锌相比其抗折能力明显增加(Mendoza et al. 1997)。

近来,随着纤维桩和简化的黏结技术的出现,一些作者研究了纤维桩黏结到根管内后的加固效果（Carvalho et al. 2005；Goncalves et al. 2006；Hayashi et al. 2006；D'Arcangelo et al. 2010）。Mangold 和 Kern （2011）研究了纤维桩对下颌前磨牙在不同程度缺损的情况下的抗折裂能力的影响。纤维桩的放置明显影响根管治疗后前磨牙的抗折能力；然而，抗折能力取决于残留冠部牙本质壁的量。当窝洞的壁少于 2 个的时候，纤维桩能明显影响其抗折能力。

总之，有证据表明纤维桩黏结后能加固残留的牙齿结构。

6.7.2 桩的合适程度对固位的影响

科斯塔（Costa）等（2012）分析了人前磨牙根管治疗后用纤维桩黏结和树脂核修复后的抗折能力。在主桩和根管壁间插入细的副桩不会增加牙齿的抗折能力。在另一项体外研究中，不考虑桩的长度，在热机械加载后，匹配的桩对抗折能力没有明显影响（Büttel et al. 2009）。佩尔迪高等（2007）研究了小锥度的桩，冠部末端直径为 1.5 mm，根尖部末端直径为 0.9 mm。桩道用稍大直径的钻来预备。桩道的直径对推出黏结强度没有明显的影响（图 6-11）。法拉利等（2012）报道用预成桩修复的患牙比用定制的桩修复的患牙 6 年失败的风险要低。

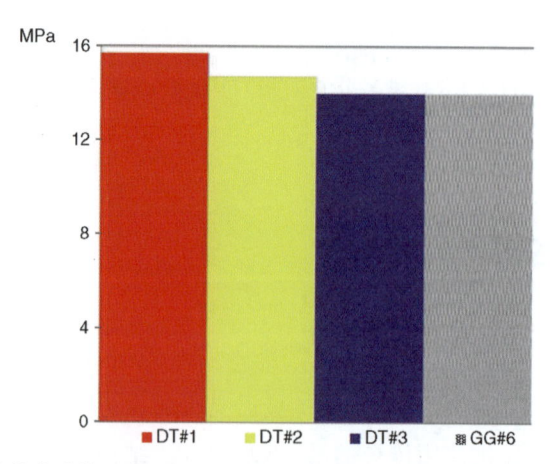

图 6-11 平均推出黏结强度（MPa）（改编自 Perdigão et al. 2007）所有实验组都使用 A D.T. Light Post size 1（Bisco，Inc.）。冠部末端直径为 1.5 mm，根尖部末端直径为 0.9 mm。黏结系统为 One-Step Adhesive（Bisco，Inc.）和 Post Cement Hi-X Self-Cured Resin Cement（Bisco，Inc.）。DT#1，#1 D.T. Drill（Bisco Inc.）；DT#2，#2 D.T. Drill（Bisco Inc.）；DT#3，#3 D.T. Drill（Bisco Inc.）；GG#6，#6 Gates-Glidden

纤维桩与根管壁的适应在桩的固位中好像不能起到明显作用。

6.7.3 冠部的修复对根管治疗后牙齿的临床成功率起着最重要的作用

如第1章所述，吉伦（Gillen）等（2011）就冠部修复质量对比根管充填质量对牙髓治疗成功率的影响做了系统性的综述。作者发现冠部修复的质量和根管充填的质量对牙髓治疗成功率有同等重要的作用。恰当的根管治疗合并恰当的修复治疗能够提高根尖周炎愈合的机会。

6.7.4 宽大的桩道可以使用宽大的桩从而可以获得比较好的桩固位

随着桩直径的增加和垂直载荷的增加根管壁的应力也会增加（Mattison 1982）。通路和根管的过度预备可以导致牙齿的折断。根管治疗后的牙齿用小直径的不锈钢桩修复的时候，其抗折能力比用较大型号的桩修复时要强（Trabert et al. 1978）。而且，金属桩直径的增加对其固位能力没有明显影响（Standlee et al. 1978）。小直径的桩可以减少根管壁的应力分布，而且可以减少桩道预备过程中牙体组织的去除量。因此，修复科医师可以有更多的牙体组织来操作，有助于在有限的牙体组织上顺利完成操作（Mattison 1982）。最近的研究显示最小直径的纤维桩有较高的弯曲强度（Zicari et al. 2013a）。

过度的桩道预备和较大的桩不会加固患牙，反而会降低牙齿的抗折能力（Trabert et al. 1978；Mattison 1982）。根管治疗后的牙齿折断可以在以下情况下发生：如在牙齿结构的缺损和在修复时通路预备产生应力的时候；在根管预备、根管荡洗和根管充填的时候；在桩道预备的时候；在冠部修复的时候；在修复时桥体选择不当的时候（Tang et al. 2010）。从业者如果在牙科治疗的时候知道可控制的以及不可控制的风险，这样会降低牙齿折断的风险。

总之，不推荐预备较宽的桩道插入较大的桩，这是因为健康牙体结构的去除会降低根管治疗后牙齿的寿命。

6.7.5 透明的纤维桩可以传导光来固化根管内的水门汀

然而，也有证据表明透明桩限制光的传播（Teixeira et al. 2006；Faria e Silva et al. 2007）。两种纤维桩，DT Light Post（Bisco Inc.）和FRC Postec

Plus（Ivoclar Vivadent）各自的传播率为 10.2%和 7.7%（Kim et al. 2009）。另一个纤维桩，SnowPost（Danville Materials）的传播率更低为 0.5%。Variolink II（Ivoclar Vivadent）的转换率从 32.78%～69.73%，这取决于桩的深度和类型（Kim et al. 2009）。

随着透明桩在根管内深度的增加，光的传播量明显减少。即使没有桩，根管内光的强度也会降低到不能聚合的水平，尤其是在根尖 1/3（dos Santos Alves Morgan et al. 2008）。

在桩道的根尖区域，透明桩不能传播足够光使树脂水门汀聚合。

6.7.6　凸凹纤维桩的固位能力比光滑桩好

固位的凹槽（锯齿状）可以降低抗疲劳强度（Grandini et al. 2005）。纤维桩的固位不受表面锯齿的影响，但是却受树脂水门汀类型的影响（Soares et al. 2012）。桩上的锯齿可能是应力集中区，使得桩变弱（Zicari et al. 2013a）。

不推荐使用锯齿状的纤维桩是因为与光滑的桩相比，这些锯齿是生理性的薄弱区。

6.7.7　根管封闭剂的类型影响根管牙本质的黏结

当桩黏结到桩道预备前已做根管充填的牙齿内时，其固位能力高于桩道预备后再行根管充填的牙齿，因为在其内部可能预留污染的牙本质（Boone et al. 2001）。封闭剂的类型、有无丁香油酚、黏结的时间对桩固位没有影响。当使用树脂基质的水门汀的时候，在机械的装备预备的时候，获得干净牙本质表面对桩的固位异常重要（Boone et al. 2001）。Kurtz et al.（2003）有学者测试了黏在根管内的桩的推出黏结强度，根管已经用含丁香油酚和不含丁香油酚的封闭剂进行了充填。二者的黏结强度没有差异。

根管充填时，根管封闭剂的成分（是否含丁香油酚）不影响用黏结剂和树脂水门汀黏结的桩的固位。

6.7.8　固化前桩的表面必须使用硅烷溶液涂布到桩的表面

使用硅烷溶液增强纤维桩的黏结特性是有争议的。虽然一些作者认为这可以增强黏结强度（Goracci et al. 2005），但大多数同行评议的研究论文认为,椅旁使用硅烷溶液不会增强纤维桩对根管牙本质的黏结能力(Perdigão et al. 2006;Bitter et al. 2007;Wrbas et al. 2007a,b;Tian et al. 2012)。由于大多数的桩由环氧树脂制成,目前口腔科使用的硅烷溶液与甲基丙烯酸甲酯基质的树脂相配,而与环氧树脂不匹配。但是,硅烷溶液可以提高使用自黏结树脂水门汀黏结纤维桩的黏附能力(Leme et al. 2013)。这种机制尚不清楚,但可能是与增加了桩表面的可湿性有关。

6.7.9 由于纤维桩在咬合情况下可以弯曲,所以根管内纤维桩的使用不能提供充分的封闭效果

根管的封闭以防止口腔中冠部细菌的渗漏是根管治疗后牙齿获得临床成功的重要因素。近来,自黏结树脂水门汀的出现使得在根管内黏结纤维桩时不需要酸蚀和黏结剂系统。体外研究在使用 RelyX Unicem (3M ESPE)黏结纤维桩时可以在根管冠方获得比传统树脂水门汀较好的封闭效果(Santos et al. 2009)(图 6-12 和图 6-13)。而且,与其他水门

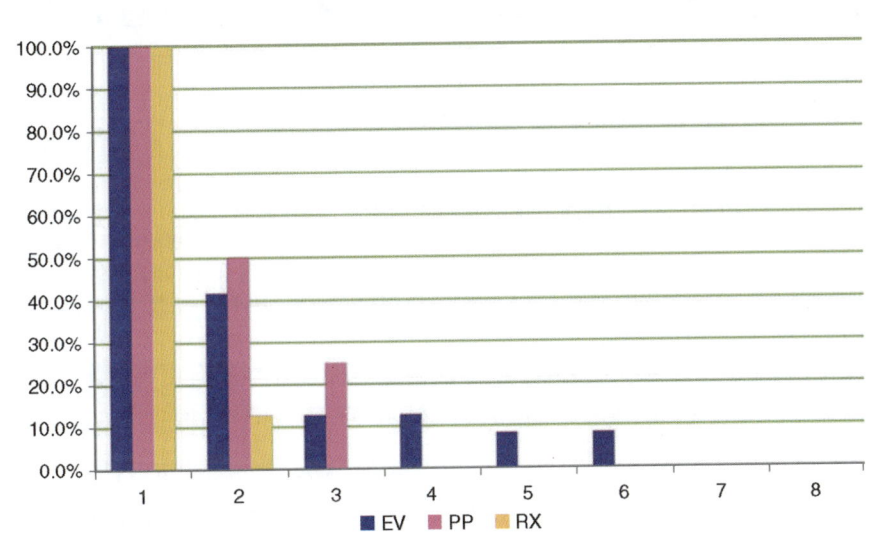

图 6-12 源自 Santos et al. (2009),图示为根管治疗后前磨牙用纤维桩修复后牙根切片伴有硝酸银渗入的百分比。样品在切片前用含氨的硝酸银处理。Disk #1 为接近冠方的切片,disk #8 为接近根方的切片。12/12 的硝酸银渗入样品都在冠方(disk #1)。EV 没有很好的封闭根管,因为银离子进入到 disk #6。RX 所允许进入的切片在 12 个中只有 2 个。RX 系统银离子只进入到 disk #2。EV, everStick POST (StickTech Ltd) + ParaCem Universal DC (Coltene);PP, ParaPost Fiber Lux (Coltene) + ParaCem Universal DC (Coltene);RX, RelyX Fiber Post (3M ESPE) + RelyX Unicem (3M ESPE)

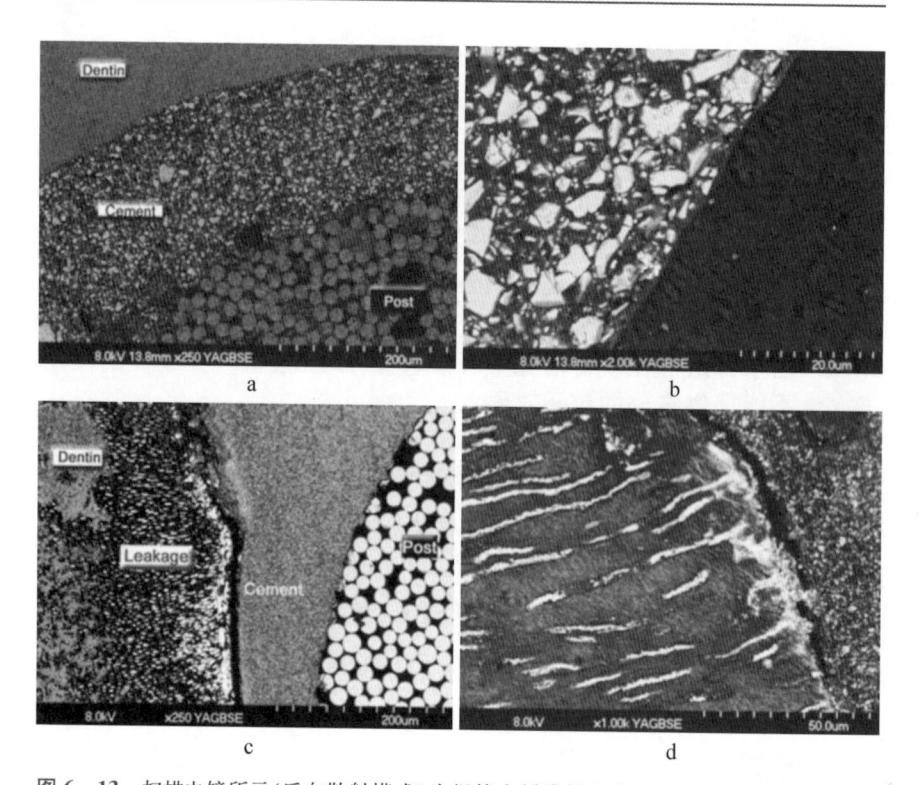

图 6-13 扫描电镜所示(反向散射模式)为根管内纤维桩黏结后的切片。按照 Santos et al. (2009)的方法,纤维桩黏结至牙根后放置含氨的硝酸银溶液中观察
a. RelyX Fiber Post (3M ESPE)用自黏结树脂水门汀黏结到根部牙本质后所形成的界面。样品中没有发现银离子的纳米渗漏,原始放大倍数 = ×250;b. 自黏结树脂水门汀与根部牙本质所形成的界面,该界面中没有发现银离子的纳米渗漏,原始放大倍数 = ×2 000;c. RelyX Fiber Post (3M ESPE)用传统的树脂水门汀和自酸蚀黏结剂所形成的界面,银离子渗入到整个界面(纳米渗漏),原始放大倍数 = ×250;d. 传统的树脂水门汀和自酸蚀黏结剂和根部牙本质所形成的界面,银离子渗入到界面和牙本质小管中。原始放大倍数 = ×1 000。

汀相比 RelyX Unicem (3M ESPE)使得桩与根管牙本质有更高的推出黏结强度(Bitter et al. 2012;Zicari et al. 2012)。在体外模拟临床情况(热和机械疲劳)下,该水门汀仍然可以在根管冠方获得很好的封闭效果(Bitter et al. 2011;Bitter et al. 2012)。这个主题会在其他章节更加详细的探讨。

6.8 纤维桩的优缺点

在过去的几十年,纤维加强型桩在根管治疗后牙齿中的使用越来多。牙科医师们已经接受纤维桩作为直接修复的步骤来保持核的形成。纤维桩的优缺点如表 6-2 和表 6-3 所示。

表 6-2 纤维桩的优点

纤维桩与牙本质的弹性模量相似(Zicari et al. 2013a)
纤维桩与根部牙本质的黏结强度比氧化锆桩高(Kurtz et al. 2003)。氧化锆桩的适应能力不足(Dietschi et al. 1997)
与金属桩和氧化锆桩相比纤维桩产生根折的可能性较低(Isidor et al. 1996；Akkayan and Gülmez 2002)
核和纤维桩吸收的力不会转移到易受损的根部结构(Isidor et al. 1996；Pegoretti et al. 2002)
与牙本质有相似弹性模量和小直径的桩会有较好的应力分布(Al-Omiri et al. 2011)
纤维桩的美观性和生物相容性可以很容易平衡
纤维桩的黏结可能会加固牙齿(Goncalves et al. 2006；Naumann et al. 2007)，尤其是在桩的表面经过喷砂处理的时候(Schmitter et al. 2006)
使用复合树脂增加薄弱牙根的厚度可以增加牙根的抗折能力(Goncalves et al. 2006)
核的成型一步完成

表 6-3 纤维桩的缺点

一些纤维桩在咬合情况下可以发生弯曲从而产生应力和界面裂隙
预成桩是圆柱形或有锥度的；不能与根管的解剖相匹配
阻射性不理想；不同品牌的阻射性也不同(图 6-5 和图 6-16)
早期纤维桩在全瓷和复合树脂修复的时候不易掩饰(Vichi et al. 2000)的时候
桩与目前树脂基质材料之间的黏结不理想

6.9 可修复性

在患者转诊至牙髓专科医师之前，受龋损和/或大面积修复累及的牙齿的可修复性必须要明确。常常一些被认为不能修复的牙齿在根管治疗后可以完成修复(图 6-14 和图 6-15)。冠部洞壁的保存是根管治疗后牙齿修复成功最重要的决定因素之一。冠部所有洞壁的缺失导致了所修

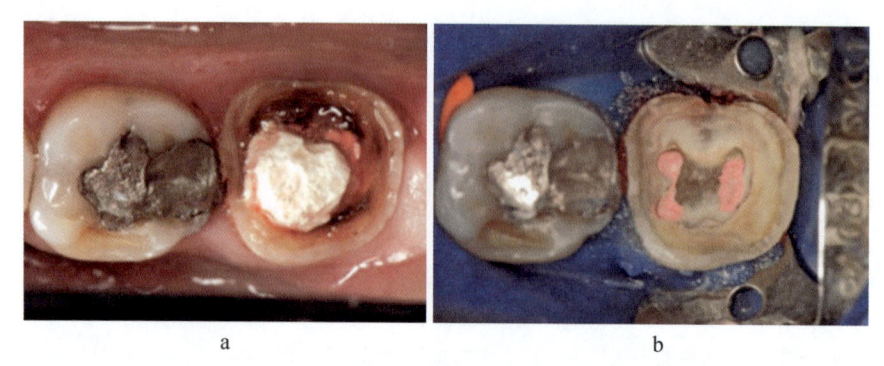

图6-14　a.伴有龋坏组织和暂封材料的根管治疗后下颌第二磨牙,判定牙齿是否可修复前所有的龋坏牙本质和残存的冠部修复材料必须去除干净;b.由于没有健康的洞壁余留,患牙不能通过纤维桩和复合树脂直接堆核来修复。

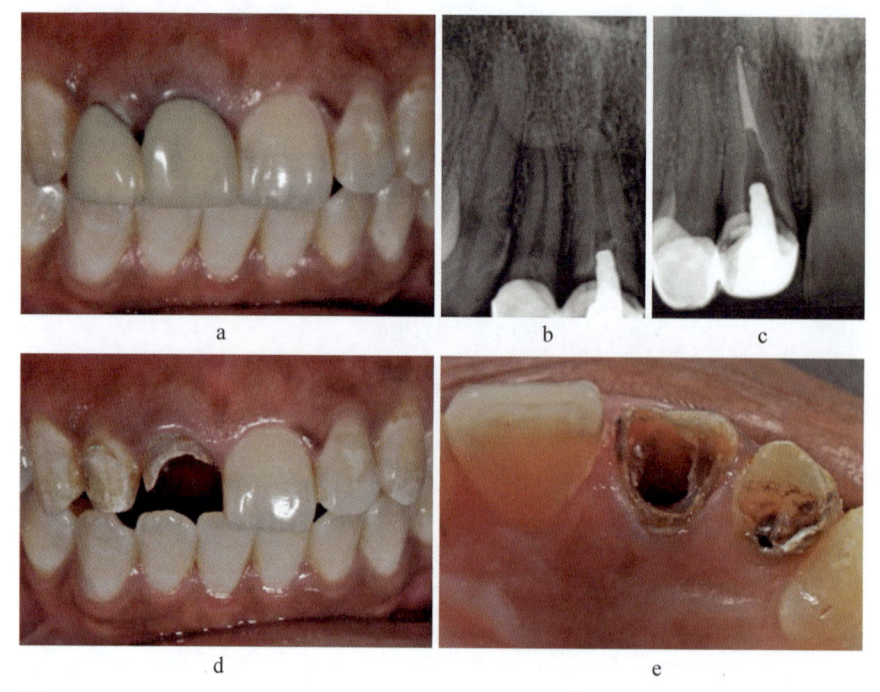

图6-15　a.1例转诊更换右侧上颌中切牙和侧切牙烤瓷熔附金属全冠FPD病例的正面观。患者最近刚刚完成右侧上颌中切牙的根管治疗打算更换2颗FPD;b.右侧上颌中切牙根管治疗前的根尖周X线片;c.右侧上颌中切牙根管治疗后的根尖周X线片。之前的FPD作为临时冠修复起来;d.去除临时冠后的正面观;e.右侧上颌中切牙的切端观。此时,该病例在这种情况下是不能修复的。

复牙齿保留最差的可能性(Cagidiaco et al. 2008；Ferrari et al. 2012)。巴拉邦(Baraban)(1967)写到"牙齿修复最基本的目标是满足其所承担

6 纤维加强型树脂桩(纤维桩)

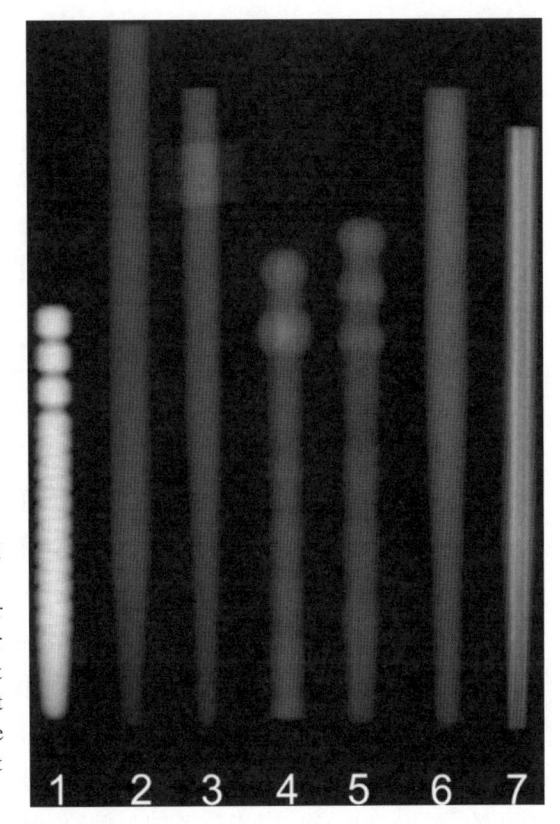

图 6-16 图 6-5 中所示的桩的 X 线片
1：Tenax (Coltene)；2：GC Fiber Post (GC Co.)；3：RelyX Fiber Post (3M ESPE)；4：Parapost Fiber Lux (Coltene)；5：Parapost Taper Lux (Coltene)；6：White Post (FGM)；7：Rebilda Post (VOCO GmbH)。

的功能和美学需求"。制订治疗计划前最首要的问题是，确定是否余留有足够健康的牙体组织以支撑核和单独的修复。如果牙齿不能保留，拔除后进行种植、固定局部义齿和可摘局部义齿的修复。

与牙本质相比，金属桩的弹性模量很高(Hicks 2008)，金属桩所致的根折和致命性失败的风险增加了(Zarone et al. 2006)。纤维桩所致的致命性失败的风险是降低的(Fernandes et al. 2003)，大多与纤维桩相关的失败是由于桩的松动和根管治疗的失败造成的(Ferrari et al. 2007；Rasimick et al. 2010)。

然而，少数的研究比较了用纤维桩和铸造金属桩修复没有余留洞壁的根管治疗后患牙。根管治疗后牙齿修复可行性的评估必须包含 4 个关键问题：

6.9.1 所有的龋坏组织去除了吗？

修复的可行性评估只有在去除现有的修复体和龋损釉质/牙本质组

织后进行(图 6 - 14)。

6.9.2 有足够的肩领来支撑基础吗?

罗森(Rosen)(1961)优美地描述其为"冠外支柱",作为"龈下金颈圈或围裙应尽可能地延伸到核龈部的冠方并完整地围绕牙颈部的周围。它是所修复的冠的延伸,能通过环抱的作用防止牙根垂直向的碎裂。"这个概念就是目前所知的肩领作用。

上颌切牙不完全的冠部肩领与更大的负载能力和断裂模式的变化相关(Naumann et al. 2006)。肩领高度从 1~1.5 mm 的增加不会明显增加纤维桩所修复的患牙的失败载荷(Akkayan 2004)。然而,当样品的肩领在 2.0 mm 高的时候,所有桩系统的断裂阈值都比较高(Akkayan 2004)。另一项研究(Tan et al. 2005)证实用铸造钉/核修复的中切牙在冠有 2 mm 一致肩领的时候,其抗折能力比没有一致肩领高度(0.5~2 mm)的中切牙要强。有 2 mm 一致肩领的组别和没有均一肩领的组别比没有肩领的组别抗折能力要强。当测试桩核设计和肩领对金属陶瓷冠修复的根管治疗后的中切牙的抗折能力的影响的时候,铸造桩核和烤瓷熔附金属冠修复的伴有 2 mm 肩领的患牙组别的折裂强度最高(Zhi-Yue and Yu-Xing 2003)。应当注意的是健康牙体组织上静止的冠部修复体对应力分布的影响大于核材料的类型或冠桩延伸长度的影响(Al-Omiri et al. 2011)。

当至少有 2 mm 肩领存在的时候临床成功率明显提高(Cagidiaco et al. 2008)。对 45 例有肩领(大于 2 mm 高)患牙和 42 例无肩领患牙(小于 2 mm 高)进行 3 年临床研究(Mancebo et al. 2010)。发现有肩领患牙的失败率为 6.7%,无肩领患牙的失败率为 26.2%。如果临床上达不到圆周肩领,与完全没有肩领相比,不完全肩领(图 6 - 17)也是更好的选择(Juloski et al. 2012)。

在不存在肩领影响的时候,铸造金属桩和纤维桩 3 年成功率统计学上相似(Sarkis-Onofre et al. 2014)。齐卡里(Zicari)等(2013)评估了体外肩领和插入纤维桩对用树脂核和焦磷酸锂冠修复的根管治疗后患牙的抗折能力,用循环疲劳加载进行试验。无论用桩与否,肩领明显增加修复后患牙的抗折能力。没有肩领和纤维桩的患牙的抗折能力最低。

6 纤维加强型树脂桩(纤维桩)

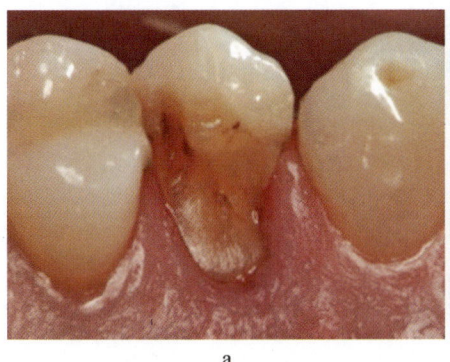

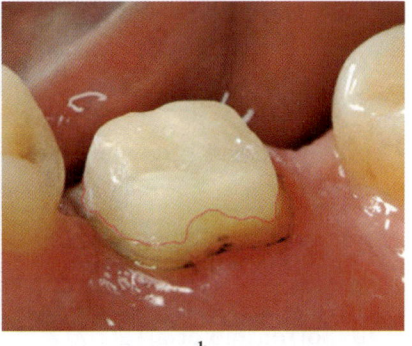

图 6-17 a. 上颌第一前磨牙折断到龈下水平。如果没有正畸牵引或冠延长术,该病例的箍效应(Rosen 1961)是不可行的;b. 预备周长的 90%存在 2 mm 高和 1 mm 厚的牙结构肩领。尽管认为有不完全的肩领,由于冠边缘没有在龈下,我们决定在修复治疗计划中没有牙牵引或冠延长术的情况下继续完成病例。

6.9.3 牙周状态评估了吗?

有学者(2011)为了未来预后调查验证了术前因素能预测需要根管治疗和冠修复的磨牙的长期预后的假说。从包含磨牙根管治疗和冠修复并有至少 4～6 年随访的临床数据库中随机挑选 42 位患者(年龄从 19～87 岁)伴有 50 例根管治疗作图分析。获得基线和随访的 X 线片,从咬翼片计算可获得的肩领。其他参数也被记录,包括附着丧失、冠延长、根分叉病变和松动度。根尖周炎的存在也被评估。影响根管治疗修复后磨牙预后的唯一的术前相关因素是术前的牙周条件(Setzer et al. 2011)。这项研究的结论很有临床意义——如果牙周条件不理想则需要牙周专科医师会诊。

重新获得颈部肩领并防止破坏生物学宽度的最常见的临床步骤之一是冠延长术。然而,当患牙没有冠部结构的时候正畸牵引应当被考虑而不是冠延长术。如果没有替代方法可以选择,证据表明很有可能出现不佳的临床效果(Juloski et al. 2012)。

6.9.4 剩余冠部洞壁的最小数目是什么?

在达 6 年的临床研究中,冠部洞壁的保存降低了根管治疗后前磨牙失败的风险(Cagidiaco et al. 2008;Ferrari et al. 2012)。

6.9.4.1 前牙

除了桩本身的失败,根管桩修复的患牙的失败与牙的位置有关;桩固位的患牙的失败主要发生在上前牙区,该部位的横向力比其他部位大(Torbjörner and Fransson 2004)。科尔曼(Colman)(1979)主张不管剩余牙体结构有多少根管治疗后都需要放置钉。放置钉的原理是预防根管治疗后患牙的颈部折断,除非患牙没有功能性的咬合关系(Colman 1979)。实际上,根管治疗后患牙修复后颈部区域受到最高的应变和应力集中(Sorrentino et al. 2007)。

根管治疗后切牙(图6-18)放置桩增加了抗折能力,改善了预后以防折断(Colman 1979;Smith and Schuman 1997)。萨拉米(Salameh)等(2008)评估了用微杂合树脂修复的上颌切牙用不同类型的全冠覆盖后,在使用或不使用纤维桩的情况下的抗折能力和失败模式。该研究的结果表明根管治疗后的前牙在使用纤维桩时能提高其抗折能力,改善了预后以防折断。存在/缺乏桩对可修复或不可修复折断的比例有明显影响。

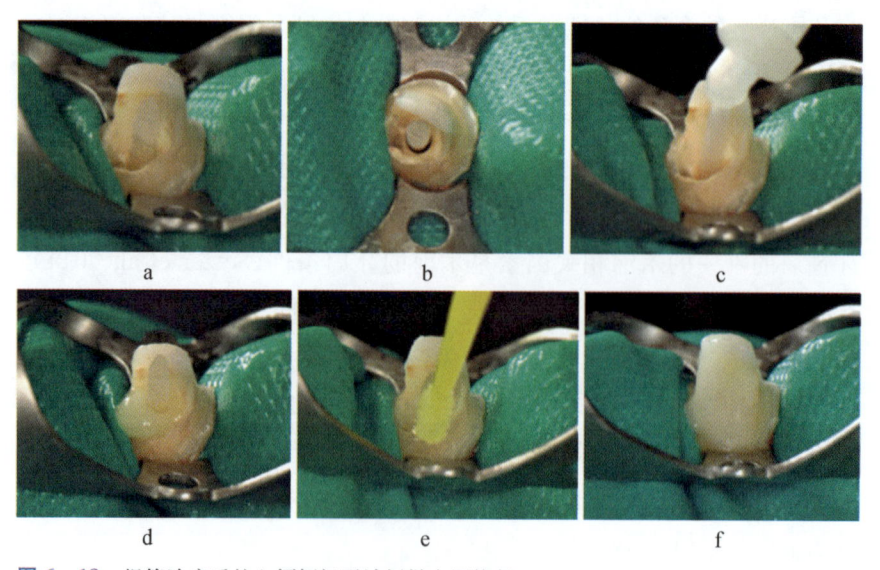

图6-18 根管治疗后的上颌侧切牙计划做全冠修复
a. 桩在修整匹配后插入就位;b. 切端观察显示纤维桩在根管内适合;c. 在这个特殊的临床病例中,根部和冠部的牙本质用35%磷酸酸蚀15秒,用水冲洗,纸尖干燥,用小毛刷涂布双固化的牙本质黏结剂。该图显示为根管内注入传统的双固化树脂水门汀;d. 纤维桩插入到双固化树脂水门汀内,多余的水门汀用毛刷去除。外部的水门汀光固化40秒;e. 涂布新一层牙本质黏结剂并固化;f. 双固化的复合树脂核材料嵌入并固化。

证据表明纤维桩能提高根管治疗后前牙修复后的抗折能力，即使在患牙全覆盖修复的情况下也是如此。

6.9.4.2 后牙

垂直折断是后牙常见的根管治疗后并发症。所修复的根管治疗后患牙必须能抵抗长期的咀嚼力，尤其是在后牙区域。曼戈尔德（Mangold）和克恩（Kern）（2011）评估了纤维桩对伴有不同程度缺损的根管治疗后前磨牙抗折能力的影响。当剩余洞壁少于 2 个时，放置纤维桩能明显影响其抗折能力，但是当 2 个或 3 个洞壁存在时没有明显影响（Mangold and Kern 2011）。近中-颌面-远中（MOD）预备代表了修复体嵌入时在折裂风险方面最差的病例（Morin et al. 1984）。与没有髓腔通路的 MOD 预备相比，在伴有髓腔通路的前磨牙的 MOD 预备中牙尖偏差明显增加（Panitvisai and Messer 1995）。与复合树脂单独修复相比，复合树脂伴有纤维桩的修复在减少伴有边缘嵴缺失的根管治疗后前磨牙的牙尖偏移方面更加有效（Acquaviva et al. 2011）。

对根管治疗后磨牙来说，当剩余洞壁少于 2 个时或边缘嵴缺失时，即使在全冠完全覆盖下，很有必要放置纤维桩提高患牙的抗折能力（Salameh et al. 2007；Mangold and Kern 2011；Acquaviva et al. 2011）。

6.10 临床研究

与冠部牙本质的黏结相比，根部牙本质的黏结挑战更大（表 6-4）。7 位私人开业者使用碳纤维桩修复了 236 例患牙，包括 130 例上颌牙和 106 例下颌牙，平均修复时间为 32 个月（在 27～41 个月内变动）。5 颗牙（2%）因与纤维桩系统不相关而拔除。牙周状况如碳纤维桩所修复患牙的菌斑堆积、牙龈健康、探诊出血、牙周袋深度与对照牙相似。临床或 X 线片所示未见移位或牙根或桩的折断。该研究发现 2～3 年临床观察效果满意（Fredriksson et al. 1998）。随后的回顾性研究利用相同的患者组评估了直达 7 年的治疗效果。前面 7 位私人开业者的 5 位参与了随访研究，病例总数减少至 138。39 例因数据不足被排除掉。剩余的 99 例从牙科病历中收集数据。平均的随访时间为 6.7 年（5 颗牙在之前的研究中已拔除）。如果桩核或 X 线片没有技术失败的指征则所观察结果为成功。

64 颗(65%)用碳纤维桩系统修复的患牙在平均 6.7 年后是成功的。32 颗患牙因折断、根尖周病损和牙周炎而被拔除。3 个病例中观察到桩移位。在平均 6.7 年后，碳纤维桩修复的患牙的生存时间比先前文件记录的铸造桩短(Segerström et al. 2006)。

表 6-4 根部牙本质的黏结——挑战性

有限的视野和通路
残余的牙胶和根管封闭剂碎片
在根管内使用和固化黏结剂困难
冲洗酸蚀剂和干燥多余的水分困难
黏结剂中的溶剂不能完全挥发掉
NaOCl 潜在的氧化影响
过多的水门汀增加来填充桩和根部牙本质壁之间的空隙
高的 C-因子(结合和未结合表面的比率)可能导致更大的聚合应力
牙本质小管密度的变化
透明牙本质的沉积

Carvalho et al. (2009)，Ree and Schwartz(2010)

碳纤维桩目前不推荐用作根管治疗后患牙的修复。

法拉利等(2000)评估了使用了 1～6 年超过 1 200 例用碳桩和玻璃纤维桩修复的根管治疗后患牙。他们发现 3.2%的失败率与桩不相关，25 例桩在去除临时修复体的时候出现了黏结失效，16 颗牙出现了根尖周病损。法拉利等(2007)评估了使用了 7～11 年的 985 例用纤维桩修复的根管治疗后患牙。他们发现 79 例失败，其中 39 例是由于根管治疗失败所致，1 例由于根折所致，1 例出现纤维桩折断，17 例出现冠松动，21 例出现桩黏结失效。力学失败与冠部牙体结构缺失有关。这两项研究中失败的病例凸显了在黏结过程中临床技术的重要性，同时根管封闭的质量也很重要，这是因为大部分失败是由于根管治疗失败、桩黏结失效和冠的松动所致。

另一项临床研究(Ferrari 等 2012)检查了剩余冠部牙本质和放置预成桩对比定制纤维桩对用全冠修复的根管治疗后前磨牙的 6 年存活率的

影响。345位患者中60颗前磨牙需要根管治疗。通过超过6年的观察期发现放置预成桩或定制桩明显有助于提高根管治疗后前磨牙的存活率。预成纤维桩比定制的"解剖"纤维桩更有效。不管修复步骤,至少保留一个冠部洞壁能明显降低失败风险。

克里格(Creugers)等(2005)进行了5年的临床研究去检测:① 铸造桩核修复体的存活率是否比直接桩核修复或无桩全树脂核修复的要好;② 这些堆砌修复体的存活受到备牙后牙本质高度的影响。18位术者在249位患者中做了319例核修复。修复体包括:① 铸造桩核修复;② 直接桩和树脂核修复;③ 无桩全树脂核修复。所有的修复体都用烤瓷熔附金属全冠单冠覆盖。桩和核的类型与存活率不相关。因素"剩余牙本质高度"对桩核修复体的存活率有明显影响。如前所述,当至少有2.0 mm的肩领存在的时候,临床成功率明显提高(Cagidiaco et al. 2008;Mancebo et al. 2010)。

在大多数临床研究中两个常见的结果是剩余牙体结构的量和箍效应对根管治疗后牙齿修复后的寿命起决定性的作用。

6.11 总结

根管治疗后牙齿修复后的成功率取决于以下几点:
1. 去净所有的龋坏组织。
2. 根管治疗和修复治疗的质量。
3. 良好的牙周和咬合条件。
4. 根部和冠部牙体组织的保存。
5. 能提供抗力形的肩领的存在。
6. 使用不转移应力到剩余牙体结构的桩。
7. 使用能黏结桩到根管牙本质和封闭根管的黏结剂。
8. 依靠科学证据一丝不苟地使用材料和技术。

致谢　特别感谢Dr. George Gomes,Dr. Virgínia Santos,and Dr. Ana Sezinando 的支持

(朱来宽　译)

参考文献

Abramovitz L, Lev R, Fuss Z, Metzger Z (2001) The unpredictability of seal after post space preparation: a fluid transport study. J Endod 27: 292–295.

Acquaviva PA, Madini L, Krokidis A, et al., Cerutti A (2011) Adhesive restoration of endodontically treated premolars: influence of posts on cuspal deflection. J Adhes Dent 13: 279–286.

Aggarwal V, Singla M, Miglani S, Kohli S (2012) Comparative evaluation of fracture resistance of structurally compromised canals restored with different dowel methods. J Prosthodont 21: 312–316.

Akkayan B (2004) An in vitro study evaluating the effect of ferrule length on fracture resistance of endodontically treated teeth restored with fiber-reinforced and zirconia dowel systems. J Prosthet Dent 92: 155–162.

Akkayan B, Gülmez T (2002) Resistance to fracture of endodontically treated teeth restored with different post systems. J Prosthet Dent 87: 431–437.

Al-Omiri MK, Rayyan MR, Abu-Hammad O (2011) Stress analysis of endodontically treated teeth restored with post-retained crowns: a finite element analysis study. J Am Dent Assoc 142: 289–300.

Antoon MK, Koenig JL, Serafini T (1981) Fourier-transform infrared study of the reversible interaction of water and a crosslinked epoxy matrix. J Polym Sci Pol Phys Ed 19: 1567–1575.

Arola D, Reprogel RK (2005) Effects of aging on the mechanical behavior of human dentin. Biomaterials 26: 4051–4061.

Asmussen E, Peutzfeldt A, Heitmann T (1999) Stiffness, elastic limit, and strength of newer types of endodontics posts. J Dent 27: 275–278.

Assif D, Oren E, Marshak BL, Aviv I (1989) Photoelastic analysis of stress transfer by endodontically treated teeth to the supporting structure using different restorative techniques. J Prosthet Dent 61: 535–543.

Balooch M, Demos SG, Kinney JH, et al., Marshall SJ (2001) Local mechanical and optical properties of normal and transparent root dentin. J Mater Sci Mater Med 12: 507–514.

Baraban DJ (1967) The restoration of pulpless teeth. Dent Clin North Am 633–653. http://www.ncbi.nlm.nih.gov/pubmed/5262486.

Bitter K, Noetzel J, Neumann K, Kielbassa AM (2007) Effect of silanization on bond strengths of fiber posts to various resin cements. Quintessence Int 38: 121–128.

Bitter K, Perdigão J, Hartwig C, Neunmann K, Kielbassa AM (2011) Nanoleakage of luting agents for bonding fi ber posts after thermo-mechanical fatigue. J Adhes Dent 13: 61–69.

Bitter K, Perdigão J, Exner M, et al., Sterzenbach G (2012) Reliability of fiber post bonding to root canal dentin after simulated clinical function in vitro. Oper Dent 37: 397–405.

Black GV (1895) An investigation of the physical characters of the human teeth in relation to their diseases and to practical dental operations, together with the physical characters of filling materials. Dent Cosmos 37: 353, 469, 553, 637, 737.

Boone KJ, Murchison DF, Schindler WG, Walker WA 3rd (2001) Post retention: the effect of sequence of post-space preparation, cementation time, and different sealers. J Endod 27: 768–771.

Büttel L, Krastl G, Lorch H, et al., Weiger R (2009) Influence of post fit and post length on fracture resistance. Int Endod J 42: 47–53.

Butz F, Lennon AM, Heydecke G, Strub JR (2001) Survival rate and fracture strength of endodontically treated maxillary incisors with moderate defects restored with different post-

and-core systems: an in vitro study. Int J Prosthodont 14: 58 – 64.

Cagidiaco MC, García-Godoy F, Vichi A, et al., Ferrari M (2008) Placement of fiber prefabricated or custom made posts affects the 3-year survival of endodontically treated premolars. Am J Dent 21: 179 – 184.

Carvalho CA, Valera MC, Oliveira LD, Camargo CHR (2005) Structural resistance in immature teeth using root reinforcements in vitro. Dent Traumatol 21: 155 – 159.

Carvalho RM, Tjäderhane L, Manso AP, et al., Carvalho CAR (2009) Dentin as a bonding substrate. Endod Topics 21: 62 – 88.

Cohen BI, Musikant BL, Deutsch AS (1992) Comparison of retentive properties of four post systems. J Prosthet Dent 68: 264 – 268.

Colman HL (1979) Restoration of endodontically treated teeth. Dent Clin North Am 23: 647 – 662.

Costa RG, De Morais EC, Campos EA, et al., Correr GM (2012) Customized fiber glass posts. Fatigue and fracture resistance. Am J Dent 25: 35 – 38.

Creugers NH, Mentink AG, Fokkinga WA, Kreulen CM (2005) 5-year follow-up of a prospective clinical study on various types of core restorations. Int J Prosthodont 18: 34 – 39.

D'Arcangelo C, De Angelis F, Vadini M (2010) Fracture resistance and deflection of pulpless anterior teeth restored with composite or porcelain veneers. J Endod 36: 153 – 156.

de Sousa Menezes M, Queiroz EC, Soares PV, Faria-e-Silva AL, Soares CJ, Martins LR (2011) Fiber post etching with hydrogen peroxide: effect of concentration and application time. J Endod 37: 398 – 402.

Dietschi D, Romelli M, Goretti A (1997) Adaptation of adhesive posts and cores to dentin after fatigue testing. Int J Prosthodont 10: 498 – 507.

Dorriz H, Alikhasi M, Mirfazaelian A, Hooshmand T (2009) Effect of ferrule and bonding on the compressive fracture resistance of post and core restorations. J Contemp Dent Pract 10: 1 – 8.

dos Santos Alves Morgan LF, Peixoto RT, de Castro Albuquerque R, et al., Pinotti MB (2008) Light transmission through a translucent fiber post. J Endod 34: 299 – 302.

Duret B, Reynaud M, Duret F (1990) Un nouveau concept de reconstitution corono-radiculaire. Le Composipost (1). Chir Dent Fr 540: 131 – 141.

Elsaka SE (2013) Influence of chemical surface treatments on adhesion of fiber posts to composite resin core materials. Dent Mater 29: 550 – 558.

Faria e Silva AL, Arias VG, Soares LE, et al., Martins LR (2007) Influence of fiber-post translucency on the degree of conversion of a dual-cured resin cement. J Endod 33: 303 – 305.

Fernandes AS, Dessai GS (2001) Factors affecting the fracture resistance of post-core reconstructed teeth: a review. Int J Prosthodont 14: 355 – 363.

Fernandes AS, Shetty S, Coutinho I (2003) Factors determining post selection: a literature review. J Prosthet Dent 90: 556 – 562.

Ferrari M, Vichi A, Mannocci F, Mason PN (2000) Retrospective study of the clinical performance of fiber posts. Am J Dent 13(Spec No): 9B – 13B.

Ferrari M, Cagidiaco MC, Goracci C, et al., Tay F (2007) Long-term retrospective study of the clinical performance of fiber posts. Am J Dent 20: 287 – 291.

Ferrari M, Vichi A, Fadda GM, et al., Goracci C (2012) A randomized controlled trial of endodontically treated and restored premolars. J Dent Res 91(7 Suppl): 72S – 78S.

Fokkinga WA, Kreulen CM, Vallittu PK, Creugers NHJ (2004) A structured analysis of in vitro failure loads and failure modes of fiber, metal, and ceramic post-and-core systems. Int J Prosthodont 17: 476 – 482.

Fredriksson M, Astbäck J, Pamenius M, Arvidson K (1998) A retrospective study of 236 patients with teeth restored by carbon fiber-reinforced epoxy resin posts. J Prosthet Dent 80: 151 – 157.

Gillen BM, Looney SW, Gu LS, et al., Pashley DH, Tay FR (2011) Impact of the quality of coronal restoration versus the quality of root canal fillings on success of root canal treatment: a systematic review and meta-analysis. J Endod 37: 895-902.

Gómez-Polo M, Llidó B, Rivero A, et al., Celemín A (2010) A 10-year retrospective study of the survival rate of teeth restored with metal prefabricated posts versus cast metal posts and cores. J Dent 38: 916-920.

Goncalves LA, Vansan LP, Paulino SM, Sousa Neto MD (2006) Fracture resistance of weakened roots restored with a transilluminating post and adhesive restorative materials. J Prosthet Dent 96: 339-344.

Goodacre CJ, Spolnik KJ (1994) The prosthodontics management of endodontically treated teeth: a literature review. Part I. Success and failure data, treatment concepts. J Prosthodont 3: 243-250.

Goodacre CJ, Spolnik KJ (1995) The prosthodontic management of endodontically treated teeth: a literature review. Part III Tooth preparation considerations. J Prosthodont 4: 122-128.

Goracci C, Raffaelli O, Monticelli F, Balleri B, Bertelli E, Ferrari M (2005) The adhesion between prefabricated FRC posts and composite resin cores: microtensile bond strength with and without post-silanization. Dent Mater 21: 437-444.

Grandini S, Goracci C, Monticelli F, et al., Ferrari M (2005) Fatigue resistance and structural characteristics of fiber posts: three-point bending test and SEM evaluation. Dent Mater 21: 75-82.

Grant T, Bradley W (1995) In-situ observations in SEM of degradation of graphite/epoxy composite materials due to seawater immersion. J Compos Mater 29: 852-867.

Gutmann JL (1992) The dentin-root complex: anatomic and biologic considerations in restoring endodontically treated teeth. J Prosthet Dent 67: 458-467.

Guzy GE, Nicholls JI (1979) In vitro comparison of intact endodontically treated teeth with and without endo-post reinforcement. J Prosthet Dent 42: 39-44.

Harris CS, Austen PH (1871) The principles and practice of dentistry: including anatomy, physiology, pathology, therapeutics, dental surgery and mechanism. 10th edn. Rev. and edited by Philip H. Austen. Philadelphia, Lindsay and Blakiston, pp. 507-520.

Hayashi M, Takahashi Y, Imazato S, Ebisu S (2006) Fracture resistance of pulpless teeth restored with post and cores and crowns. Dent Mater 22: 477-485.

Helfer AR, Melnick S, Schilder H (1972) Determination of the moisture content of vital and pulpless teeth. Oral Surg Oral Med Oral Pathol 34: 661-670.

Hicks N (2008) Esthetic fiber reinforced composite posts. Smile Dental J 3: 43-48. Available at http: //www.smile-mag.com/? pid = artd&artid = 38&magid = 9. Last accessed 12 Oct 2014 Huang TJ, Schilder H, Nathanson D (1992) Effects of moisture content and endodontic treatment on some mechanical properties of human dentin. J Endod 18: 209-215.

Hunter AJ, Feiglin B, Williams JF (1989) Effects of post placement on endodontically treated teeth. J Prosthet Dent 162: 166-172.

Isidor F, Odman P, Brøndum K (1996) Intermittent loading of teeth restored using prefabricated carbon fiber posts. Int J Prosthodont 9: 131-136.

Jameson MW, Hood JA, Tidmarsh BG (1993) The effects of dehydration and rehydration on some mechanical properties of human dentine. J Biomech 26: 1055-1065.

Johnson JK, Sakumura JS (1978) Dowel form and tensile force. J Prosthet Dent 40: 645-649.

Juloski J, Radovic I, Goracci C, et al., Ferrari M (2012) Ferrule effect: a literature review. J Endod 38: 11-19.

Kahler B, Swain MV, Moule A (2003) Fracture-toughening mechanisms responsible for differences in work to fracture of hydrated and dehydrated dentine. J Biomech 36: 229-337.

Kantor ME, Pines MS (1977) A comparative study of restorative techniques for pulpless teeth. J Prosthet Dent 38: 405-412.

Kim YK, Kim SK, Kim KH, Kwon TY (2009) Degree of conversion of dual-cured resin cement light-cured through three fibre posts within human root canals: an ex vivo study. Int Endod J 42: 667-674.

King PA, Setchell DJ (1990) An in vitro evaluation of a prototype CFRC prefabricated post developed for the restoration of pulpless teeth. J Oral Rehabil 17: 599-609.

Kinney JH, Nalla RK, Pople JA, et al., Ritchie RO (2005) Age-related transparent root dentin: mineral concentration, crystallite size, and mechanical properties. Biomaterials 26: 3363-3376.

Kurtz JS, Perdigão J, Geraldeli S, et al., Bowles WR (2003) Bond strengths of tooth-colored posts, effect of sealer, dentin adhesive, and root region. Am J Dent 16(Spec No): 31A-36A.

Lang H, Korkmaz Y, Schneider K, Raab WH (2006) Impact of endodontic treatments on the rigidity of the root. J Dent Res 85: 364-368.

Lassila LV, Tanner J, Le Bell AM, et al., Vallittu PK (2004) Flexural properties of fiber reinforced root canal posts. Dent Mater 20: 29-36.

Leary JM, Aquilino SA, Svare CW (1987) An evaluation of post length within the elastic limits of dentin. J Prosthet Dent 57: 277-281.

Lee MC, Peppas NA (1993) Models of moisture transport and moisture-induced stresses in epoxy composites. J Compos Mater 27: 1146-1171.

Leme AA, Pinho AL, de Gonçalves L, et al., Sinhoreti MA (2013) Effects of silane application on luting fiber posts using self-adhesive resin cement. J Adhes Dent 15: 269-274.

Mancebo JC, Jiménez-Castellanos E, Cañadas D (2010) Effect of tooth type and ferrule on the survival of pulpless teeth restored with fiber posts: a 3-year clinical study. Am J Dent 23: 351-356.

Mangold JT, Kern M (2011) Influence of glass-fiber posts on the fracture resistance and failure pattern of endodontically treated premolars with varying substance loss: an in vitro study. J Prosthet Dent 105: 387-393.

Mannocci F, Ferrari M, Watson TF (1999) Intermittent loading of teeth restored using quartz fiber, carbon-quartz fiber, and zirconium dioxide ceramic root canal post. J Adhes Dent 1: 153-158.

Mattison GD (1982) Photoelastic stress analysis of cast-gold endodontic posts. J Prosthet Dent 48: 407-411.

Mazzitelli C, Ferrari M, Toledano M, et al., Osorio R (2008) Surface roughness analysis of fiber post conditioning processes. J Dent Res 87: 186-190.

Mazzitelli C, Papacchini F, Monticelli F, et al., Ferrari M (2012) Effects of post surface treatments on the bond strength of self-adhesive cements. Am J Dent 25: 159-164.

Mendoza DB, Eakle WS, Kahl EA, Ho R (1997) Root reinforcement with a resin-bonded preformed post. J Prosthet Dent 78: 10-14.

Monticelli F, Toledano M, Tay FR, et al., Ferrari M (2006) Post-surface conditioning improves interfacial adhesion in post/core restorations. Dent Mater 22: 602-609.

Morgano SM (1996) Restoration of pulpless teeth: application of traditional principles in present and future contexts. J Prosthet Dent 75: 375-380.

Morin D, De Long R, Douglas WH (1984) Cusp reinforcement by the acid-etch technique. J Dent Res 63: 1075-1078.

Murray PE, Hafez AA, Windsor LJ, Smith AJ, Cox CF (2002) Comparison of pulp responses following restoration of exposed and non-exposed cavities. J Dent 30: 213-222.

Nalbandian J, Gonzales F, Sognnaes RF (1960) Sclerotic age changes in root dentin of human teeth as observed by optical, electron, and X-ray microscopy. J Dent Res 39: 598-607.

Naumann M, Preuss A, Rosentritt M (2006) Effect of incomplete crown ferrules on load capacity of endodontically treated maxillary incisors restored with fiber posts, composite build-ups, and all-ceramic crowns: an in vitro evaluation after chewing simulation. Acta Odontol Scand 64: 31–36.

Naumann M, Preuss A, Frankenberger R (2007) Reinforcement effect of adhesively luted fiber reinforced composite versus titanium posts. Dent Mater 23: 138–144.

Panitvisai P, Messer HH (1995) Cuspal deflection in molars in relation to endodontic and restorative procedures. J Endod 21: 57–61.

Pashley DH (1996) Dynamics of the pulpo-dentin complex. Crit Rev Oral Biol Med 7: 104–133.

Pegoretti A, Fambri L, Zappini G, Bianchetti M (2002) Finite element analysis of a glass fibre reinforced composite endodontic post. Biomaterials 23: 2667–2682.

Perdigão J, Gomes G, Lee IK (2006) The effect of silane on the bond strengths of fiber posts. Dent Mater 22: 752–758.

Perdigão J, Gomes G, Augusto V (2007) The effect of dowel space on the bond strengths of fiber posts. J Prosthodont 16: 154–164.

Prati C, Chersoni S, Mongiorgi R, et al., Pashley DH (1999) Thickness and morphology of resin-infiltrated dentin layer in young, old, and sclerotic dentin. Oper Dent 24: 66–72.

Randow K, Glantz PO (1986) On cantilever loading of vital and non-vital teeth. An experimental clinical study. Acta Odontol Scand 44: 271–277.

Rasimick BJ, Wan J, Musikant BL, Deutsch AS (2010) A review of failure modes in teeth restored with adhesively luted endodontic dowels. J Prosthodont 19: 639–646.

Ree M, Schwartz RS (2010) The endo-restorative interface: current concepts. Dent Clin North Am 54: 345–374.

Rosen H (1961) Operative procedures on mutilated endodontically treated teeth. J Prosthet Dent 11: 973–986.

Safavi KE, Dowden WE, Langeland K (1987) Influence of delayed coronal permanent restoration on endodontic prognosis. Endod Dent Traumatol 3: 187–191.

Salameh Z, Sorrentino R, Ounsi HF, et al., Ferrari M (2007) Effect of different all-ceramic crown system on fracture resistance and failure pattern of endodontically treated maxillary premolars restored with and without glass fiber posts. J Endod 33: 848–851.

Salameh Z, Sorrentino R, Ounsi HF, et al., Ferrari M (2008) The effect of different full-coverage crown systems on fracture resistance and failure pattern of endodontically treated maxillary incisors restored with and without glass fiber posts. J Endod 34: 842–846.

Santos V, Perdigão J, Gomes G, Silva AL (2009) Sealing ability of three fiber dowel systems. J Prosthodont 18: 566–576.

Santos AF, Meira JB, Tanaka CB, et al., Versluis A (2010) Can fiber posts increase root stresses and reduce fracture? J Dent Res 89: 587–591.

Sarkis-Onofre R, Jacinto Rde C, Boscato N, et al., Pereira-Cenci T (2014) Cast metal vs. glass fibre posts: a randomized controlled trial with up to 3 years of follow up. J Dent 42: 582–587.

Schmage P, Ozcan M, McMullan-Vogel C, Nergiz I (2005) The fit of tapered posts in root canals luted with zinc phosphate cement: a histological study. Dent Mater 21: 787–793.

Schmitter M, Huy C, Ohlmann B, et al., Rammelsberg P (2006) Fracture resistance of upper and lower incisors restored with glass fiber reinforced posts. J Endod 32: 328–330.

Schwartz RS, Robbins JW (2004) Post placement and restoration of endodontically treated teeth: a literature review. J Endod 30: 289–301.

Seefeld F, Wenz HJ, Ludwig K, Kern M (2007) Resistance to fracture and structural characteristics of different fiber reinforced post systems. Dent Mater 23: 265–271.

Segerström S, Astbäck J, Ekstrand KD (2006) A retrospective long term study of teeth restored with prefabricated carbon fiber reinforced epoxy resin posts. Swed Dent J 30: 1–8.

Setzer FC, Boyer KR, Jeppson JR, et al., Kim S (2011) Long-term prognosis of endodontically treated teeth: a retrospective analysis of preoperative factors in molars. J Endod 37: 21-25.

Shillingburg HT, Kessler JC, Wilson EL (1982) Root dimensions and dowel size. CDA J 10: 43-49.

Smith CT, Schuman N (1997) Restoration of endodontically treated teeth: a guide for the restorative dentist. Quintessence Int 28: 457-462.

Smith CT, Schuman NJ, Wasson W (1998) Biomechanical criteria for evaluating prefabricated post-and-core systems: a guide for the restorative dentist. Quintessence Int 29: 305-312.

Soares CJ, Pereira JC, Valdivia AD, Novais VR, Meneses MS (2012) Influence of resin cement and post configuration on bond strength to root dentine. Int Endod J 45: 136-145.

Sorenson JA, Martinoff JT (1984) Intracoronal reinforcement and coronal coverage: a study of endodontically treated teeth. J Prosthet Dent 51: 780-784.

Sornkul E, Stannard JG (1992) Strength of roots before and after endodontic treatment and restoration. J Endod 18: 440-443.

Sorrentino R, Aversa R, Ferro V, et al., Apicella A (2007) Three-dimensional finite element analysis of strain and stress distributions in endodontically treated maxillary central incisors restored with different post, core and crown materials. Dent Mater 23: 983-993.

Standlee JP, Caputo AA, Hanson EC (1978) Retention of endodontic dowels: effects of cement, dowel length, diameter, and design. J Prosthet Dent 39: 400-405.

Tan PL, Aquilino SA, Gratton DG, et al., Dawson D (2005) In vitro fracture resistance of endodontically treated central incisors with varying ferrule heights and configurations. J Prosthet Dent 93: 331-336.

Tang W, Wu Y, Smales RJ (2010) Identifying and reducing risks for potential fractures in endodontically treated teeth. J Endod 36: 609-617.

Teixeira EC, Teixeira FB, Piasick JR, Thompson JY (2006) An in vitro assessment of prefabricated fiber post systems. J Am Dent Assoc 137: 1006-1012.

Tian Y, Mu Y, Setzer FC, et al., Yu Q (2012) Failure of fiber posts after cementation with different adhesives with or without silanization investigated by pullout tests and scanning electron microscopy. J Endod 38: 1279-1282.

Tidmarsh BG (1976) Restoration of endodontically treated posterior teeth. J Endod 2: 374-375.

Torbjörner A, Fransson B (2004) Biomechanical aspects of prosthetic treatment of structurally compromised teeth. Int J Prosthodont 17: 135-141.

Torbjörner A, Karlsson S, Syverud M, Hensten-Pettersen A (1996) Carbon fiber reinforced root canal posts. Mechanical and cytotoxic properties. Eur J Oral Sci 104: 605-611.

Trabert KC, Caput AA, Abou-Rass M (1978) Tooth fracture-a comparison of endodontic and restorative treatments. J Endod 4: 341-345.

Trope M, Maltz DO, Tronstad L (1985) Resistance to fracture of restored endodontically treated teeth. Endod Dent Traumatol 1: 108-111.

Vallittu P (2000) Effect of 180-week water storage on the flexural properties of E-glass and silica fiber acrylic resin composite. Int J Prosthodont 13: 334-339.

Vichi A, Ferrari M, Davidson CL (2000) Influence of ceramic and cement thickness on the masking of various types of opaque posts. J Prosthet Dent 83: 412-417.

Wandscher VF, Bergoli CD, Limberger IF, et al., Valandro LF (2014) Preliminary results of the survival and fracture load of roots restored with intracanal posts: weakened vs nonweakened roots. Oper Dent 39: 541-555.

Wrbas KT, Altenburger MJ, Schirrmeister JF, et al., Kielbassa AM (2007a) Effect of adhesive resin cements and post surface silanization on the bond strengths of adhesively inserted fiber posts. J Endod 33: 840-843.

Wrbas KT, Schirrmeister JF, Altenburger MJ, et al., Hellwig E (2007b) Bond strength between fibre posts and composite resin cores: effect of post surface silanization. Int Endod J 40: 538 – 543.

Yenisey M, Kulunk S (2008) Effects of chemical surface treatments of quartz and glass fiber posts on the retention of a composite resin. J Prosthet Dent 99: 38 – 45.

Zarone F, Sorrentino R, Apicella D, et al., Apicella A (2006) Evaluation of the biomechanical behavior of maxillary central incisors restored by means of endocrowns compared to a natural tooth: a 3D static linear finite elements analysis. Dent Mater 22: 1035 – 1044.

Zhi-Yue L, Yu-Xing Z (2003) Effects of post-core design and ferrule on fracture resistance of endodontically treated maxillary central incisors. J Prosthet Dent 89: 368 – 373.

Zhou L, Wang Q (2013) Comparison of fracture resistance between cast posts and fiber posts: a meta-analysis of literature. J Endod 39: 11 – 15.

Zicari F, De Munck J, Scotti R, et al., Van Meerbeek B (2012) Factors affecting the cement-post interface. Dent Mater 28: 287 – 297.

Zicari F, Coutinho E, Scotti R, et al., Naert I (2013a) Mechanical properties and micro-morphology of fiber posts. Dent Mater 29: e45 – e52.

Zicari F, Van Meerbeek B, Scotti R, Naert I (2013b) Effect of ferrule and post placement on fracture resistance of endodontically treated teeth after fatigue loading. J Dent 41: 207 – 215.

根管牙本质黏结：一项具有挑战性的任务

7

亚历山德拉·里斯（Alessandra Reis）
爱丽丝·多拉杜·洛古尔齐（Alessandro Dourado Loguercio）
克斯廷·比特（Kerstin Bitter）
乔奇·佩尔迪高（Jorge Perdigão）

摘　要

玻璃纤维桩的放置是提高修复体固位力的方法，严重缺损牙齿的治疗通常会包含这一步骤。玻璃纤维桩在根管内的黏结是一项极具挑战性的工作，其最终结果会受到多种因素的影响。本章将阐述① 一些依赖于临床医师专业知识的，能够显著影响黏结效果甚至导致失败的限制性因素；② 临床治疗中如何克服这些因素。

在根管内或者髓腔内应用黏结材料的主要目的是提高复合树脂直接修复体或者是增加冠方严重破坏牙齿内桩核的固位力。

纤维桩黏结技术涉及牙本质黏结系统的使用，通过该黏结系统，牙本质基质和树脂水门汀形成混合层并黏结根管壁与纤维桩。目前有两种可用的黏结对策：需要传统的磷酸酸蚀并冲洗的全酸蚀黏结技术以及自酸蚀黏结系统。由于光固化灯的光线很难进入根管的根中 1/3 和根尖 1/3，因此，传统上一般选择双固化树脂水门汀。此外，临床上有时使用自黏结树脂作为酸蚀-冲洗和自酸蚀黏结系统的替代方案。

不考虑材料的类型和/或所用的技术，根部牙本质与冠部牙本质有着相同的黏结步骤。然而，Bouillaguet 等人（Bouillaguet et al. 2003）的一项体外研究结果显示，桩在根管系统内的黏结力要弱于对修整平坦的牙根表面牙本质的黏结力。

这种差异是需要临床医师更加关注以减少黏结失败发生的诸多限制性因素中的一个例子。本章节将讨论为何根管内黏结是一项具有挑战性任务的原因，及临床医师该如何合理地进行黏结操作。

7.1 牙根内的解剖

为了规避桩道预备过程中发生长轴偏移或者根管壁侧穿等并发症的风险,临床医师必须熟悉不同牙齿根管的解剖。

7.1.1 牙根解剖

上颌前牙根管横截面的形态在颈 1/3 为椭圆形而在根尖 1/3 则趋向于圆形。在下颌前牙,有 40% 是双根管,其横截面往往是圆形。如果是单根管型,其横断面形态一般是唇舌径宽、近远中径窄的圆形。这种根管解剖形态可能存在较高的侧穿风险,因此桩道预备的适应证应严格控制在严重牙冠缺损的病例。

尖牙是单根牙且绝大多数情况下为单根管。其根尖 1/3 是根管治疗过程中发生侧穿的高风险区,但值得欣慰的是桩道预备并不会涉及该区域。

与上颌第二双尖牙通常为拥有宽广颊腭径单根管的单根牙,与之不同的是,62% 的上颌第一双尖牙有两个牙根,且绝大多数为双根管。下颌双尖牙通常是单根,根管拥有宽广的颊舌径。

磨牙的桩道应该预备在最粗和最直的根管内,一般是上颌磨牙的腭根管和下颌磨牙的远中根管。

7.1.2 牙本质基质

根部牙本质和冠部牙本质的相似性是临床医师普遍关心的一个问题。根据一篇综述的报道(Schwartz 2006),虽然相关研究数量很少,但研究结果一致认为两种牙本质存在少量的差异。

根部牙本质中的牙本质小管起自牙髓止于牙骨质,也有管间牙本质和管周牙本质。靠近根尖方向牙本质内,牙本质小管的数量急剧下降,因此根尖 1/3 和根冠 1/3 牙本质内管周牙本质和管间牙本质的比例不同(Ferrari et al. 2000；Mjor et al. 2001)。

根尖 1/3 的牙本质内牙本质小管数量较少(Ferrari et al. 2000；Mjor et al. 2001；Mannocci et al. 2004),排列不规则甚至是缺如(Mjor et al. 2001)。即使存在牙本质小管,也往往被与管周牙本质来源相似的矿物盐所填满（Paque et al. 2006），表现为硬化和类透明牙本质样。

冠部牙本质和根部牙本质之间轻微的差异似乎并不会对根部牙本质黏结造成影响，因此，冠部与根部牙本质基质黏结的差异可能是来自其他一些因素，这些因素会在下文解释说明。

7.2 玷污层

7.2.1 根管治疗来源的玷污层

根管预备时，无论使用的是手用还是机动旋转器械，均能产生大量粉末状而非条块状的牙本质碎屑玷污层，玷污层紧密附着于预备后的根管壁表面，很难被水冲去或者擦拭除去（Pashley et al. 1988；Breschi et al. 2009）。

这种由于根管预备所形成的玷污层具有双层结构：外层厚度为 1～2 μm，由有机物和牙本质颗粒组成，内层主要有牙本质碎屑组成，并向牙本质小管延伸超过 10 μm，形成管塞（smear plugs）（Mader et al. 1984）。玷污层的组成依赖于牙齿本身的基质组成、根管预备的器械以及根管冲洗的方式，差异很大。举例而言，在根管预备的早期由于根管内存在牙髓或者炎症、坏死组织，此时所形成的玷污层有机物含量颇高（Violich and Chandler 2010）。

玷污层的存在会如屏障一般，阻碍根管封闭剂向牙本质小管的黏附和渗透（Goracci et al. 2005；Breschi et al. 2009）。在根管治疗的过程中有必要去除玷污层。因此，在根管预备后就需要用能够溶解有机物和无机物的冲洗液冲洗根管。

次氯酸钠（NaOCl）和乙二胺四乙酸（EDTA）具有杀菌、溶解和螯合的作用，因而被广泛地应用于玷污层的去除。氯己定可以吸附在牙本质表面发挥长效抗菌作用，因而也是一种临床常用的根管冲洗液，但是其不具备 NaOCl 和 EDTA 所有的溶解有机质和去除玷污层的能力（Violich and Chandler 2010）。本章后续会讨论根管冲洗液对于根管内纤维桩的最终黏结效果的作用和影响。

7.2.2 二次玷污层

在一篇 2009 年的文献综述中，Breschi 等人（Breschi et al. 2009）认

为除了在使用手用或者机动旋转器械预备根管壁时会产生玷污层，在桩道预备过程中也会产生玷污层，其厚度甚至会超过前者。这种玷污层主要由牙本质碎屑以及硬化的牙胶和根管封闭剂组成（Breschi et al. 2009），会抑制黏结剂的渗透和化学反应，从而严重影响纤维桩的黏结（Goracci et al. 2005）。为了提高桩的黏结效果提升固位力，在桩黏结之前必须对桩道进行仔细的清洁（Goracci and Ferrari 2011），这一点尤为重要。

目前桩道的预备通常使用的是纤维桩厂商提供的配套硬质合金钻。之所以使用硬质合金钻很可能是基于一些冠部牙本质的研究结果，这些研究报道指出，与金刚砂钻针相比，硬质合金钻切割预备后能够获得更高的黏结力（Sekimoto et al. 1999；Dias et al. 2004；Yiu et al. 2008）。然而现实可能要令大家失望了，硬质合金钻针切割根管壁牙本质后所产生的玷污层比金刚砂所产生的更难以被磷酸酸蚀溶解去除（Gomes et al. 2012）。

冠部牙本质和根管壁牙本质切割后所产生的玷污层，其组成存在差异。事实上钻针在去除根充材料预备桩道的过程中会产生一层新的玷污层，富含根管封闭剂和牙胶尖残留物，由于桩道预备过程中缺少水的冲洗，这些组分会被钻针摩擦产生的高热塑化。这会阻碍黏结剂中的成分渗透和发生化学反应，从而影响纤维桩的黏结效果（图 7-1）。临床医师必须重视这个问题。应对该问题的方法将在下一章节详细介绍。

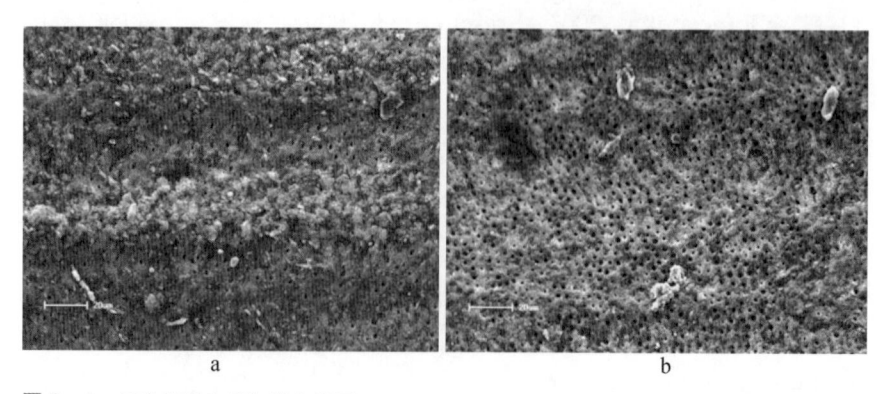

a

b

图 7-1 根尖部牙本质扫描电镜图
a. 根充后的根管以硬质合金钻针预备桩道并使用 37% 磷酸酸蚀处理。仍有大约 50% 的牙本质小管为玷污层所封闭，阻碍后续的有效黏结；b. 根充后的根管先以硬质合金钻针预备桩道，再用金刚砂车针糙化牙本质表面并用 37% 磷酸酸蚀。仅有少量牙本质小管为玷污层封闭，说明金刚砂车针预备所产生的牙本质表层更适合黏结操作（Gomes et al. 2012）。

7.3 根管治疗过程中的化学预备

纤维桩脱胶是纤维桩修复最常见的失败类型（Weston et al. 2007；Cagidiaco et al. 2008；Dietschi et al. 2008）。考虑到桩是通过黏结而被动地固位于根管内，黏结的效果直接关系到修复体的总体临床效果。因此，了解那些可能阻碍黏结水门汀和根管牙本质之间形成牢固黏结的因素就显得十分重要。根管治疗中所使用的一些根管冲洗液可能会对根管壁牙本质黏结产生不利的影响。

7.3.1 次氯酸钠和其他氧化性溶液

有报道指出，一些根管治疗术中常规使用的根管冲洗液会对根管壁牙本质的黏结强度产生不利影响。次氯酸钠是一种被广泛应用于根管治疗的根管冲洗液，然而因其具有强氧化性，可能会抑制树脂基质材料的聚合。研究报道，次氯酸钠处理后会在牙本质表面形成一层富氧层，这层富氧层会显著降低牙本质的黏结强度（Nikaido et al. 1999；Saleh and Ettman 1999；Perdigao et al. 2000；Morris et al. 2001；Ari et al. 2003；Erdemir et al. 2004；Ozturk and Ozer 2004；Marques et al. 2014）。

同样的，其他的一些用于根管治疗的氧化性材料，诸如主要成分为过氧化脲的 RC-prep，也会在根管壁牙本质表层形成富氧层，从而阻碍黏结（Nikaido et al. 1999；Morris et al. 2001；Erdemir et al. 2004）。使用10%的抗坏血酸或者10%抗坏血酸钠处理至少1分钟可以逆转这种黏结力的下降（Morris et al. 2001；Weston et al. 2007）。

研究显示（Rocha et al. 2012；Vilanova et al. 2012），当使用次氯酸钠作为根管冲洗液时，树脂基质的根充材料与根管壁之间的封闭性也会受到影响。

7.3.2 EDTA

临床上经常将 EDTA 与次氯酸钠联合应用以脱矿和溶解有机质。不过，若二者联合应用作用时间超过1分钟，就会因为过度脱矿而在牙本质表面形成一个侵蚀面（Calt and Serper 2002），妨碍牙本质与黏结系统特别是自酸蚀黏结系统形成强效黏结（Hayashi et al. 2005）。因此，临床上应避免用 EDTA 长时间冲洗根管。

7.3.3 氯己定

葡萄糖酸氯己定具有一定的杀菌效果而被用作根管治疗术中的辅助根管冲洗液。其优点是不会妨碍树脂和根管壁牙本质的黏结（Erdemir et al. 2004），缺点是不能作为独立的根管冲洗液替代次氯酸钠和 EDTA。此外，氯己定可能会在脱矿牙本质表面形成不容易降解的黏结界面（Cecchin et al. 2011，2014；Martinho et al. 2015），这一点将会在下个章节中详细展开。

7.3.4 氢氧化钙

氢氧化钙糊剂因其抗菌效果而时常被用作约诊间根管内封药。有报道指出，由于封药后很难被完全去净（Lambrianidis et al. 1999；Maalouf et al. 2013），残留的氢氧化钙就可能成为黏结剂发挥黏结作用的物理屏障（Lee et al. 2014）。另外，Breschi 等人（Breschi et al. 2009）曾报道，氢氧化钙具有高 pH，其强碱性可能会中和自酸蚀黏结剂中的酸/底胶，不过，该观点有待进一步研究的证实。

7.3.5 根管封闭剂

关于根管封闭剂对黏结效果的影响存在一定的争议。一些学者报道，根管封闭剂的类型会影响纤维桩与根管牙本质之间的黏结效果。另一项研究则显示，预成根管桩在根管内的固位效果与根管是否已行根充有关而与根管封闭剂的类型无关，且根充后根管内的固位效果弱于未根充的根管（Hagge et al. 2002）。因此，体外研究评估纤维桩与根管牙本质黏结强度时要考虑根管封闭剂的影响。

一些学者报道，使用含丁香油酚的根管封闭剂会削弱后续桩的黏结固位效果（Tjan and Nemetz 1992；Burns et al. 2000；Alfredo et al. 2006；Aleisa et al. 2012；AlEisa et al. 2013）。其理论基础是，与其他酚类化合物相似，丁香油酚能够阻碍树脂基质材料的聚合。与之相反，其他的一些研究并不支持这一观点，认为根管封闭剂中丁香油酚的存在与否并不影响桩的固位（Mannocci et al. 2001；Hagge et al. 2002；Kurtz et al. 2003；Davis and O'Connell 2007）。

这些相互矛盾的结果可能与根充后行纤维桩黏结的时间有关。有学者（Menezes et al. 2008）研究了根充后即刻和根充后 1 周黏结根管桩的效果差异，结果发现，同样使用含有丁香油酚的根管封闭剂，后者的黏结效果强于前者。对于矛盾结果的另一个可能的解释是桩道预备过程中牙本质的去除量。桩的直径越粗大，桩道预备过程中去除的被含丁香油酚根管封闭剂污染的牙本质就越多，桩道表面就越清洁，根管桩黏结后的固位力也就越强（Izadi et al. 2013）。

使用树脂基质而不是含有丁香油酚的根管封闭剂能够提升根管桩的黏结固位效果。其原理可能是使用树脂基质根管封闭剂与黏结剂具有相似的化学组分且管牙本质未受丁香油酚的污染（Aleisa et al. 2012；AlEisa et al. 2013）。

实验室研究结果提示临床医师要尽量避免根充后即刻黏结根管桩，同时，根管桩的直径应当适当的扩大。应当指出的是，后者需要临床医师仔细的术前评估以降低根折和根管壁侧穿的风险。

研究也显示，传统的 3 步法酸蚀-冲洗黏结系统，酸蚀冲洗的步骤能够去除绝大部分含丁香油酚玷污层，因而能够提升丁香油酚污染的牙本质表面的黏结效果（Peutzfeldt and Asmussen 1999；Wolanek et al. 2001）。自酸蚀黏结系统会保留富含丁香油酚的玷污层并与之混杂形成混合层，临床医师应当慎用。

7.4 黏结剂之间的不相容性

临床上有各种类型的黏结系统可供选择。除了传统的 3 步法酸蚀-冲洗黏结系统（3-step ER）和自酸蚀黏结系统（2-step SE），还有简化的 2-step ER 和 1-step SE，后者因其操作简便而被临床医师广泛接受和使用。

但是有研究结果显示，简化的黏结系统（2-step ER 和 1-step SE）与化学固化或双固化复合树脂存在不相容性（Sanares et al. 2001；Cheong et al. 2003；Tay et al. 2003a，2004a，b）。然而这种现象并未出现在传统的 ER（Cheong et al. 2003；Tay et al. 2003b）或 SE 黏结系统（Tay et al. 2002），其原因可能是在黏结固化的过程中形成了一层额外的疏水性树脂层。因此,造成这种不相容性的原理可能是黏结系统的酸度(化学不相容性)(Sanares et al. 2001; Suh et al. 2003)或者黏结剂所形成的亲水性黏结层攫取其下方牙本质内的水至表层而阻碍了黏结剂与树脂水门汀的紧密接触(物理不相容性)(Tay et al. 2003a)(图 7-2)。

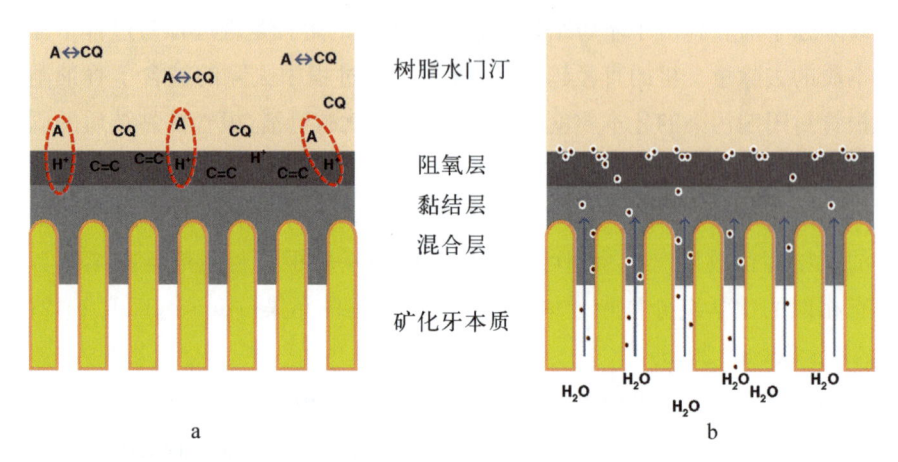

图 7-2 酸性黏结剂和树脂水门汀之间的化学不相容性和物理不相容性
a. 化学不相容性。来自于酸性单体的质子(H)与阻氧层中的樟脑醌(CQ)竞争叔胺(A);
b. 物理不相容性,深层牙本质中的水可以方便地穿过亲水性黏结层。这些在黏结剂表面集聚的水阻碍了黏结剂和树脂水门汀的紧密结合。

化学不相容发生过程中,在未完全聚合的酸性树脂单体与阻氧层之间发生了不利的化学作用,而化学固化或者双固化树脂中的碱性叔胺催化剂可能是罪魁祸首(Sanares et al. 2001)。基于同样的原理,在化学固化和双固化树脂之后,使用延迟固化技术固化的光固化树脂也被发现存在相似的不相容性(Tay et al. 2001,2003b)。

对于物理不相容性,阻氧层的出现造成了一个高渗环境,黏结面的含水牙本质中的水被攫取并透过亲水的黏结剂层(Tay et al. 2003a,2004b)。由于简化的黏结系统缺少不含溶剂的树脂包被,这些被攫取的水会在黏结剂内部和表面积聚,形成水树(Tay and Pashley 2003),阻碍树脂与黏结剂的良好紧密接触。

7.5 聚合时光照强度不够

由于光线无法穿透桩道的全长,根管内牙科材料的光照固化十分困

7 根管牙本质黏结：一项具有挑战性的任务

难(Wu et al. 2009；Ho et al. 2011；Moazzami et al. 2012)。穿透纤维桩或者甚至在没有纤维桩的情况下进入根管内的光线强度会随着根管深度的增加而呈现几何数量级的衰减，给根管全长实现良好的黏结效果带来了挑战(Goracci et al. 2008；Wu et al. 2009；Ho et al. 2011；Moazzami et al. 2012)(图7-3)。这也是为什么一些研究报道指出使用光固化黏结系统时，根尖区域的黏结效果不尽如人意(Bouillaguet et al. 2003；Goracci et al. 2004；Akgungor and Akkayan 2006；Aksornmuang et al. 2007；Mallmann et al. 2007)。

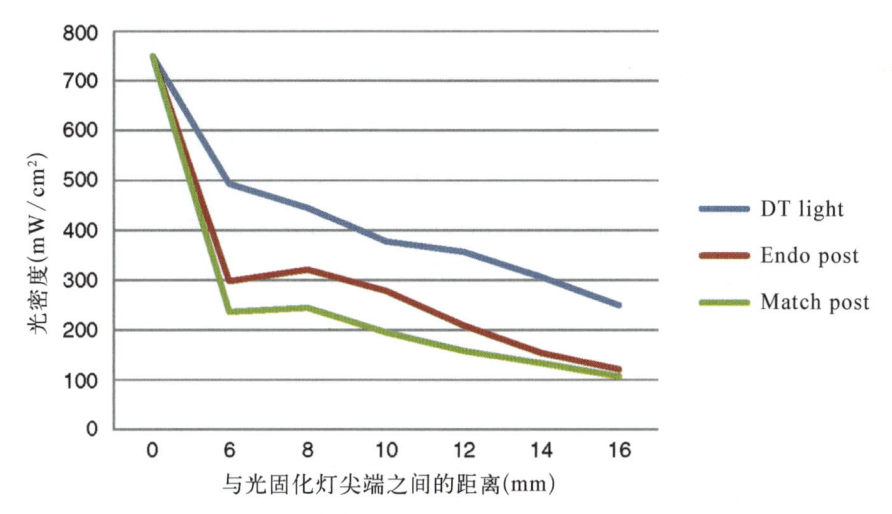

图7-3 3种纤维桩系统内光线的衰减
0 mm代表中切牙的切端区域，该区域的光密度为100%(图片来源Moazzami et al. 2012并做修改)。

光线在根管内行进深度的限制导致可聚合二甲基丙烯酸树脂单体的不完全固化。当根管长度增加，固化的树脂单体就越少(Le Bell et al. 2003；Hayashi and Ebisu 2008)。

最近的研究显示，即使采用透光的根管桩，透射到达根尖区域的光线量仍不足以使树脂水门汀完全固化(Goracci et al. 2008)。这种情况不单发生在碳纤维桩，甚至是玻璃纤维桩也会显著地阻碍光线的透射(Goracci et al. 2008；Ho et al. 2011)。

7.6 术者的经验

纤维桩的黏结具有相当的技术敏感性,黏结效果对术者的经验有着较强的依赖性。有研究证实,术者的经验能够影响冠方牙本质的黏结效果(Sano et al. 1998；Miyazaki et al. 2000)。

最新的研究结果显示,当使用传统或者简化的酸蚀-冲洗黏结系统时,术者的经验显著影响纤维桩黏结的效果(Gomes et al. 2013),而相似的情况却并未出现在使用自酸蚀黏结系统黏结纤维桩时。

未能按照厂商的说明书操作,对影响根管牙本质黏结效果的诸多操作因素的不熟悉是缺乏临床经验的医师使用酸蚀-冲洗黏结系统临床失败的主要原因。而简化的操作步骤和无须在黏结剂涂布前保持牙本质湿润是自酸蚀黏结系统对临床医师操作技术敏感性不高的主要原因。因此,对于临床经验不丰富的医师,减少黏结的操作步骤是获得更为可靠和优良的树脂和根管牙本质黏结效果的重要保证。

7.7 C 因素

甲基丙烯酸基质树脂聚合时,树脂单体会相互靠近,缩小单体分子间的间距,这就导致了足以造成材料从根管壁牙本质脱胶的收缩应力的产生。从临床角度而言,这种应力的产生会降低根管桩钉的固位力,产生间隙并且在黏结面产生细菌渗漏。

Feilzer 等人(Feilzer et al. 1987)提出收缩应力与 C 因素相关。C 因素指的是修复体黏结面数量与非黏结面数量之比。黏结面积越大,收缩应力越大,对树脂水门汀机械性能的影响也就越大(Jongsma et al. 2012)。根管内部几何形态决定了没有足够的非黏结面来释放收缩应力,因而不利于黏结修复的远期效果。

如果换算成可比的数值,冠部充填体的 C 因素介于 1～5,那么根管桩的 C 因素将超过 200(Bouillaguet et al. 2003；Breschi et al. 2009)。最小化 C 因素的方法之一就是降低黏结树脂水门汀的层厚使其局限在根管内不能流动释放应力。采用技术降低根管内黏结材料的量(诸如直接或间接解剖式根管桩）可以降低聚合收缩带来的不良后果从而获得更好的纤维桩对根管壁牙本质的黏结效果。这样做还可以减少牙本质-树脂水门汀界面裂隙的产生（Gomes et al. 2014）。

由于圆形的纤维桩与大多数根管椭圆形的形状或者过度预备的根管在形态上不匹配，临床上要减少树脂水门汀的用量可能是一件困难的事（图7-4）。黏结之前先在体外完成预成桩的复合树脂重衬可能是一个有效的临床对策（Faria-e-Silva et al. 2009；Macedo et al. 2010；Gomes et al. 2014）。

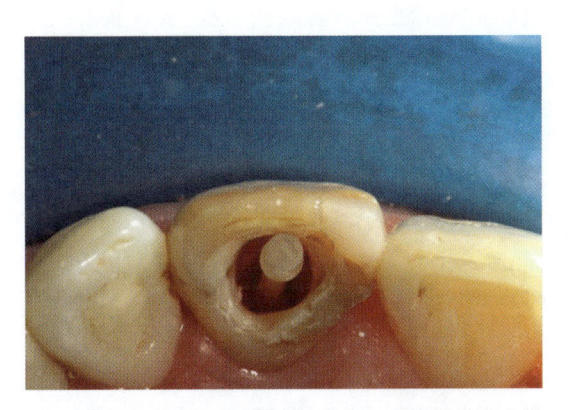

图7-4 过度预备的根管与市售最粗玻璃纤维桩之间存在不匹配

为了减小过量树脂水门汀引起的聚合收缩应力所带来的不利影响，临床上有时采用直接或间接玻璃纤维桩。

（梁景平 刘斌 译）

参考文献

Akgungor G, Akkayan B (2006) Influence of dentin bonding agents and polymerization modes on the bond strength between translucent fiber posts and three dentin regions within a post space. J Prosthet Dent 95：368-378.

Aksornmuang J, Nakajima M, Foxton RM, Tagami J (2007) Mechanical properties and bond strength of dual-cure resin composites to root canal dentin. Dent Mater 23：226-234.

Aleisa K, Alghabban R, Alwazzan K, Morgano SM (2012) Effect of three endodontic sealers on the bond strength of prefabricated fiber posts luted with three resin cements. J Prosthet Dent 107：322-326.

AlEisa K, Al-Dwairi ZN, Lynch E, Lynch CD (2013) In vitro evaluation of the effect of different endodontic sealers on retentive strength of fiber posts. Oper Dent 38：539-544.

Alfredo E, de Souza ES, Marchesan MA, et al., Sousa-Neto MD (2006) Effect of eugenol-based endodontic cement on the adhesion of intraradicular posts. Braz Dent J 17: 130–133.

Ari H, Yasar E, Belli S (2003) Effects of NaOCl on bond strengths of resin cements to root canal dentin. J Endod 29: 248–251.

Bouillaguet S, Troesch S, Wataha JC, et al., Pashley DH (2003) Microtensile bond strength between adhesive cements and root canal dentin. Dent Mater 19: 199–205.

Breschi L, Mazzoni A, Dorigo ES, Ferrari M (2009) Adhesion to intraradicular dentin: a review. J Adhes Sci Technol 23: 1053–1083.

Burns DR, Moon PC, Webster NP, Burns DA (2000) Effect of endodontic sealers on dowels luted with resin cement. J Prosthodont 9: 137–141.

Cagidiaco MC, Goracci C, Garcia-Godoy F, Ferrari M (2008) Clinical studies of fiber posts: a lit-erature review. Int J Prosthodont 21: 328–336.

Calt S, Serper A (2002) Time-dependent effects of EDTA on dentin structures. J Endod 28: 17–19 Cecchin D, de Almeida JF, Gomes BP, Zaia AA, Ferraz CC (2011) Effect of chlorhexidine and ethanol on the durability of the adhesion of the fiber post relined with resin composite to the root canal. J Endod 37: 678–683.

Cecchin D, Farina AP, Giacomin M, et al., Ferraz CC (2014) Influence of chlorhexidine application time on the bond strength between fiber posts and dentin. J Endod 40: 2045–2048.

Cheong C, King NM, Pashley DH, et al., Tay FR (2003) Incompatibility of self-etch adhesives with chemical/dual-cured composites: two-step vs one-step systems. Oper Dent 28: 747–755.

Davis ST, O'Connell BC (2007) The effect of two root canal sealers on the retentive strength of glass fibre endodontic posts. J Oral Rehabil 34: 468–473.

Dias WR, Pereira PN, Swift EJ Jr (2004) Effect of bur type on microtensile bond strengths of self-etching systems to human dentin. J Adhes Dent 6: 195–203.

Dietschi D, Duc O, Krejci I, Sadan A (2008) Biomechanical considerations for the restoration of endodontically treated teeth: a systematic review of the literature, part II (evaluation of fatigue behavior, interfaces, and in vivo studies). Quintessence Int 39: 117–129.

Erdemir A, Ari H, Gungunes H, Belli S (2004) Effect of medications for root canal treatment on bonding to root canal dentin. J Endod 30: 113–116.

Faria-e-Silva AL, Pedrosa-Filho Cde F, Menezes Mde S, et al., Martins LR (2009) Effect of relining on fiber post retention to root canal. J Appl Oral Sci 17: 600–604.

Feilzer AJ, De Gee AJ, Davidson CL (1987) Setting stress in composite resin in relation to con-figuration of the restoration. J Dent Res 66: 1636–1639.

Ferrari M, Mannocci F, Vichi A, et al., Mjor IA (2000) Bonding to root canal: structural characteristics of the substrate. Am J Dent 13: 255–260.

Gomes OMM, Gomes GM, Rezende EC, et al., Reis A (2012) Influence of the rotating device used for root canal preparation. J Dent Res 91: Abstract 1429.

Gomes GM, Gomes OM, Reis A, et al., Calixto AL (2013) Effect of operator experience on the outcome of fiber post cementation with different resin cements. Oper Dent 38: 555–564.

Gomes GM, Gomes OM, Gomes JC, et al., Reis A (2014) Evaluation of different restorative techniques for filling flared root canals: fracture resistance and bond strength after mechanical fatigue. J Adhes Dent 16: 267–276.

Goracci C, Ferrari M (2011) Current perspectives on post systems: a literature review. Aust Dent J 56(Suppl 1): 77–83.

Goracci C, Tavares AU, Fabianelli A, Monticelli F, Raffaelli O, Cardoso PC, Tay F, Ferrari M (2004) The adhesion between fiber posts and root canal walls: comparison between microtensile and push-out bond strength measurements. Eur J Oral Sci 112: 353–361.

Goracci C, Sadek FT, Fabianelli A, Tay FR, Ferrari M (2005) Evaluation of the adhesion of fiber posts to intraradicular dentin. Oper Dent 30: 627-635.

Goracci C, Corciolani G, Vichi A, Ferrari M (2008) Light-transmitting ability of marketed fiber posts. J Dent Res 87: 1122-1126.

Hagge MS, Wong RD, Lindemuth JS (2002) Retention strengths of five luting cements on prefabricated dowels after root canal obturation with a zinc oxide/eugenol sealer: 1. Dowel space preparation/cementation at one week after obturation. J Prosthodont 11: 168-175.

Hayashi M, Ebisu S (2008) Key factors in achieving firm adhesion in post — core restorations. Jpn Dent Sci Rev 44: 22-28.

Hayashi M, Takahashi Y, Hirai M, Iwami Y, Imazato S, Ebisu S (2005) Effect of endodontic irriga-tion on bonding of resin cement to radicular dentin. Eur J Oral Sci 113: 70-76.

Ho YC, Lai YL, Chou IC, et al., Lee SY (2011) Effects of light attenuation by fibre posts on polymerization of a dual-cured resin cement and microleakage of post-restored teeth. J Dent 39: 309-315.

Izadi A, Azarsina M, Kasraei S (2013) Effect of eugenol-containing sealer and post diameter on the retention of fiber reinforced composite posts. J Conserv Dent 16: 61-64.

Jongsma LA, Kleverlaan CJ, Pallav P, Feilzer AJ (2012) Influence of polymerization mode and C-factor on cohesive strength of dual-cured resin cements. Dent Mater 28: 722-728.

Kurtz JS, Perdigao J, Geraldeli S, et al., Bowles WR (2003) Bond strengths of tooth-colored posts, effect of sealer, dentin adhesive, and root region. Am J Dent 16(Special Issue A): 31-36 Lambrianidis T, Margelos J, Beltes P (1999) Removal efficiency of calcium hydroxide dressing from the root canal. J Endod 25: 85-88.

Le Bell AM, Tanner J, Lassila LV, et al., Vallittu PK (2003) Depth of light-initiated polymerization of glass fiber-reinforced composite in a simulated root canal. Int J Prosthodont 16: 403-408.

Lee BS, Lin YC, Chen SF, et al., Chang CC (2014) Influence of calcium hydroxide dressing and acid etching on the push-out bond strengths of three luting resins to root canal dentin. Clin Oral Investig 18: 489-498.

Maalouf L, Zogheib C, Naaman A (2013) Removal efficiency of calcium hydroxide dressing from the root canal without chemically active adjuvant. J Contemp Dent Pract 14: 188-192.

Macedo VC, Faria e Silva AL, Martins LR (2010) Effect of cement type, relining procedure, and length of cementation on pull-out bond strength of fiber posts. J Endod 36: 1543-1546.

Mader CL, Baumgartner JC, Peters DD (1984) Scanning electron microscopic investigation of the smeared layer on root canal walls. J Endod 10: 477-483.

Mallmann A, Jacques LB, Valandro LF, Muench A (2007) Microtensile bond strength of photoactivated and autopolymerized adhesive systems to root dentin using translucent and opaque fiber-reinforced composite posts. J Prosthet Dent 97: 165-172.

Mannocci F, Ferrari M, Watson TF (2001) Microleakage of endodontically treated teeth restored with fiber posts and composite cores after cyclic loading: a confocal microscopic study. J Prosthet Dent 85: 284-291.

Mannocci F, Pilecki P, Bertelli E, Watson TF (2004) Density of dentinal tubules affects the tensile strength of root dentin. Dent Mater 20: 293-296.

Marques EF, Bueno CE, Veloso HH, Almeida G, Pinheiro SL (2014) Influence of instrumentation techniques and irrigating solutions on bond strength of glass fiber posts to root dentin. Gen Dent 62: 50-53.

Martinho FC, Carvalho CA, Oliveira LD, et al., Pucci CR (2015) Comparison of different dentin pretreatment protocols on the bond strength of glass fiber post using self-etching adhesive. J Endod 41: 83-87.

Menezes MS, Queiroz EC, Campos RE, et al., Soares CJ (2008) Influence of endodontic sealer cement on fibreglass post bond strength to root dentine. Int Endod J 41: 476-484 Miyazaki M, Onose H, Moore BK (2000) Effect of operator variability on dentin bond strength of two-step bonding systems. Am J Dent 13: 101-104.

Mjor IA, Smith MR, Ferrari M, Mannocci F (2001) The structure of dentine in the apical region of human teeth. Int Endod J 34: 346-353.

Moazzami SM, Kazemi R, Alani M, et al., Shahrokh H (2012) Light conduction capability of different light-transmitting FRC posts. J Dent Mater Technol 1: 40-46.

Morris MD, Lee KW, Agee KA, et al., Pashley DH (2001) Effects of sodium hypochlorite and RC-prep on bond strengths of resin cement to endodontic surfaces. J Endod 27: 753-757 Nikaido T, Takano Y, Sasafuchi Y, Burrow MF, Tagami J (1999) Bond strengths to endodontically-treated teeth. Am J Dent 12: 177-180.

Ozturk B, Ozer F (2004) Effect of NaOCl on bond strengths of bonding agents to pulp chamber lateral walls. J Endod 30: 362-365.

Paque F, Luder HU, Sener B, Zehnder M (2006) Tubular sclerosis rather than the smear layer impedes dye penetration into the dentine of endodontically instrumented root canals. Int Endod J 39: 18-25.

Pashley DH, Tao L, Boyd L, et al., Horner JA (1988) Scanning electron microscopy of the substructure of smear layers in human dentine. Arch Oral Biol 33: 265-270.

Perdigao J, Lopes M, Geraldeli S, et al., Garcia-Godoy F (2000) Effect of a sodium hypochlorite gel on dentin bonding. Dent Mater 16: 311-323.

Peutzfeldt A, Asmussen E (1999) Influence of eugenol-containing temporary cement on efficacy of dentin-bonding systems. Eur J Oral Sci 107: 65-69.

Rocha AW, de Andrade CD, Leitune VC, et al., dos Santos RB (2012) Influence of endodontic irrigants on resin sealer bond strength to radicu-lar dentin. Bull Tokyo Dent Coll 53: 1-7.

Saleh AA, Ettman WM (1999) Effect of endodontic irrigation solutions on microhardness of root canal dentine. J Dent 27: 43-46.

Sanares AM, Itthagarun A, King NM, et al., Pashley DH (2001) Adverse surface interactions between one-bottle light-cured adhesives and chemical-cured composites. Dent Mater 17: 542-556.

Sano H, Kanemura N, Burrow MF, et al., Tagami J (1998) Effect of operator variabil-ity on dentin adhesion: students vs. dentists. Dent Mater J 17: 51-58.

Schwartz RS (2006) Adhesive dentistry and endodontics. Part 2: bonding in the root canal system-the promise and the problems: a review. J Endod 32: 1125-1134.

Sekimoto T, Derkson GD, Richardson AS (1999) Effect of cutting instruments on permeability and morphology of the dentin surface. Oper Dent 24: 130-136.

Suh BI, Feng L, Pashley DH, Tay FR (2003) Factors contributing to the incompatibility between simplified-step adhesives and chemically-cured or dual-cured composites. Part III. Effect of acidic resin monomers. J Adhes Dent 5: 267-282.

Tay FR, Pashley DH (2003) Water treeing-a potential mechanism for degradation of dentin adhe-sives. Am J Dent 16: 6-12.

Tay FR, King NM, Suh BI, Pashley DH (2001) Effect of delayed activation of light-cured resin composites on bonding of all-in-one adhesives. J Adhes Dent 3: 207-225.

Tay FR, Pashley DH, Suh BI, et al., Itthagarun A (2002) Single-step adhesives are perme-able membranes. J Dent 30: 371-382.

Tay FR, Pashley DH, Peters MC (2003a) Adhesive permeability affects composite coupling to dentin treated with a self-etch adhesive. Oper Dent 28: 610-621.

Tay FR, Suh BI, Pashley DH, et al., Li F (2003b) Factors contributing to the incom-patibility between simplified-step adhesives and self-cured or dual-cured composites. Part II. Single-bottle, total-etch adhesive. J Adhes Dent 5: 91-105.

Tay FR, Frankenberger R, Krejci I, et al., Lai CN (2004a) Single-bottle adhesives behave as permeable membranes after polymerization. I. In vivo evi-dence. J Dent 32: 611-621.

Tay FR, Pashley DH, Suh B, et al., Miller M (2004b) Single-step, self-etch adhesives behave as permeable membranes after polymerization. Part I. Bond strength and morphologic evidence. Am J Dent 17: 271-278.

Tjan AH, Nemetz H (1992) Effect of eugenol-containing endodontic sealer on retention of prefab-ricated posts luted with adhesive composite resin cement. Quintessence Int 23: 839-844.

Vilanova WV, Carvalho-Junior JR, Alfredo E, et al., Silva-Sousa YT (2012) Effect of intracanal irrigants on the bond strength of epoxy resin-based and methacrylate resin-based sealers to root canal walls. Int Endod J 45: 42-48.

Violich DR, Chandler NP (2010) The smear layer in endodontics — a review. Int Endod J 43: 2-15 Weston CH, Ito S, Wadgaonkar B, Pashley DH (2007) Effects of time and concentration of sodium ascorbate on reversal of NaOCl-induced reduction in bond strengths. J Endod 33: 879-881.

Wolanek GA, Loushine RJ, Weller RN, et al., Volkmann KR (2001) In vitro bacterial penetration of endodontically treated teeth coronally sealed with a dentin bonding agent. J Endod 27: 354-357.

Wu H, Hayashi M, Okamura K, et al., Ebisu S (2009) Effects of light penetration and smear layer removal on adhesion of post-cores to root canal dentin by self-etching adhesives. Dent Mater 25: 1484-1492.

Yiu CK, Hiraishi N, King NM, Tay FR (2008) Effect of dentinal surface preparation on bond strength of self-etching adhesives. J Adhes Dent 10: 173-182.

延长根管壁牙本质黏结寿命的方法　　8

爱丽丝・多拉杜・洛尔古乔（Alessandro Dourado Loguercio）
塞萨尔・奥古斯托・拉雷（César Augusto Arrais）
亚历山德拉・里斯（Alessandra Reis）

> **摘　要**
>
> 无论使用何种黏结方法，纤维桩与根管壁牙本质的黏结力都会随时间推移而减弱，这是纤维桩在临床上发生脱落的原因之一。了解黏结力变弱的原理对临床医师采取措施防止纤维桩脱落，延长纤维桩的使用寿命是非常关键的。本章节将对根管壁牙本质与纤维桩的黏结力下降的机制以及临床上可采取的延长纤维桩根管壁牙本质黏结寿命的方法进行描述。

8.1　引文

在临床上，大多数纤维桩修复后的根管治疗牙失败原因为黏结失败（Aksornmuang et al. 2004），临床研究显示，黏结失败所致的脱胶可以毫无症状的随时发生（Rasimick et al. 2010）。牙本质的解剖和组织（结构牙本质小管的走向以及不均匀分布）可能影响根管壁牙本质与纤维桩的黏结力，影响黏结力的其他因素在本书其他章节也有讨论。尽管存在这些缺点，但是与传统黏结相比，根管壁牙本质与纤维桩黏结能够有效降低微渗漏（Bachicha et al. 1998；Reid et al. 2003）以及提高黏结力（Junge et al. 1998；Hedlund et al. 2003；Schwartz and Robbins 2004）。因此，良好的黏结是保证纤维桩黏结修复后修复体成功的关键因素。

根管内黏结的持久性与混合层成分的内在降解易感性密切相关（Van Meerbeek et al. 2003；Breschi et al. 2008）。虽然混合层降解的确切机制尚不明晰(Breschi et al. 2008；Vaidyanathan and Vaidyanathan 2009)，但其内在的降解抵抗力很大程度上依赖于树脂单体对脱矿根管牙本质的完全渗透，以及单体向聚合体实现最佳的转化，这是桩在根管内长期固位的保证(Perdigao et al. 2013；Reis et al. 2013)。因此，发生在黏结材料和根管牙本质间所形成的黏结界面中混合层降解的机制是临床医师必须理解的重要知识。本章节将详述在纤维桩黏固前，黏结系统应用到根管壁后两者间形成的混合层的降解机制，以及各种延长黏结寿命的临床策略。

8.2 与根管壁牙本质黏结老化相关的影响因素

混合层由牙本质有机基质、残余羟基磷灰石晶体、树脂单体以及溶剂组成，老化可能发生在每个单独的成分，也可能是几种成分协同老化(Breschi et al. 2008)。因此，混合层主要成分的降解将被单独介绍。

8.2.1 聚合物网络的降解

绝大多数商品化的黏结剂中都含有易水解成分，如酯类、尿烷、羟基、羧基以及磷酸基；因此，水的存在会影响这些成分的机械性能(Ferracane 2006)。事实上，由于含有易水解成分，这些产品非常容易吸收水分而发生降解(Malacarne et al. 2006；Reis et al. 2007b)。由此所导致的结果是，即使经过了光固化，黏结树脂在亲水特性的驱使下仍会使持续性吸收外界水分，树脂单体被水取代进而发生水解(Tay et al. 2004；Malacarne et al. 2006)。换句话说，黏结剂在混合层中所形成的亲水层会持续性吸水，脆化和削弱聚合物网络(Shono et al. 1999；Tanaka et al. 1999；Abdalla and Feilzer 2008)，最终导致黏结力随时间推移而下降(De Munck et al. 2003；Abdalla and Feilzer 2008)。

8.2.1.1 酸蚀-冲洗(ER)黏结系统

在全酸蚀湿黏结技术中，水在单体渗透进入脱矿牙本质中扮演至关重要的角色，因此，该技术中树脂水解的问题就需要引起加倍重视。全酸蚀湿黏结技术要求先酸蚀牙本质使牙本质表层脱矿，暴露一薄层胶原纤维网为树脂渗透提供空间。酸蚀后以流水将酸蚀剂冲洗干净。必须注意

8 延长根管壁牙本质黏结寿命的方法

的是,冲洗后的干燥不能过度,要求黏结界面微微润湿维持胶原纤维不发生塌陷,以利于树脂单体的渗透(Kanca 1992,1996)(图 8-1)。为了实现这一目的,黏结系统中加入了有机溶剂。有机溶剂能够加速残余水分与有机溶剂的共同挥发(Carvalho et al. 2003;Yiu et al. 2005b;Reis et al. 2013)。

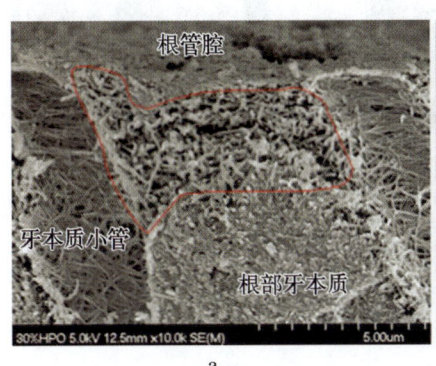

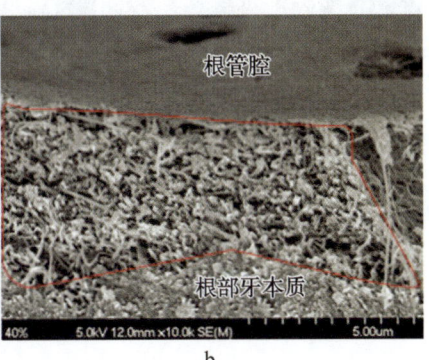

图 8-1 牙本质酸蚀后的扫描电镜图
a. 30%磷酸酸蚀 15 秒后;b. 40%磷酸酸蚀 15 秒后。注意红线标注的脱矿区域。

虽然绝大多数牙科黏结剂厂商均推荐了促进溶剂挥发的方法,但是要完全去除溶剂是非常困难的,尤其是高亲水性的配方中的溶剂(Pashley et al. 1998;Carvalho et al. 2003;Yiu et al. 2005b)。结果是,黏结面残留水分和溶剂的存在可能会阻止黏结剂和牙面的黏结,使混合层的交联反应更加困难(图 8-2、图 8-3)(Paul et al. 1999;Ye et al. 2007;Loguercio et al. 2009)。

因此,在聚合过程中,聚合物网络与剩余有机溶剂相关的自由空间大大增加而非形成优化的大分子堆积密度。当水分摄取的程度与速度由黏结系统的化学组成决定时(Ito et al. 2005a;Malacarne et al. 2006;Malacarne-Zanon et al. 2009;Reis et al. 2013),聚合不全的树脂最终会加快水分的吸收,进而破坏黏结剂-牙本质界面的远期完整性(Reis et al. 2013)。

尽管根部牙本质和冠部牙本质的黏结机制相似(Mannocci et al. 1999;Ferrari et al. 2000;Breschi et al. 2009),但发生在根部牙本质的黏结层的退化与其他任何区域相比更加具有不确定性(Mannocci et al. 1999;Ferrari et al. 2000;Breschi et al. 2009)。如前所述,根管的解剖

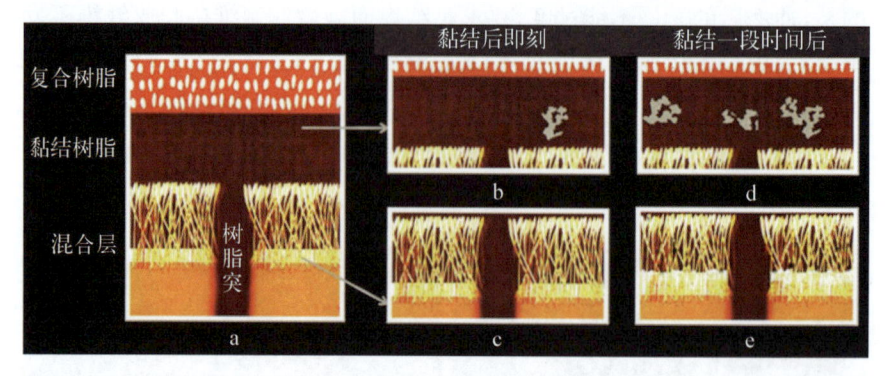

图 8-2 树脂牙本质黏结界面随时间推移而发生退化（改编自 Perdigao et al. 2013）
a. 树脂牙本质黏结界面；b. 灰色的区域代表黏结层中存在水分或树脂未完全聚合；c. 在混合层的基底部可以见到被剥蚀的胶原纤维和未完全渗透的树脂单体，这些胶原纤维更加容易受到蛋白酶的分解作用；d. 随着时间的推移，黏结层的灰色区域扩大了。这是由于水分的吸附，树脂聚合物会分解释放未与聚合物主链交联的寡聚物和残余单体；e. 树脂未渗透的胶原区域随着时间推移而增加。

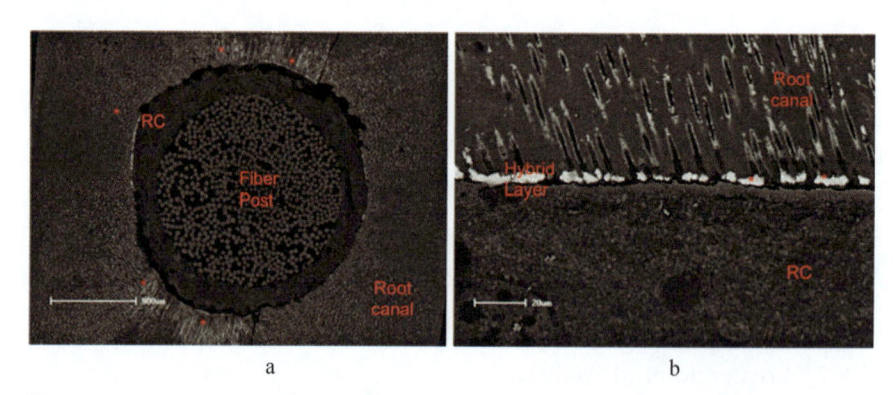

图 8-3 电镜下观察以简化酸蚀-冲洗黏结系统和双固化树脂黏固的根管桩根尖段
a. 殆面观可以看到在根管桩和根管壁之间有较多的微渗漏（红色箭头所指）；b. 更大的放大倍数的图片显示混合层内存在纳米渗漏。

特点决定了在使用酸蚀-冲洗黏结系统时，磷酸的彻底去除和黏结面的干燥难以实现（Breschi et al. 2009），因此，牙根中上部脱矿牙本质中会残留更多的水分（Thitthaweerat et al. 2013）。

由于受到牙根解剖形态的影响而发生的光固化灯光线衰减可能会进一步降低牙根中上部黏结剂和树脂水门汀的单体转化率（Roberts et al. 2004；Faria e Silvaet al. 2007）。由此引起的聚合不良叠加较多水分和溶剂的残留会造成根管中下部的黏结面比根管上部更易发生水解，最终导致较差的近期和远期黏结强度(Foxton et al. 2003；Monticelli et al. 2006)。

8.2.1.2 自酸蚀(SE)黏结系统

使用自酸蚀黏结剂进行纤维桩的黏固可以避免全酸蚀湿黏结的技术敏感问题。相较于全酸蚀-黏结系统，自酸蚀黏结剂自带酸性单体，使用自酸蚀黏结剂形成的混合层包含一部分污染层(Watanabe et al. 1994；Nakabayashi and Saimi 1996)。在黏结过程中，自酸蚀黏结剂中的酸性单体能够穿透玷污层、管塞及下方的牙本质。因此，自酸蚀黏结剂形成的玷污层同时包含黏结剂树脂、胶原纤维以及矿物。鉴于此原因，自酸蚀黏结剂不需要提前使用磷酸酸蚀和湿黏结，这使临床医师能更方便快捷地进行临床黏结操作。

然而，由于自酸蚀黏结剂中含有大量的高度亲水物质和溶剂，所以自酸蚀黏结系统较酸蚀-冲洗黏结系统更加亲水，也更加容易发生水解(Breschi et al. 2008；Reis et al. 2013)。这导致水解后混合层不单水分可以渗入，牙本质小管中的氟离子也能进入混合层。此外，根管桩黏结时使用的双固化树脂的化学成分与自酸蚀黏结剂中的酸性单体成分存在冲突(Sanares et al. 2001；Tay et al. 2003b；Arrais et al. 2009)。因为根管口照射进根管内的光难以抵达根尖区，那么根尖区树脂的固化依赖于化学固化，然而自酸蚀黏结剂或二步法自酸蚀黏结剂中的酸性单体会干扰树脂聚合过程(Sanares et al. 2001；Arrais et al. 2009)。自酸蚀黏结剂与双固化树脂之间化学组成的冲突会导致黏结层更多的水解和退化，通透性更大(Tay et al. 2003b)。

8.2.1.3 自黏结树脂水门汀

近年来，为了进一步简化操作，厂商制造了不用黏结剂即能完成黏结的树脂，这些树脂的配方中含有酸官能化单体，如4-甲基丙烯酰氧基乙基偏苯三酸酐(4-methacryloxyethyl trimellitic anhydride, 4-META)和1,2,4,5-苯四酸甘油二甲基丙烯酸酯(pyromellitic glycerol dimethacrylate, PMGDM)，或是磷酸基团与2-甲基丙烯酰氧基乙基苯基磷酸氢盐(2-methacryloxyethyl phenyl hydrogen phosphate, phenyl-P)、10-甲基丙烯酰氧基癸基二氢磷酸酯(10-methacryloy-loxydecyl dihydrogen phosphate, MDP)、2-甲基丙烯酰氧乙基酸式磷酸酯(2-methacryloxyethyl acid phosphate，BMP)以及二季戊四醇五丙烯酸酯单磷酸酯(dipentaerythritol pentaacrylate monophosphate，Penta-P)，以利于牙齿表面的脱矿和黏结(Ferracane et al. 2011)。

当自黏结树脂水门汀混合后,其酸性单体能够将 pH 降至 1.5～3,使釉质和牙本质轻度脱矿。酸性基团与羟基磷灰石中的钙结合,在甲基丙烯酸酯网络与牙本质之间形成稳定的离子键。从酸溶性填料中释放的离子会中和剩余的酸性基团并形成一个螯合增强的三维甲基丙烯酸酯网络。在黏结初期,树脂水门汀变得相当亲水,因此允许牙齿表面有适度的湿润。

自黏结树脂中的酸性成分与羟基磷灰石释放的钙以及树脂离子可浸出填料中释放的阳离子反应,结合形成疏水化合物(Ferracane et al. 2011)。因此,与简化的酸蚀-冲洗黏结系统和自酸蚀黏结系统形成的黏结层相比,自黏结树脂形成的黏结层更加不容易发生水解。尽管短期实验显示自黏结树脂的黏结强度较传统的双固化树脂高,然而,最近的长期研究显示,自黏结树脂黏固的桩,其黏结强度随着时间推移而下降。研究者们认为这是由于水引发的树脂聚合物塑化导致的黏结强度降低,也就是说,自黏结树脂的黏结层并未变得如预计的那样疏水(Mazzoni et al. 2009a；Goracci and Ferrari 2011；Marchesi et al. 2013)。

总体而言,水解降解可能是黏结系统应用于冠方牙本质后黏结强度随时间推移而降低的主要原因和机制(Breschi et al. 2008，2009；Perdigao et al. 2013；Reis et al. 2013)。有研究认为,黏结过程中沿牙本质小管流向黏结面的小管液与应用酸蚀-冲洗黏结系统进行湿黏时残留的水分或者黏结剂中的水/溶剂一起,导致了混合层的水解降解(Breschi et al. 2008，2009；Perdigao et al. 2013；Reis et al. 2013)。然而,根部牙本质小管内并未观察到液体的流动。此外,临床上一旦完成了桩的黏结,一般会即刻行树脂充填或者冠修复,避免桩与根管牙本质间的黏结面直接暴露于口腔,口腔内的液体并不会与桩-根管牙本质黏结区域直接接触(Vano et al. 2006；Ferrari et al. 2008)。

事实上,只有在极端情况下,例如冠方修复体无法保证边缘封闭性且口腔内的液体直接接触桩-牙本质黏结面,才会出现黏结面聚合体加速降解的情况。因此，虽然水的确会对酸蚀-冲洗黏结系统、自酸蚀黏结系统甚至是自黏结树脂水门汀的黏结面聚合体产生明显的影响，但是牙本质小管内的水分不应该被视作根部牙本质黏结面随时间推移而降解的主要原因（Breschi et al. 2009）。

8.2.2 胶原纤维的降解

在根管治疗和桩道预备后，根管壁内侧牙本质在组成和结构上与冠部牙本质相似（Ferrari et al. 2000）。根管壁牙本质中牙本质小管由内侧壁向周围呈放射状（Ferrari et al. 2000），存在管间牙本质和管周牙本质。因此，桩-根管壁黏结面内胶原纤维的退化与在牙冠牙本质内观察到的胶原纤维退化类似（Breschi et al. 2009）。

蛋白酶参与了牙本质龋（Tjaderhane et al. 1998；van Strijp et al. 2003）和牙周病（Lee et al. 1995）发病过程中胶原基质的降解。近年来，有研究报道，这些酶类可能在树脂-牙本质黏结面的降解中过程中发挥了一定的作用（Pashley et al. 2004）。具体而言，牙本质胶原纤维内含有未激活形式的蛋白水解酶，称为基质金属蛋白酶（matrix metalloproteinases，MMPs），以酶原形式分泌，在成牙本质细胞、矿化或未矿化的牙本质中均可检出（Bourd-Boittin et al. 2005；Mazzoni et al. 2007；Sulkala et al. 2007）。在人类矿化牙本质中可以发现多种MMPs，以未激活的形式存在，包括MMP-8胶原酶（Sulkala et al. 2007），MMP-2和MMP-9明胶酶（Mazzoni et al. 2007，2009b），以及MMP-20釉质溶解素（Sulkala et al. 2002）。尽管MMP-2和MMP-9被归类为明胶酶，但是有学者观察到这两种酶具有胶原酶活性（Aimes and Quigley 1995；Garnero et al. 2003）。

MMPs会被蛋白酶和一些化学成分如活性氧族激活。也就是说，在黏结过程中MMPs暴露于酸性试剂而被激活。如果与基质结合并被活化的MMPs未被黏结树脂完全渗透，这些MMPs可能会缓慢地降解树脂-牙本质黏结面内的胶原纤维（Carrilho et al. 2007）。因此，胶原纤维的降解与树脂单体是否完全浸润以及MMPs的激活有关（Carrilho et al. 2007）。

例如，混合层的厚度以及树脂突的密度随黏结面距根管口的距离增加而减少。有学者发现，在根管中上段，黏结剂在牙本质小管内渗透完全的占总黏结面积的三分之二，而根尖段只有三分之一（Mannocci et al. 2003）。

将黏结剂用于酸蚀过的牙齿表面时，树脂单体沿着胶原纤维的空隙渗透，距离黏结面越远，树脂单体浓度越低，这样就形成了一个下行浓度梯度（Wang and Spencer 2002）。而在混合层的基底部，树脂单体无法完全渗透，树脂固化后位于基底部的酸蚀后的胶原纤维将直接暴露（Wang and Spencer 2002；Hashimoto et al. 2003；Spencer et al. 2004）。也就是说，树脂渗透能力和酸蚀脱矿程度的不一致使混合层基底部始终存在一个脱矿区域，位于脱矿区域的胶原纤维不被树脂包裹（图8-2,8-3）（Spencer and Swafford 1999；Pioch et al. 2001）。有意思的是，有学者在混合层基底部检测到高浓度的活化 MMP-2 和 MMP-9（De Munck et al. 2009；Breschi et al. 2010）。

相反，使用自酸蚀黏结系统进行黏结时，酸蚀脱矿和树脂单体渗入同时进行，玷污层部分或全部与黏结面融合。因此，研究者们目前认为使用自酸蚀黏结系统获得同步进行的酸蚀脱矿和树脂单体渗入将克服酸蚀-冲洗黏结中牙本质酸蚀脱矿程度与树脂浸润能力不一致的缺点，即黏结混合层与牙本质之间将不存在未被树脂单体渗透的胶原纤维层。然而，研究者在自酸蚀黏结中仍观察到混合层基底部存在纳米级的渗透不全区域，其原因是黏结过程中存在纳米级渗漏（Tay et al. 2002；Tay and Pashley 2003），水经由这些纳米级的管道渗入黏结面。无论是自酸蚀黏结过程形成的纳米级脱矿区域还是酸蚀-冲洗黏结时形成的混合层基底部脱矿区域，MMPs 都会被黏结剂激活并降解Ⅰ型胶原纤维（Mazzoni et al. 2006；Carrilho et al. 2009）。

如本章之前所述，无论采用何种简化的黏结策略（两步法酸蚀-冲洗黏结系统和一步法自酸蚀黏结系统），通过将亲水的离子树脂单体添加到黏合剂中，黏结面都将受益于不可溶解的疏水树脂涂层。黏结所形成的混合层不仅对来自口腔环境的水具有渗透性，对于来自牙本质小管的水分也具有渗透性（Chersoni et al. 2004；Tay et al. 2004；Hashimoto et al. 2004b）。因此，简化黏结策略所形成的黏结面被认为是半透膜。本章接下来将对覆盖牙面的疏水树脂层进行讨论。

混合层内易水解不稳定聚合物中树脂成分的洗脱会导致胶原纤维的进一步暴露(Perdigao et al. 2013)。因此,当冠方封闭物损坏或者黏结时过于潮湿,水分将侵入混合层,激活的 MMPs 也将作用于混合层中暴露的胶原纤维,使其水解。此外,近年来的研究显示根管封闭剂(Huang et al. 2008)和根管内细菌的分解产物也会激活 MMP-2 和 MMP-9 (Itoh et al. 2009),这两种酶会水解混合层基底部暴露的胶原纤维(Mazzoni et al. 2007,2009b)。另外,在正常的根管牙本质中存在 TIMPs,TIMPs 会调节抑制 MMP 的活性(Reynolds and Meikle 1997;Malemud 2006),然而在牙髓摘除后以及根管充填后,根管壁牙本质内的 TIMPs 将很快耗尽。

除了 MMPs 外,牙髓组织、成牙本质细胞中还存在并在牙本质中表达不同种类的半胱氨酸组织蛋白酶(Tersariol et al. 2010)。组织蛋白酶能作用于龋坏或者健康牙本质(Tersariol et al. 2010;Nascimento et al. 2011),分解绝大多数细胞外基质,如胶原纤维、黏连蛋白以及糖蛋白(Turk et al. 1997;Dickinson 2002),组织蛋白酶能被酸性环境激活(Dickinson 2002),一些学者发现组织蛋白酶能被黏结剂中的酸性单体激活(Zhang et al. 2014),他们认为黏结剂中的酸性单体会使牙本质脱矿并暴露激活牙本质内部的组织蛋白酶,导致混合层胶原纤维的退化。也就是说,组织蛋白酶和 MMPs 一样,可能是混合层胶原纤维退化的原因,进而影响牙本质的黏结持久性(Liu et al. 2011;Tjaderhan et al. 2013b)。

总而言之,为了达到更加持久的黏结,在进行黏结时,必须使树脂尽可能多的包裹脱矿后暴露的胶原纤维,才能避免酶的分解作用。此外,还应尽量清除残存的水分和溶剂,在光固化时尽可能使光线进入根管的深部以保证树脂聚合达到最大化。然而,受限于根管的解剖结构,必要时还需要用一些辅助方法。

8.3 如何提升树脂-牙本质黏结的稳定性

如前所述,树脂黏结的质量决定于黏结面树脂突渗入胶原纤维的程度和树脂突是否完全包裹胶原纤维形成树脂聚合物。有学者研究了如何使用不同改良方法进行黏结以便于获得更加不易退化的黏结面。

然而，目前的研究大多针对冠部牙本质，关于根管内牙本质黏结的研究较少。考虑到牙冠牙本质结构和根管牙本质结构的相似，那么提高牙冠牙本质黏结质量的方法应同样能提高根管壁牙本质与桩的远期和近期黏结效果。

概括而言，提高黏结效果的原理包括：① 提高树脂突渗入脱矿或未脱矿牙本质的能力。② 提高黏结系统形成的聚合体的强度。③ 提高胶原纤维抵抗酶水解的能力。接下来介绍的一些临床方法可能同时使用了 2 种或 3 种原理，但是为了便于教学和分类，这些方法将会被分为以上 3 类中的一类。

8.3.1 提高树脂渗入脱矿或未脱矿牙本质的能力

8.3.1.1 使用金刚砂车针预备根管

磷酸酸蚀由硬质合金钻预备的桩道，得到的是一个脱矿不连续的根管壁牙本质面。这个不连续的牙本质面由脱矿的管间牙本质、开放的牙本质小管口，以及被牙本质碎屑、玷污层、牙胶尖和/或残留的根管封闭剂覆盖的区域间杂交替组成。想要以化学溶解的方法对这些区域进行清洁十分困难(Serafino et al. 2004；Breschi et al. 2009)。与之相反，金刚砂车针预备后的根管壁牙本质，酸蚀能够更有效地去除表面的玷污层，从而暴露更多的牙本质小管开放区域(Gomes et al. 2012)。

目前市面上并没有专用于根管壁预备的金刚砂车针，因此，临床上可先用硬质合金钻完成根管桩道预备，然后使用同直径的金刚砂车针再次进行根管壁的清理预备。这样可以将硬质合金钻预备产生的不易被酸蚀清除的玷污层变得易于酸蚀清除。

8.3.1.2 使用液体型酸蚀剂

如前所述，使用磷酸凝胶不能高效溶解清除所有的根管壁玷污层。有研究报道，根管经过预备、充填和桩道预备后，借助扫描电镜可以在根管壁和桩之间的间隙内发现大范围被玷污层、牙本质碎屑以及根管封闭剂/牙胶尖残余所覆盖的区域。这些区域不能被黏结，也不能黏固纤维桩(Serafino et al. 2004)。

在凝胶型酸蚀剂中，由于酸性物质无法自由移动，常无法与牙本质面自由接触。近年来的一些研究发现，使用酸蚀-冲洗黏结系统时以根管冲洗针头将液态的磷酸注入根管进行酸蚀能够更加彻底去除玷污层,从而获得更强的黏结力(Salas et al. 2011;Scotti et al. 2013)。

8.3.1.3 用力涂布黏结剂

由于根管内的湿润程度很难控制,因此在使用简化的酸蚀-冲洗黏结系统时,若黏结剂涂布的力量过小会导致树脂单体(特别是大分子量单体)难以完全渗透进入脱矿的根部牙本质。而如果用力涂布黏结剂,那么黏结剂能够更好地渗透进入牙本质胶原网(Jacobsen and Soderholm 1998;Reis et al. 2007a),加速溶剂的蒸发扩散,提高混合层树脂单体的交联度。

最近,一些学者(2014)对3种简化的酸蚀-冲洗黏结系统分别在有超声设备辅助(模拟用力涂布黏结剂)和没有超声设备辅助下进行根管内黏结的黏结效果进行了评估。结果发现,使用超声设备辅助可以提高黏结强度,提升黏结效果并降低根尖段的纳米渗漏。

当超声设备辅助应用于自酸蚀黏结时,也能有效提高黏结的效果(未发表的数据)。其原理在于,用力涂布自酸蚀黏结剂能够使更多新鲜的酸性树脂单体渗透进入脱矿牙本质的基底层,拓展牙本质的脱矿深度,进而促进更多的树脂与玷污层和位于玷污层下方的牙本质相接触,形成更加紧密的黏结。

8.3.1.4 多层黏结技术

研究显示,无论使用酸蚀-冲洗黏结系统还是自酸蚀黏结系统,多层黏结都能够获得更高的黏结力(Hashimoto et al. 2004a;Ito et al. 2005b),且黏结面更加不易发生水解(Reis et al. 2008)。对上述两类黏结系统而言,多层黏结在促进溶剂挥发的同时有利于提高混合层树脂单体的饱和度。此外,额外的未聚合的自酸蚀黏结剂共聚单体层能够促进酸性单体渗透至混合层的基底部以替换被牙本质中和的酸性单体,因而能提高自酸蚀黏结剂的酸蚀能力(Camps and Pashley 2000)。

这种方法对于根管牙本质黏结的影响虽然尚无报道,不过我们有理由猜测,该方法在根部牙本质应该能够获得与应用于冠部牙本质相似的效果。因此多层黏结也能提高根管壁牙本质的黏结力。值得注意的是,多层涂布黏结剂会增加黏结层的厚度,过厚的黏结层可能会影响桩的就位,使用纸尖清除多余的黏结剂有助于避免这种情况的发生。

8.3.2 提高黏结层聚合物的强度

8.3.2.1 疏水性树脂覆盖

有一种降低黏结剂亲水性的方法是在已聚合的黏结层表面再涂布一层疏水性树脂，这样做可以明显降低黏结层水分和溶剂的残留，降低黏结后黏结层内的液体流动率，使黏结层更加平整，但是会增加黏结层的厚度（King et al. 2005；de Andrade e Silva et al. 2009）。

在黏结层表面涂布疏水树脂层可以消除自酸蚀黏结剂与化学固化树脂之间的理化不相容性（King et al. 2005；Van Landuyt et al. 2006）。无论是三步法的酸蚀-冲洗黏结系统还是两步法的自酸蚀黏结系统，使用这种方法都可以提高树脂的聚合度，降低对水的渗透性（Cadenaro et al. 2005；Breschi et al. 2007）。

如果在一步法自酸蚀黏结层表面涂布一层疏水树脂层，那么这种简单化的黏结将转变成为更加稳定的两步法自酸蚀黏结。同理，在两步法酸蚀-冲洗黏结系统形成的黏结面上涂布一层疏水树脂层，将会把两步法黏结转化为更加稳定的三步法酸蚀-冲洗黏结。来自额外的疏水性树脂层的疏水性单体能够增加黏结层的密实度（Breschi et al. 2008；Lombardo et al. 2008），其结果是形成了一个更为稳定的树脂-牙本质黏结面（Reis et al. 2008）。这种方法将单层黏结转变成为多层黏结，区别在于在黏结时具有亲水性的树脂层位于内层且已固化，而疏水性的树脂层位于外层。

通过减少底漆层和黏结层间未反应的树脂单体，混合层会变得更加致密（de Andrade e Silva et al. 2009）。然而使用这种方法要注意黏结层的厚度，避免黏结层过厚导致的桩无法就位。

8.3.2.2 乙醇湿黏结

如前所述，由于简化的酸蚀-冲洗黏结系统和自酸蚀黏结系统内含有亲水性单体，易吸潮和发生水解。然而，疏水的树脂如 Bis－GMA\TEGDMA 等无法渗透湿润的牙本质。乙醇湿黏结的原理是使用乙醇取代水润湿牙本质胶原纤维，以便于树脂能渗透脱矿牙本质形成混合层（Breschi et al. 2007；Sadek et al. 2008）。

疏水性树脂几乎不会从牙本质中吸潮（Sadek et al. 2008）。使用乙醇湿黏结技术产生的黏结面其吸水率相较传统树脂黏结剂黏结面下降5倍(Yiu et al. 2004；Ito et al. 2005a；Malacarne et al. 2006)。同时，MMPs在缺水的时候无法激活，使用乙醇取代水在某种程度上增强了远期的黏结效果。乙醇湿黏结技术提高了即刻黏结强度(Tjaderhane et al. 2013a)，降低了根管壁牙本质黏结面的纳米渗漏(Duan et al. 2011；Pei et al. 2012)。有体外研究结果显示，乙醇湿黏结技术同时提高了6个月和12个月的根部牙本质黏结强度(Bitter et al. 2014；Ekambaram et al. 2014)。然而，发现有待更多实验结果和支持(Cecchin et al. 2011)。

乙醇湿黏结技术要求使用一系列浓度逐渐升高的乙醇处理黏结面，耗时3～4分钟，操作烦琐，技术敏感性高(Osorio et al. 2010)。最近的一项研究显示，使用较高浓度的乙醇润湿牙本质60秒也能获得较高的黏结强度，而且也大大降低了技术敏感性和操作门槛(Sauro et al. 2010)。

8.3.2.3 提高根管内树脂的聚合程度

尽管厂商为自酸蚀黏结系统和酸蚀-黏结系统提供了独立包装的含有化学三元催化剂的激活剂，在使用前与黏结剂混合可以催化黏结剂固化。然而，只有光照才能达到最大程度的固化(Faria-e-Silva et al. 2008)。

相似地，双固化树脂在光照后可以获得更好的机械性能(Pegoraro et al. 2007；Manso et al. 2011)。因此，使用双固化树脂进行黏结时也要保证光照(Caughman et al. 2001；Goracci et al. 2008；Breschi et al. 2009；Wu et al. 2009)。为了保证在根管狭小的空间内能得到足够的光照，临床医师应尽量使用光线强的光源进行照射，同时延长照射时间以提高黏结剂和树脂对根管壁牙本质的黏结(Akgungor and Akkayan 2006；Aksornmuang et al. 2008；Teixeira et al. 2009；Miguel-Almeida et al. 2012)。

延长光照时间能有效提高根部牙本质的黏结强度(Aksornmuang et al. 2006)。而使用透明纤维桩对黏结强度影响却不大，主要原因是透明的纤维桩并不能让足够的光线透射进入根管根尖段(Teixeira et al. 2006；dos Santos Alves Morgan et al. 2008；Goracci et al. 2008)。其他方法,如使用光导纤维或透明的光导装置将光线投射到根尖的最深部也可以作为潜在的选择(Goracci and Ferrari 2011)。

8.3.2.4 使用含有草酸的脱敏剂

使用简化系统黏结有一个缺点,即黏结面会表现为允许来自其深部牙本质水分渗透的半透性界面。有报道称使用含有草酸成分的脱敏剂处理根管壁牙本质能显著降低牙本质对水分的通透性(Gillam et al. 2001; Tay et al. 2003a; Garcia et al. 2010)。在酸蚀处理后,牙本质的玷污层被完全去除,牙本质通透性会显著增加,此时如果使用脱敏剂处理,会显著降低树脂黏结层对水分的通透性。使用这种方法还能增加树脂层和黏结层的结合,有效降低树脂层和黏结层的物理不相容性。

使用磷酸酸蚀牙本质会耗尽牙本质表面的钙离子,那么脱敏剂中的草酸只有移动到牙本质小管的深层才会和牙本质中解离出来的钙离子反应形成草酸钙(Tay et al. 2003a)。此外,草酸(pH2.3)本身就能酸蚀牙本质,释放牙本质中的钙离子并与之反应形成草酸钙。新形成的草酸钙会堵塞牙本质小管,减少牙本质小管中的水分向黏结层的渗透,从而降低黏结层中的水分残留量。

尽管这项技术很好地处理了树脂和黏结剂的物理相容性的问题,但是这项技术仅限于酸蚀-冲洗黏结系统,因为草酸只能作用于酸蚀后的牙本质。此外,如果含草酸成分的脱敏剂和含氟的黏结剂或pH小于2.8的黏结剂一同使用可能会造成草酸盐晶体的溶解(Yiu et al. 2005a)。

8.3.3 提高胶原纤维的抗酶解能力

8.3.3.1 氯己定

尽管氯己定过去一直在口腔修复和牙体牙髓治疗中被用作消毒剂和抗菌剂,尤其是在根管治疗时,氯己定常被用作最后的根管冲洗剂(Mohammadi and Abbott 2009; Gomes et al. 2013)。近年来的研究发现,氯己定具有抑制牙本质中MMPs(Pashley et al. 2004)和半胱氨酸组织蛋白酶的作用(Tersariol et al. 2010)。

无论是自酸蚀黏结系统还是酸蚀-冲洗黏结系统,在黏结过程中使用氯己定水溶液处理黏结面均不会对黏结效果造成影响(Lindblad et al.

2010；Pelegrine et al. 2010）。然而，若使用氯己定来保持混合层的黏结强度和其长期完整性仍存在一定的争议。有研究结果显示，使用氯己定处理黏结面能维持桩与根管壁的黏结强度（Cecchin et al. 2011；Bitter et al. 2014；Toman et al. 2014），而另一些研究则显示经过12个月的水中保存，氯己定处理组与对照组的黏结强度没有任何差异（Leitune et al. 2010；Cecchin et al. 2011；Bitter et al. 2014；Ekambaram et al. 2014）。研究结果出现争议原因可能在于研究中所使用的黏结系统和树脂的种类和品牌以及实验方法不同。

研究结果显示低浓度的氯己定足以抑制MMPs和组织蛋白酶（Gendron et al. 1999；Scaffa et al. 2012），但根管治疗中仍推荐使用2%的氯己定溶液作为最后的根管冲洗液，其原因在于2%的氯己定溶液比低浓度的氯己定溶液有着更强的抗菌活性（Mohammadi and Abbott 2009）和对根管壁牙本质的亲和力（Basrani and Lemonie 2005），这些特性还有助于降低根管发生远期再感染的概率（Roach et al. 2001；Rosenthal et al. 2004），也未观察到有任何长期不良影响。因此，使用2%的氯己定可以作为维持树脂远期黏结强度的方法。

有学者报道用含氯己定的磷酸代替2%浓度的氯己定溶液（Stanislawczuk et al. 2009，2011）。虽然尚无研究评估氯己定溶液对于根管壁牙本质黏结效果的影响，但已有研究结果显示，使用2%氯己定处理2年后，冠部牙本质的黏结强度仍保持稳定（Stanislawczuk et al. 2009，2011）。因此在使用酸蚀-冲洗黏结系统时，可以考虑引入用氯己定处理根管壁牙本质以期获得更持久的黏结。

8.3.3.2 EDTA

EDTA是根管机械预备中最常使用的冲洗剂之一，同时也被广泛地应用于牙周手术中（Hulsmann et al. 2003）。EDTA能够使玷污层覆盖的牙本质表层脱钙，但其作用有自限性。EDTA是一种螯合剂，能与牙本质羟基磷灰石中的钙离子进行反应，形成可溶的钙盐（Hulsmann et al. 2003）。由于EDTA是一种高效的锌离子和钙离子螯合剂，因而能够抑制MMP的活性（Osorio et al. 2011a；Thompson et al. 2012）。事实上，EDTA处理1～5分钟就能够有效抑制人牙本质中MMP-2和MMP-9的活性（Osorio et al. 2011a；Thompson et al. 2012）。

因此，EDTA 被用作牙本质黏结预处理剂。研究显示，使用 EDTA 处理牙面较磷酸或其他牙本质表面处理剂能获得更高的黏结强度（Torii et al. 2003；Jacques and Hebling 2005；Sauro et al. 2010）。体外研究结果显示，使用 EDTA 处理牙面能够更好地维持牙本质树脂黏结面的长久稳定（Sauro et al. 2010）。

EDTA 应用的问题是，EDTA 能够被水冲洗去除，牙本质表面没有残留的 EDTA 也就失去了抑制 MMPs 活性的能力（Osorio et al. 2011a；Thompson et al. 2012）。有学者观察到 EDTA 脱钙牙本质中的胶原对 MMP 降解敏感，类似于经磷酸酸蚀的牙本质中的胶原（Osorio et al. 2011b）。因此，EDTA 对混合层的保护是因为牙本质浅层脱矿的结果还是源于对 MMP 的抑制，目前尚不清楚。

8.3.3.3 交联剂

牙本质基质的抗性和寿命的基础是其固有的分子间和微纤维间的交联。因此，有学者认为在黏结前提高胶原纤维的交联度能提高黏结面的稳定性和持久性（Liu et al. 2011；Bedran-Russo et al. 2014）。

在黏结前使用胶原纤维交联剂处理脱矿后的牙本质面，可以增强胶原纤维层的机械性能（Bedran-Russo et al. 2014）。最新的研究发现，交联剂还具有抗 MMP 的能力（Liu et al. 2011；Bedran-Russo et al. 2014），主要是通过变构沉默胶原蛋白水解酶或通过改变胶原分子中的酶结合位点来降低胶原的酶解（Tjaderhane 2015）。最近有研究评估了不同种类的交联剂（Perdigao et al. 2013；Bedran-Russo et al. 2014）。其中牙科应用特别感兴趣的是原花色素，它们是天然存在的化合物且没有细胞毒性（Bedran-Russo et al. 2014）。

使用交联剂的主要问题在于，要达到理想治疗效就需要花费大量的时间，这在临床上缺乏可行性（Castellan et al. 2010，2011）。不过，厂商已经开发出了一些简化的方案，例如将原花色素掺入酸蚀剂和黏结剂中（Green et al. 2010；Epasinghe et al. 2012；Liu et al. 2013，2014）。遗憾的是，关于交联剂应用于根管牙本质的报道很少，缺乏充分的评估。到目前为止，只有一项研究评估了在使用树脂基质根管封闭剂根充之前使用原花青素处理根管的效果。结果显示，在水中保存 3 个月后，花青素处理提升了根管封闭剂的持久性（Kalra et al. 2013）。

8.3.3.4 苯扎氯铵

使用苯扎氯铵水溶液或含有苯扎氯铵的酸或黏结剂可能是抑制基质内 MMP 活性的另一种更简单的方法（Tezvergil-Mutluay et al. 2011；Sabatini and Patel 2013），因为在冠部牙本质的应用中，它能够随时间产生更稳定的键（Sabatini et al. 2015；Sabatini and Pashley 2015）。这种方法尚未在根部牙本质上进行研究，但是由于冠状冠部牙本质和根部牙本质的相似性，因而可能会得到类似的良好结果。

8.4 自黏结树脂水门汀

一项近期的 Meta 分析显示，与使用黏结传统树脂的自酸蚀黏结系统或酸蚀-冲洗黏结系统黏结纤维桩相比，使用自黏结树脂水门汀黏结纤维桩能取得更好的固位（Sarkis-Onofre et al. 2014）。但是，绝大部分研究只评估了某一品牌黏结系统的即时黏结效果（Radovic et al. 2008；Ferracane et al. 2011）。只有少数实验研究了自黏结树脂的远期效果，部分研究认为传统的自酸蚀黏结系统或酸蚀-冲洗黏结系统黏结纤维桩能获得较好的黏结效果（Mazzoni et al. 2009a；Marchesi et al. 2013），而另外一些研究则认为使用自黏结树脂水门汀黏结效果更佳（Leme et al. 2011；Bitter et al. 2012）。

使用 MMP 抑制剂并不能提高自黏结水门汀的远期黏结效果（Luhrs et al. 2013），其原因可能是自黏结水门汀和牙本质之间仅有表面接触（Radovic et al. 2008；Ferracane et al. 2011）。也就是说，这些黏结系统的降解模式更多地与其中单体成分的亲水性相关。由于氯己定可能会影响某些材料的即刻黏结力，因此当使用自酸蚀黏结剂时，不建议使用氯己定作为最后的根管冲洗液（Hiraishi et al. 2009；Luhrs et al. 2013）。

8.5 总结

最后，我们将分别介绍使用传统树脂和黏结系统（自酸蚀和酸蚀-冲洗）以及自黏结树脂水门汀进行黏结的方法，以便于综合讲解本章所涉及的所有临床操作技术以及其细节。

8.5.1 玷污层的预备

在使用厂商推荐的器械完成根管预备后,使用金刚砂车针粗糙化根管壁牙本质表层并获得更加容易酸蚀清除的玷污层,使用大量清水冲洗(图8-4)。

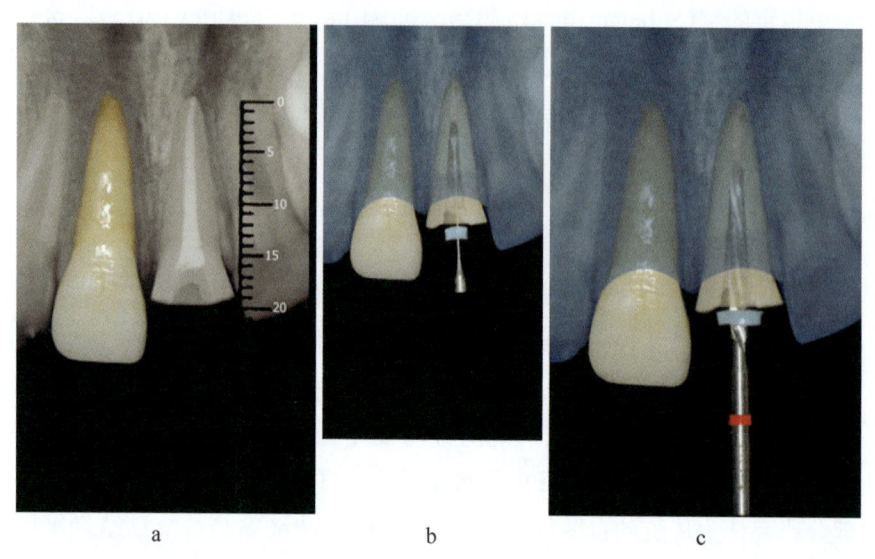

图8-4 桩道预备
a. 术前使用X线片测量牙根长度;b. 使用P钻去除冠方的牙胶;c. 使用厂商提供的硬质合金钻进行桩道预备。之后可以使用相同直径的金刚砂车针重新预备根管以获得更加容易酸蚀的和去除的玷污层。
以上方法仅适用于使用酸蚀-冲洗黏结剂和传统树脂进行黏结时。
(临床病例来自 Prof. Leonardo Muniz; Muniz 2010)

8.5.2 磷酸酸蚀

参考第12章中所述,酸蚀之前需要完成试桩和纤维桩的切割(图8-5)。使用浓度为34%~38%的磷酸对根管壁进行酸蚀,酸蚀时从根管根尖段开始注入磷酸并向根管冠段后退,注射时辅以轻轻搅动(Salas et al. 2011; Scotti et al. 2013)(图8-6a)。最好使用流动性好且含有苯扎氯铵和氯己定的酸蚀剂,目前市场上已经有相关产品销售。使用流水冲洗时,无论磷酸是否完全去除,应保证冲洗时间在15秒以上(图8-6b)。之后使用纸尖吸干根管(图8-6c),注意纸尖上是否有残余的磷酸,尤其是当使用凝胶型酸蚀剂和半凝胶型酸蚀剂(图8-6d)。

8 延长根管壁牙本质黏结寿命的方法 | 171

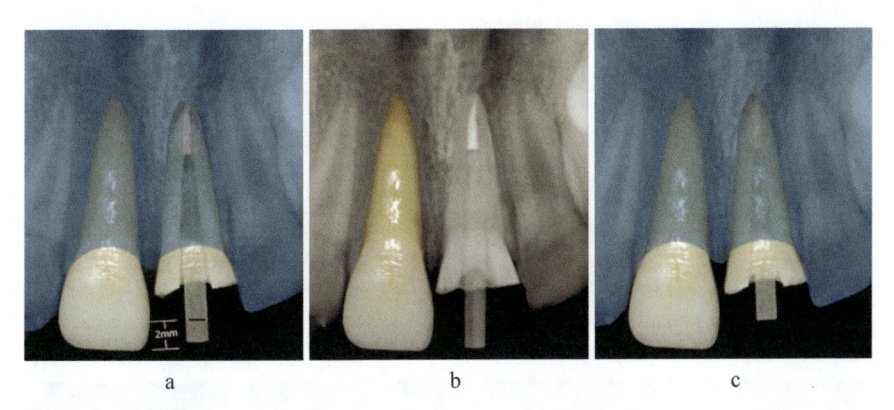

图 8-5 桩的预备
a. 试桩,检查纤维桩是否完全就位,可以拍摄牙片以确保纤维桩贯穿桩道的全长;b. 按照第 12 章所述切断纤维桩。
(临床病例来自 Prof. Leonardo Muniz;Muniz 2010)

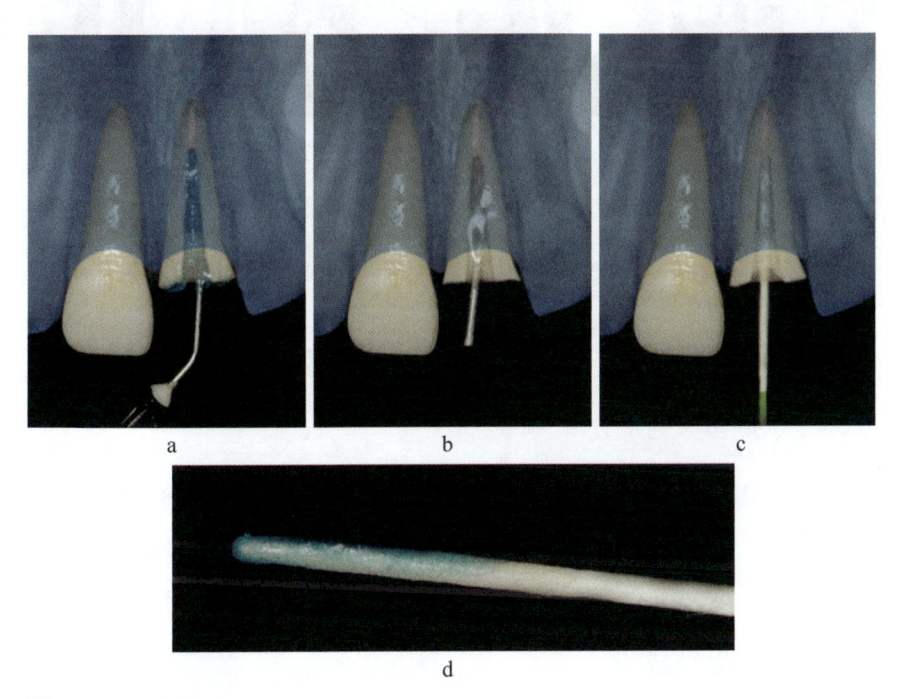

图 8-6 桩道的酸蚀
a. 酸蚀,最好使用液态的含有氯己定和苯扎氯铵的磷酸;b. 使用纸尖吸干根管内的水分;c. 在吸干根管内多余水分的同时观察纸尖上是否有残余的磷酸;d. 这些操作仅限于使用酸蚀-冲洗黏结剂进行黏结时。
(临床病例来自 Prof. Leonardo Muniz;Muniz 2010)

8.5.3 在黏结剂中添加酶抑制剂

2%的氯己定溶液冲洗根管60秒(Cecchin et al. 2011；Bitter et al. 2014；Toman et al. 2014)，干燥根管(图8-7)。如果使用传统树脂和酸蚀-冲洗黏结系统进行黏结，且酸蚀剂中含有苯扎氯铵或氯己定，可以省略此步骤。如果使用的是自黏结树脂水门汀，则应避免使用氯己定冲洗，因为氯己定会降低自黏结树脂的即刻黏结强度(Hiraishi et al. 2009；Luhrs et al. 2013)。

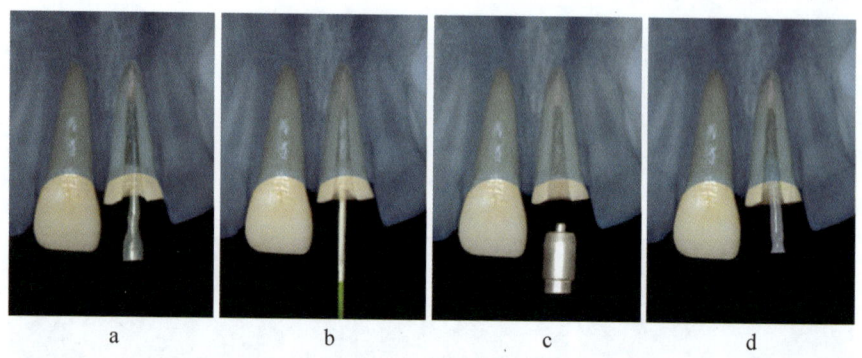

图8-7 乙醇和氯己定溶液的使用
a.使用2%浓度的氯己定溶液冲洗根管60秒。注意自黏结水门汀不能和氯己定溶液冲洗一同使用，因为氯己定溶液冲洗会降低自黏结水门汀的即刻黏结强度；b.使用纸尖吸干根管下段多余的水分；c.使用气枪轻吹干燥根管上段；d.使用浓度为95%~100%的乙醇浸泡根管1分钟，按照之前的步骤去除根管内多余的酒精。
(临床病例来自Prof. Leonardo Muniz；Muniz 2010)

8.5.4 去除多余的水分

位于根管中上段的多余水分可以通过气枪轻吹去除(图8-7c)，但是应注意防止牙本质脱水。而位于根管中下段的多余水分只能通过纸尖吸除(Souza et al. 2007；Thitthaweerat et al. 2013)(图8-7b)。

8.5.5 乙醇黏结技术

乙醇湿黏结技术需要使用95%~100%的乙醇处理黏结面1分钟(Bitter et al. 2014；Ekambaram et al. 2014)，去除根管内多余乙醇的方法与去除多余水分类似(图8-7d)。

8.5.6 涂布黏结剂

如果使用的是自黏结树脂,则可以省略此步骤。严格按照要求涂布黏结剂,如果使用的是 3 步法酸蚀-冲洗黏结系统或 2 步法自酸蚀黏结系统,尽量使用双固化模式的黏结。如果使用的是简化黏结法(2 步法酸蚀-冲洗黏结系统和一步法自酸蚀黏结系统)在黏结剂表层可以再涂布一层疏水树脂。为了达到上述目的,将任意 3 步法酸蚀-冲洗黏结系统或 2 步法自酸蚀黏结系统中的黏结剂、流动树脂或封闭剂涂布在黏结面表面都可以有产生一个疏水层的效果。

涂布黏结剂时不要使用长头毛刷,应使用圆头毛刷(Souza et al. 2007)(图 8-8a)。黏结剂一般反复涂 2~3 次,每次涂 10~15 秒。根尖区多余的黏结剂使用纸尖吸除,而根中上段多余的黏结剂则需使用气枪轻柔地吹干(Souza et al. 2007;Thitthaweerat et al. 2013)(图 8-8b、c)。

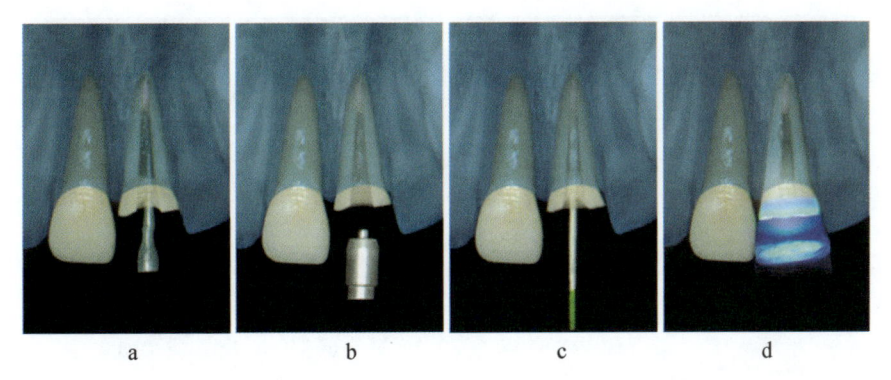

图 8-8 黏结剂的使用
a. 使用圆头的小毛刷涂布黏结剂,黏结剂中最好含有疏水树脂成分,例如 3 步法酸蚀-冲洗黏结剂和 2 步法自酸蚀黏结剂。至少涂 2 次黏结剂,每次涂 10~15 秒,如果使用的是自黏结树脂,则可以省略整个黏结剂使用的步骤;b. 使用气枪轻轻吹干去除多余的黏结剂;c. 使用纸尖去除根尖段和根中段的黏结剂;d. 光固化时延长光照时间 20~40 秒,同时使用高强度的光固化灯(高于 1 000 mW/cm^2)。
(临床病例来自 Prof. Leonardo Muniz;Muniz 2010)

有多种方法可以促进黏结剂溶剂的挥发(Souza et al. 2007;Aziz et al. 2014)。Souza 推荐使用纸尖去除根尖段的多余溶剂,而根中上段的多余溶剂可以通过气枪轻吹去除多余的溶剂。最近,有学者(2014)认为使用一次性塑料尖可以更有效地去除多余的溶剂，然而这需要专门的器械。无论使用何种方法，促进溶剂蒸发是黏结中的重要步骤，应认真操作。

8.5.7 黏结剂的光固化

在光固化前检查纤维桩是否完全就位，在纤维桩就位前先使用光固化灯光照 20～40 秒（Aksornmuang et al. 2006；Thitthaweerat et al. 2012）。使用高强度光源进行光照。即使使用双固化黏结剂，也应进行光照，因为双固化树脂在缺乏光照的情况下聚合不完全。

8.5.8 涂布树脂黏结剂

使用厂商提供的长头毛刷在根管内涂布黏结剂，也可以使用其他能将树脂水门汀注射到根管深部的器械（Michida et al. 2010）（图 8 - 9a、b）。

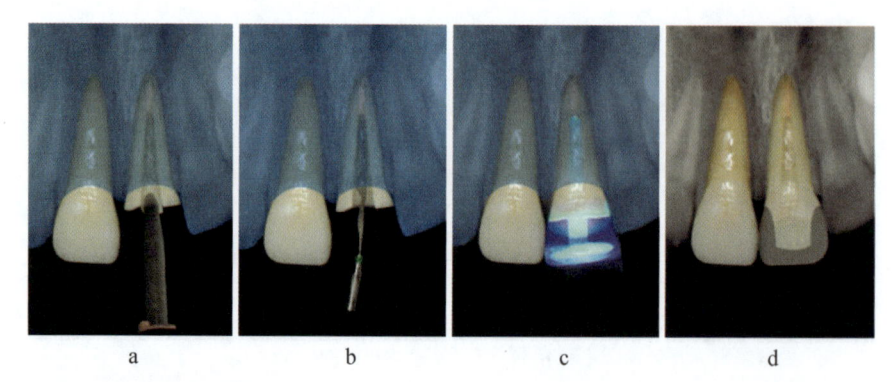

图 8 - 9 纤维桩的黏结
a. 使用厂商提供的长头毛刷在根管内涂布树脂黏结剂，也可以使用装置将树脂黏结剂注射进入根管深处；b. 使用光强在 1 000 mW/cm² 以上的光源进行光固化，延长光照时间；c. 按照第 11 章所述方法黏结修复体。
（临床病例来自 Prof. Leonardo Muniz；Muniz 2010）

8.5.9 树脂水门汀的光固化

应保证光照时间在 40 秒以上，光源的光强大于 1 000 mW/cm²（图 8 - 9c），而修复体的预备和最终黏结将在第 12 章中讨论。

（梁景平　刘斌　译）

参考文献

Abdalla AI, Feilzer AJ (2008) Four-year water degradation of a total-etch and two self-etching adhesives bonded to dentin. J Dent 36: 611-617.

Aimes RT, Quigley JP (1995) Matrix metalloproteinase-2 is an interstitial collagenase. Inhibitor- free enzyme catalyzes the cleavage of collagen fibrils and soluble native type I collagen gener-ating the specific 3/4-and 1/4-length fragments. J Biol Chem 270: 5872-5876.

Akgungor G, Akkayan B (2006) Influence of dentin bonding agents and polymerization modes on the bond strength between translucent fiber posts and three dentin regions within a post space. J Prosthet Dent 95: 368-378.

Aksornmuang J, Foxton RM, Nakajima M, Tagami J (2004) Microtensile bond strength of a dual-cure resin core material to glass and quartz fibre posts. J Dent 32: 443-450.

Aksornmuang J, Nakajima M, Foxton RM, Tagami J (2006) Effect of prolonged photo-irradiation time of three self-etch systems on the bonding to root canal dentine. J Dent 34: 389-397.

Aksornmuang J, Nakajima M, Foxton RM, et al., Tagami J (2008) Regional bond strengths and failure analysis of fiber posts bonded to root canal dentin. Oper Dent 33: 636-643.

Arrais CA, Giannini M, Rueggeberg FA (2009) Effect of sodium sulfinate salts on the polymeriza-tion characteristics of dual-cured resin cement systems exposed to attenuated light-activation. J Dent 37: 219-227.

Aziz TM, Anwar MN, El-Askary FS (2014) Push-out bond strength of fiber posts to root canal dentin using a one-step self-etching adhesive: the effect of solvent removal and light-curing methods. J Adhes Dent 16: 79-86.

Bachicha WS, DiFiore PM, Miller DA, et al., Pashley DH (1998) Microleakage of endodontically treated teeth restored with posts. J Endod 24: 703-708.

Basrani B, Lemonie C (2005) Chlorhexidine gluconate. Aust Endod J 31: 48-52.

Bedran-Russo AK, Pauli GF, Chen SN, et al., Leme AA (2014) Dentin biomodification: strategies, renewable resources and clinical applications. Dent Mater 30: 62-76.

Bitter K, Perdigao J, Exner M, et al., Sterzenbach G (2012) Reliability of fiber post bonding to root canal dentin after simulated clinical function in vitro. Oper Dent 37: 397-405.

Bitter K, Aschendorff L, Neumann K, et al., Sterzenbach G (2014) Do chlorhexidine and ethanol improve bond strength and durability of adhesion of fiber posts inside the root canal? Clin Oral Investig 18: 927-934.

Bourd-Boittin K, Fridman R, Fanchon S, et al., Menashi S (2005) Matrix metalloproteinase inhibition impairs the processing, formation and mineralization of dental tissues during mouse molar development. Exp Cell Res 304: 493-505.

Breschi L, Cadenaro M, Antoniolli F, et al., Di Lenarda R (2007) Polymerization kinetics of dental adhesives cured with LED: correlation between extent of conversion and permeability. Dent Mater 23: 1066-1072.

Breschi L, Mazzoni A, Ruggeri A, et al., De Stefano Dorigo E (2008) Dental adhesion review: aging and stability of the bonded interface. Dent Mater 24: 90-101.

Breschi L, Mazzoni A, De Stefano ED, Ferrari M (2009) Adhesion to intraradicular dentin: a review. J Adhes Sci Technol 23: 1053-1083.

Breschi L, Martin P, Mazzoni A, et al., Pashley DH (2010) Use of a specific MMP-inhibitor (galardin) for preservation of hybrid layer. Dent Mater 26: 571-578.

Cadenaro M, Antoniolli F, Sauro S, et al., Breschi L (2005) Degree of conversion and permeability of dental adhesives. Eur J Oral Sci 113: 525-530.

Camps J, Pashley DH (2000) Buffering action of human dentin in vitro. J Adhes Dent 2: 39-50.
Carrilho MR, Geraldeli S, Tay F, et al., Pashley D (2007) In vivo preservation of the hybrid layer by chlorhexi-dine. J Dent Res 86: 529-533.
Carrilho MR, Tay FR, Donnelly AM, et al., Pashley DH (2009) Host-derived loss of dentin matrix stiffness associated with solubilization of collagen. J Biomed Mater Res B Appl Biomater 90: 373-380.
Carvalho RM, Mendonca JS, Santiago SL, et al., Pashley DH (2003) Effects of HEMA/solvent combinations on bond strength to dentin. J Dent Res 82: 597-601.
Castellan CS, Pereira PN, Grande RH, Bedran-Russo AK (2010) Mechanical characterization of proanthocyanidin-dentin matrix interaction. Dent Mater 26: 968-973.
Castellan CS, Bedran-Russo AK, Karol S, Pereira PN (2011) Long-term stability of dentin matrix following treatment with various natural collagen cross-linkers. J Mech Behav Biomed Mater 4: 1343-1350.
Caughman WF, Chan DC, Rueggeberg FA (2001) Curing potential of dual-polymerizable resin cements in simulated clinical situations. J Prosthet Dent 86: 101-106.
Cecchin D, de Almeida JF, Gomes BP, et al., Ferraz CC (2011) Influence of chlorhexidine and ethanol on the bond strength and durability of the adhesion of the fiber posts to root dentin using a total etching adhesive system. J Endod 37: 1310-1315.
Chersoni S, Suppa P, Breschi L, et al., Prati C (2004) Water movement in the hybrid layer after different dentin treatments. Dent Mater 20: 796-803.
Cuadros-Sanchez J, Szesz A, Hass V, et al., Loguercio AD (2014) Effects of sonic application of adhesive systems on bonding fiber posts to root canals. J Endod 40: 1201-1205.
de Andrade e Silva SM, Carrilho MR, Marquezini Junior L, et al., de Carvalho RM (2009) Effect of an additional hydrophilic versus hydrophobic coat on the quality of dentinal sealing provided by two-step etch-and-rinse adhesives. J Appl Oral Sci 17: 184-189.
De Munck J, Van Meerbeek B, Yoshida Y, et al., Vanherle G (2003) Four-year water degradation of total-etch adhesives bonded to dentin. J Dent Res 82: 136-140.
De Munck J, Van den Steen PE, Mine A, et al., Van Meerbeek B (2009) Inhibition of enzymatic degradation of adhesive-dentin interfaces. J Dent Res 88: 1101-1106.
Dickinson DP (2002) Cysteine peptidases of mammals: their biological roles and potential effects in the oral cavity and other tissues in health and disease. Crit Rev Oral Biol Med 13: 238-275.
dos Santos Alves Morgan LF, Peixoto RT, de Castro Albuquerque R, Santos Correa MF, de Abreu Poletto LT, Pinotti MB (2008) Light transmission through a translucent fiber post. J Endod 34: 299-302.
Duan SS, Ouyang XB, Pei DD, et al., Huang C (2011) Effects of ethanol-wet bonding technique on root dentine adhesion. Chin J Dent Res 14: 105-111.
Ekambaram M, Yiu CK, Matinlinna JP, et al., King NM (2014) Effect of chlorhexidine and ethanol-wet bonding with a hydrophobic adhesive to intraradicular dentine. J Dent 42: 872-882.
Epasinghe DJ, Yiu CK, Burrow MF, Tay FR, King NM (2012) Effect of proanthocyanidin incorporation into dental adhesive resin on resin-dentine bond strength. J Dent 40: 173-180.
Faria e Silva AL, Arias VG, Soares LE, et al., Martins LR (2007) Influence of fiber-post translucency on the degree of conversion of a dual-cured resin cement. J Endod 33: 303-305.
Faria-e-Silva AL, Casselli DS, Lima GS, et al., Martins LR (2008) Kinetics of conversion of two dual-cured adhesive systems. J Endod 34: 1115-1118.
Ferracane JL (2006) Hygroscopic and hydrolytic effects in dental polymer networks. Dent Mater 22: 211-222.

Ferracane JL, Stansbury JW, Burke FJ (2011) Self-adhesive resin cements — chemistry, properties and clinical considerations. J Oral Rehabil 38: 295-314.

Ferrari M, Mannocci F, Vichi A, et al., Mjor IA (2000) Bonding to root canal: structural characteristics of the substrate. Am J Dent 13: 255-260.

Ferrari M, Coniglio I, Magni E, et al., Breschi L (2008) How can droplet formation occur in endodontically treated teeth during bonding procedures? J Adhes Dent 10: 211-218.

Foxton RM, Nakajima M, Tagami J, Miura H (2003) Bonding of photo and dual-cure adhesives to root canal dentin. Oper Dent 28: 543-551.

Garcia EJ, Reis A, Arana-Correa BE, et al., Loguercio AD (2010) Reducing the incompatibility between two-step adhesives and resin composite luting cements. J Adhes Dent 12: 373-379.

Garnero P, Ferreras M, Karsdal MA, et al., Delaisse JM (2003) The type I collagen fragments ICTP and CTX reveal distinct enzymatic pathways of bone collagen degradation. J Bone Miner Res 18: 859-867.

Gendron R, Grenier D, Sorsa T, Mayrand D (1999) Inhibition of the activities of matrix metallo-proteinases 2, 8, and 9 by chlorhexidine. Clin Diagn Lab Immunol 6: 437-439.

Gillam DG, Mordan NJ, Sinodinou AD, et al., Gibson IR (2001) The effects of oxalate-containing products on the exposed dentine surface: an SEM investigation. J Oral Rehabil 28: 1037-1044.

Gomes OMM, Gomes GM, Rezende EC, Ruiz LM, Gomes JC, Loguercio AD, Reis A (2012) Influence of the rotating device used for root canal preparation. J Dent Res 91: Abstract 1429.

Gomes BP, Vianna ME, Zaia AA, et al., Ferraz CC (2013) Chlorhexidine in endodontics. Braz Dent J 24: 89-102.

Goracci C, Ferrari M (2011) Current perspectives on post systems: a literature review. Aust Dent J 56(Suppl 1): 77-83.

Goracci C, Corciolani G, Vichi A, Ferrari M (2008) Light-transmitting ability of marketed fiber posts. J Dent Res 87: 1122-1126.

Green B, Yao X, Ganguly A, et al., Wang Y (2010) Grape seed proantho-cyanidins increase collagen biodegradation resistance in the dentin/adhesive interface when included in an adhesive. J Dent 38: 908-915.

Hashimoto M, Ohno H, Sano H, Kaga M, Oguchi H (2003) In vitro degradation of resin-dentin bonds analyzed by microtensile bond test, scanning and transmission electron microscopy. Biomaterials 24: 3795-3803.

Hashimoto M, De Munck J, Ito S, et al., Pashley DH (2004a) In vitro effect of nanoleakage expression on resin-dentin bond strengths analyzed by microtensile bond test, SEM/EDX and TEM. Biomaterials 25: 5565-5574.

Hashimoto M, Ito S, Tay FR, et al., Pashley DH (2004b) Fluid movement across the resin-dentin interface during and after bonding. J Dent Res 83: 843-848.

Hedlund SO, Johansson NG, Sjogren G (2003) Retention of prefabricated and individually cast root canal posts in vitro. Br Dent J 195: 155-158; discussion 147.

Hiraishi N, Yiu CK, King NM, Tay FR (2009) Effect of 2% chlorhexidine on dentin microtensile bond strengths and nanoleakage of luting cements. J Dent 37: 440-448.

Huang FM, Yang SF, Chang YC (2008) Up-regulation of gelatinases and tissue type plasminogen activator by root canal sealers in human osteoblastic cells. J Endod 34: 291-294.

Hulsmann M, Heckendorff M, Lennon A (2003) Chelating agents in root canal treatment: mode of action and indications for their use. Int Endod J 36: 810-830.

Ito S, Hashimoto M, Wadgaonkar B, Svizero N, Carvalho RM, Yiu C, Rueggeberg FA, Foulger S, Saito T, Nishitani Y, Yoshiyama M, Tay FR, Pashley DH (2005a) Effects of resin hydrophilicity on water sorption and changes in modulus of elasticity. Biomaterials 26:

6449-6459.
Ito S, Tay FR, Hashimoto M, Yoshiyama M, Saito T, Brackett WW, Waller JL, Pashley DH (2005b) Effects of multiple coatings of two all-in-one adhesives on dentin bonding. J Adhes Dent 7: 133-141.
Itoh T, Nakamura H, Kishi J, Hayakawa T (2009) The activation of matrix metalloproteinases by a whole-cell extract from Prevotella nigrescens. J Endod 35: 55-59.
Jacobsen T, Soderholm KJ (1998) Effect of primer solvent, primer agitation, and dentin dryness on shear bond strength to dentin. Am J Dent 11: 225-228.
Jacques P, Hebling J (2005) Effect of dentin conditioners on the microtensile bond strength of a conventional and a self-etching primer adhesive system. Dent Mater 21: 103-109.
Junge T, Nicholls JI, Phillips KM, Libman WJ (1998) Load fatigue of compromised teeth: a com- parison of 3 luting cements. Int J Prosthodont 11: 558-564.
Kalra M, Iqbal K, Nitisusanta LI, et al., Fawzy AS (2013) The effect of proanthocy-anidins on the bond strength and durability of resin sealer to root dentine. Int Endod J 46: 169-178.
Kanca J 3rd (1992) Improving bond strength through acid etching of dentin and bonding to wet dentin surfaces. J Am Dent Assoc 123: 35-43.
Kanca J 3rd (1996) Wet bonding: effect of drying time and distance. Am J Dent 9: 273-276.
King NM, Tay FR, Pashley DH, et al., Sunico M (2005) Conversion of one-step to two-step self-etch adhesives for improved efficacy and extended application. Am J Dent 18: 126-134.
Lee W, Aitken S, Sodek J, McCulloch CA (1995) Evidence of a direct relationship between neutrophil collagenase activity and periodontal tissue destruction in vivo: role of active enzyme in human periodontitis. J Periodontal Res 30: 23-33.
Leitune VC, Collares FM, Werner Samuel SM (2010) Influence of chlorhexidine application at longitudinal push-out bond strength of fiber posts. Oral Surg Oral Med Oral Pathol Oral Radiol Endod 110: e77-e81.
Leme AA, Coutinho M, Insaurralde AF, Scaffa PM, da Silva LM (2011) The influence of time and cement type on push-out bond strength of fiber posts to root dentin. Oper Dent 36: 643-648.
Lindblad RM, Lassila LV, Salo V, et al., Tjaderhane L (2010) Effect of chlorhexidine on initial adhesion of fiber-reinforced post to root canal. J Dent 38: 796-801.
Liu Y, Tjaderhane L, Breschi L, et al., Tay FR (2011) Limitations in bonding to dentin and experimental strategies to prevent bond degradation. J Dent Res 90: 953-968.
Liu Y, Chen M, Yao X, et al., Wang Y (2013) Enhancement in dentin collagen's biological stability after proanthocyanidins treatment in clinically relevant time periods. Dent Mater 29: 485-492.
Liu Y, Dusevich V, Wang Y (2014) Addition of grape seed extract renders phosphoric acid a collagen-stabilizing etchant. J Dent Res 93: 821-827.
Loguercio AD, Loeblein F, Cherobin T, et al., Reis A (2009) Effect of solvent removal on adhesive properties of simplified etch-and-rinse systems and on bond strengths to dry and wet dentin. J Adhes Dent 11: 213-219.
Lombardo GH, Souza RO, Michida SM, et al., Valandro LF (2008) Resin bonding to root canal dentin: effect of the application of an experimental hydrophobic resin coating after an all-in-one adhesive. J Contemp Dent Pract 9: 34-42.
Luhrs AK, De Munck J, Geurtsen W, Van Meerbeek B (2013) Does inhibition of proteolytic activity improve adhesive luting? Eur J Oral Sci 121: 121-131.
Malacarne J, Carvalho RM, de Goes MF, et al., Carrilho MR (2006) Water sorption/solubility of dental adhesive resins. Dent Mater 22: 973-980.
Malacarne-Zanon J, Pashley DH, Agee KA, et al., Carrilho MR (2009) Effects of ethanol addition on the water sorption/solubility and percent conversion of comonomers in model dental adhesives. Dent Mater 25: 1275-1284.

Malemud CJ (2006) Matrix metalloproteinases (MMPs) in health and disease: an overview. Front Biosci 11: 1696-1701.

Mannocci F, Innocenti M, Ferrari M, Watson TF (1999) Confocal and scanning electron micro-scopic study of teeth restored with fiber posts, metal posts, and composite resins. J Endod 25: 789-794.

Mannocci F, Bertelli E, Watson TF, Ford TP (2003) Resin-dentin interfaces of endodontically-treated restored teeth. Am J Dent 16: 28-32.

Mannocci F, Pilecki P, Bertelli E, Watson TF (2004) Density of dentinal tubules affects the tensile strength of root dentin. Dent Mater 20: 293-296.

Manso AP, Silva NR, Bonfante EA, et al., Carvalho RM (2011) Cements and adhesives for all-ceramic restorations. Dent Clin North Am 55: 311-332, ix.

Marchesi G, Mazzoni A, Turco G, et al., Breschi L (2013) Aging affects the adhesive interface of posts luted with self-adhesive cements: a 1-year study. J Adhes Dent 15: 173-180.

Mazzoni A, Pashley DH, Nishitani Y, et al., Tay FR (2006) Reactivation of inactivated endogenous proteolytic activities in phosphoric acid-etched dentine by etch-and-rinse adhesives. Biomaterials 27: 4470-4476.

Mazzoni A, Mannello F, Tay FR, et al., Breschi L (2007) Zymographic analysis and characterization of MMP-2 and -9 forms in human sound dentin. J Dent Res 86: 436-440.

Mazzoni A, Marchesi G, Cadenaro M, et al., Breschi L (2009a) Push-out stress for fibre posts luted using different adhesive strategies. Eur J Oral Sci 117: 447-453.

Mazzoni A, Pashley DH, Tay FR, et al., Breschi L (2009b) Immunohistochemical identification of MMP-2 and MMP-9 in human dentin: correlative FEI-SEM/TEM analysis. J Biomed Mater Res A 88: 697-703.

Michida SM, Souza RO, Bottino MA, Valandro LF (2010) Cementation of fiber post: influence of the cement insertion techniques on the bond strength of the fiber post-root dentin and the quality of the cement layer. Minerva Stomatol 59: 633-636.

Miguel-Almeida ME, Azevedo ML, Rached-Junior FA, et al., Messias DC (2012) Effect of light-activation with different light-curing units and time intervals on resin cement bond strength to intraradicular dentin. Braz Dent J 23: 362-366.

Mohammadi Z, Abbott PV (2009) Antimicrobial substantivity of root canal irrigants and medica-ments: a review. Aust Endod J 35: 131-139.

Monticelli F, Osorio R, Albaladejo A, et al., Toledano M (2006) Effects of adhesive systems and luting agents on bonding of fiber posts to root canal dentin. J Biomed Mater Res B Appl Biomater 77: 195-200.

Muniz L (2010) Reabilitação estética em dentes tratados endodonticamente. Santos, São Paulo, p. 296 [in Portuguese].

Nakabayashi N, Saimi Y (1996) Bonding to intact dentin. J Dent Res 75: 1706-1715.

Nascimento FD, Minciotti CL, Geraldeli S, Carrilho MR, Pashley DH, Tay FR, Nader HB, Salo T, Tjaderhane L, Tersariol IL (2011) Cysteine cathepsins in human carious dentin. J Dent Res 90: 506-511.

Osorio E, Toledano M, Aguilera FS, et al., Osorio R (2010) Ethanol wet-bonding technique sensitivity assessed by AFM. J Dent Res 89: 1264-1269.

Osorio R, Yamauti M, Osorio E, Roman JS, Toledano M (2011a) Zinc-doped dentin adhesive for collagen protection at the hybrid layer. Eur J Oral Sci 119: 401-410.

Osorio R, Yamauti M, Osorio E, et al., Toledano M (2011b) Effect of dentin etching and chlorhexidine application on metalloproteinase-mediated collagen degradation. Eur J Oral Sci 119: 79-85.

Pashley EL, Zhang Y, Lockwood PE, et al., Pashley DH (1998) Effects of HEMA on water evaporation from water-HEMA mixtures. Dent Mater 14: 6-10.

Pashley DH, Tay FR, Yiu C, et al., Ito S (2004) Collagen degradation by host-derived

enzymes during aging. J Dent Res 83: 216-221.
Paul SJ, Leach M, Rueggeberg FA, Pashley DH (1999) Effect of water content on the physical properties of model dentine primer and bonding resins. J Dent 27: 209-214.
Pegoraro TA, da Silva NR, Carvalho RM (2007) Cements for use in esthetic dentistry. Dent Clin North Am 51: 453-471, x.
Pei D, Huang X, Huang C, et al., Zhang J (2012) Ethanol-wet bonding may improve root dentine bonding performance of hydrophobic adhesive. J Dent 40: 433-441.
Pelegrine RA, De Martin AS, Cunha RS, et al., da Silveira Bueno CE (2010) Influence of chemical irrigants on the tensile bond strength of an adhesive system used to cement glass fiber posts to root dentin. Oral Surg Oral Med Oral Pathol Oral Radiol Endod 110: e73-e76.
Perdigao J, Reis A, Loguercio AD (2013) Dentin adhesion and MMPs: a comprehensive review. J Esthet Restor Dent 25: 219-241.
Pioch T, Staehle HJ, Duschner H, Garcia-Godoy F (2001) Nanoleakage at the composite-dentin interface: a review. Am J Dent 14: 252-258.
Radovic I, Monticelli F, Goracci C, et al., Ferrari M (2008) Self-adhesive resin cements: a literature review. J Adhes Dent 10: 251-258.
Rasimick BJ, Wan J, Musikant BL, Deutsch AS (2010) A review of failure modes in teeth restored with adhesively luted endodontic dowels. J Prosthodont 19: 639-646.
Reid LC, Kazemi RB, Meiers JC (2003) Effect of fatigue testing on core integrity and post micro-leakage of teeth restored with different post systems. J Endod 29: 125-131.
Reis A, Pellizzaro A, Dal-Bianco K, et al., Loguercio AD (2007a) Impact of adhesive application to wet and dry dentin on long-term resin-dentin bond strengths. Oper Dent 32: 380-387.
Reis AF, Giannini M, Pereira PN (2007b) Influence of water-storage time on the sorption and solu-bility behavior of current adhesives and primer/adhesive mixtures. Oper Dent 32: 53-59.
Reis A, Albuquerque M, Pegoraro M, et al., Loguercio AD (2008) Can the durability of one-step self-etch adhesives be improved by double application or by an extra layer of hydrophobic resin? J Dent 36: 309-315.
Reis A, Carrilho M, Breschi L, Loguercio AD (2013) Overview of clinical alternatives to minimize the degradation of the resin-dentin bonds. Oper Dent 38: E1-E25.
Reynolds JJ, Meikle MC (1997) The functional balance of metalloproteinases and inhibitors in tissue degradation: relevance to oral pathologies. J R Coll Surg Edinb 42: 154-160.
Roach RP, Hatton JF, Gillespie MJ (2001) Prevention of the ingress of a known virulent bacterium into the root canal system by intracanal medications. J Endod 27: 657-660.
Roberts HW, Leonard DL, Vandewalle KS, et al., Charlton DG (2004) The effect of a trans-lucent post on resin composite depth of cure. Dent Mater 20: 617-622.
Rosenthal S, Spangberg L, Safavi K (2004) Chlorhexidine substantivity in root canal dentin. Oral Surg Oral Med Oral Pathol Oral Radiol Endod 98: 488-492.
Sabatini C, Pashley DH (2015) Aging of adhesive interfaces treated with benzalkonium chloride and benzalkonium methacrylate. Eur J Oral Sci 123: 102-107.
Sabatini C, Patel SK (2013) Matrix metalloproteinase inhibitory properties of benzalkonium chlo-ride stabilizes adhesive interfaces. Eur J Oral Sci 121: 610-616.
Sabatini C, Ortiz PA, Pashley DH (2015) Preservation of resin-dentin interfaces treated with ben-zalkonium chloride adhesive blends. Eur J Oral Sci 123: 108-115.
Sadek FT, Pashley DH, Nishitani Y, et al., Tay FR (2008) Application of hydrophobic resin adhesives to acid-etched dentin with an alternative wet bonding technique. J Biomed Mater Res A 84: 19-29.
Salas MM, Bocangel JS, Henn S, et al., Demarco FF (2011) Can viscosity of acid etchant influence the adhesion of fibre posts to root canal dentine? Int Endod J 44: 1034-1040.

Sanares AM, Itthagarun A, King NM, et al., Pashley DH (2001) Adverse surface interactions between one-bottle light-cured adhesives and chemical-cured composites. Dent Mater 17: 542-556.

Sarkis-Onofre R, Skupien JA, Cenci MS, et al., Pereira-Cenci T (2014) The role of resin cement on bond strength of glass-fiber posts luted into root canals: a systematic review and meta-analysis of in vitro studies. Oper Dent 39: E31-E44.

Sauro S, Toledano M, Aguilera FS, Mannocci F, Pashley DH, Tay FR, Watson TF, Osorio R (2010) Resin-dentin bonds to EDTA-treated vs. acid-etched dentin using ethanol wet-bonding. Dent Mater 26: 368-379.

Scaffa PM, Vidal CM, Barros N, et al., Carrilho MR (2012) Chlorhexidine inhibits the activity of dental cysteine cathepsins. J Dent Res 91: 420-425.

Schwartz RS, Robbins JW (2004) Post placement and restoration of endodontically treated teeth: a literature review. J Endod 30: 289-301.

Scotti N, Scansetti M, Rota R, et al., Berutti E (2013) Active appli-cation of liquid etching agent improves adhesion of fibre posts to intraradicular dentine. Int Endod J 46: 1039-1045.

Serafino C, Gallina G, Cumbo E, Ferrari M (2004) Surface debris of canal walls after post space preparation in endodontically treated teeth: a scanning electron microscopic study. Oral Surg Oral Med Oral Pathol Oral Radiol Endod 97: 381-387.

Shono Y, Terashita M, Shimada J, et al., Pashley DH (1999) Durability of resin-dentin bonds. J Adhes Dent 1: 211-218.

Souza RO, Lombardo GH, Michida SM, et al., Valandro LF (2007) Influence of brush type as a carrier of adhesive solutions and paper points as an adhesive-excess remover on the resin bond to root dentin. J Adhes Dent 9: 521-526.

Spencer P, Swafford JR (1999) Unprotected protein at the dentin-adhesive interface. Quintessence Int 30: 501-507.

Spencer P, Wang Y, Katz JL (2004) Identification of collagen encapsulation at the dentin/adhesive interface. J Adhes Dent 6: 91-95.

Stanislawczuk R, Amaral RC, Zander-Grande C, et al., Loguercio AD (2009) Chlorhexidine-containing acid conditioner preserves the longevity of resin-dentin bonds. Oper Dent 34: 481-490.

Stanislawczuk R, Reis A, Loguercio AD (2011) A 2-year in vitro evaluation of a chlorhexidine-containing acid on the durability of resin-dentin interfaces. J Dent 39: 40-47.

Sulkala M, Larmas M, Sorsa T, et al., Tjaderhane L (2002) The localization of matrix metallo-proteinase-20 (MMP-20, enamelysin) in mature human teeth. J Dent Res 81: 603-607.

Sulkala M, Tervahartiala T, Sorsa T, et al., Tjaderhane L (2007) Matrix metalloprotein-ase-8 (MMP-8) is the major collagenase in human dentin. Arch Oral Biol 52: 121-127.

Tanaka J, Ishikawa K, Yatani H, et al., Suzuki K (1999) Correlation of dentin bond durability with water absorption of bonding layer. Dent Mater J 18: 11-18.

Tay FR, Pashley DH (2003) Water treeing-a potential mechanism for degradation of dentin adhe-sives. Am J Dent 16: 6-12.

Tay FR, King NM, Chan KM, Pashley DH (2002) How can nanoleakage occur in self-etching adhesive systems that demineralize and infiltrate simultaneously? J Adhes Dent 4: 255-269.

Tay FR, Pashley DH, Mak YF, et al., Suh BI (2003a) Integrating oxalate desensitizers with total-etch two-step adhesive. J Dent Res 82: 703-707.

Tay FR, Pashley DH, Yiu CK, Sanares AM, Wei SH (2003b) Factors contributing to the incompatibility between simplified-step adhesives and chemically-cured or dual-cured composites. Part I. Single-step self-etching adhesive. J Adhes Dent 5: 27-40.

Tay FR, Lai CN, Chersoni S, et al., King NM (2004) Osmotic blistering in enamel bonded with one-step self-etch adhesives. J Dent Res 83: 290-295.

Teixeira EC, Teixeira FB, Piasick JR, Thompson JY (2006) An in vitro assessment of prefabricated fiber post systems. J Am Dent Assoc 137: 1006–1012.

Teixeira CS, Silva-Sousa YT, Sousa-Neto MD (2009) Bond strength of fiber posts to weakened roots after resin restoration with different light-curing times. J Endod 35: 1034–1039.

Tersariol IL, Geraldeli S, Minciotti CL, et al., Tjaderhane L (2010) Cysteine cathepsins in human dentin-pulp complex. J Endod 36: 475–481.

Tezvergil-Mutluay A, Mutluay MM, Gu LS, et al., Pashley DH (2011) The anti-MMP activity of benzalkonium chloride. J Dent 39: 57–64.

Thitthaweerat S, Nakajima M, Foxton RM, Tagami J (2012) Effect of waiting interval on chemical activation mode of dual-cure one-step self-etching adhesives on bonding to root canal dentin. J Dent 40: 1109–1118.

Thitthaweerat S, Nakajima M, Foxton RM, Tagami J (2013) Effect of solvent evaporation strategies on regional bond strength of one-step self-etch adhesives to root canal dentine. Int Endod J 46: 1023–1031.

Thompson JM, Agee K, Sidow SJ, et al., Pashley DH (2012) Inhibition of endogenous dentin matrix metalloproteinases by ethylenediaminetetraacetic acid. J Endod 38: 62–65.

Tjaderhane L (2015) Dentin bonding: can we make it last? Oper Dent 40: 4–18.

Tjaderhane L, Larjava H, Sorsa T, et al., Salo T (1998) The activation and function of host matrix metalloproteinases in dentin matrix breakdown in caries lesions. J Dent Res 77: 1622–1629.

Tjaderhane L, Nascimento FD, Breschi L, et al., Pashley DH (2013a) Strategies to prevent hydrolytic degradation of the hybrid layer-a review. Dent Mater 29: 999–1011.

Tjaderhane L, Nascimento FD, Breschi L, et al., Pashley DH (2013b) Optimizing dentin bond durabil-ity: control of collagen degradation by matrix metalloproteinases and cysteine cathepsins. Dent Mater 29: 116–135.

Toman M, Toksavul S, Tamac E, et al., Karagozoglu I (2014) Effect of chlorhexidine on bond strength between glass-fiber post and root canal dentine after six month of water storage. Eur J Prosthodont Restor Dent 22: 29–34.

Torii Y, Hikasa R, Iwate S, et al., Yoshiyama M (2003) Effect of EDTA conditioning on bond strength to bovine dentin promoted by four current adhesives. Am J Dent 16: 395–400.

Turk B, Turk V, Turk D (1997) Structural and functional aspects of papain-like cysteine protein-ases and their protein inhibitors. Biol Chem 378: 141–150.

Vaidyanathan TK, Vaidyanathan J (2009) Recent advances in the theory and mechanism of adhe-sive resin bonding to dentin: a critical review. J Biomed Mater Res B Appl Biomater 88: 558–578.

Van Landuyt KL, Peumans M, De Munck J, et al., Van Meerbeek B (2006) Extension of a one-step self-etch adhesive into a multi-step adhesive. Dent Mater 22: 533–544.

Van Meerbeek B, De Munck J, Yoshida Y, et al., Vanherle G (2003) Buonocore memorial lecture. Adhesion to enamel and dentin: current status and future challenges. Oper Dent 28: 215–235.

van Strijp AJ, Jansen DC, DeGroot J, ten Cate JM, Everts V (2003) Host-derived proteinases and degradation of dentine collagen in situ. Caries Res 37: 58–65.

Vano M, Goracci C, Monticelli F, Tognini F, Gabriele M, Tay FR, Ferrari M (2006) The adhesion between fibre posts and composite resin cores: the evaluation of microtensile bond strength following various surface chemical treatments to posts. Int Endod J 39: 31–39.

Vichi A, Grandini S, Davidson CL, Ferrari M (2002) An SEM evaluation of several adhesive sys-tems used for bonding fiber posts under clinical conditions. Dent Mater 18: 495–502.

Wang Y, Spencer P (2002) Quantifying adhesive penetration in adhesive/dentin interface using confocal Raman microspectroscopy. J Biomed Mater Res 59: 46–55.

Watanabe I, Nakabayashi N, Pashley DH (1994) Bonding to ground dentin by a phenyl-P self-etching primer. J Dent Res 73: 1212-1220.

Wu H, Hayashi M, Okamura K, et al., Ebisu S (2009) Effects of light penetration and smear layer removal on adhesion of post-cores to root canal dentin by self-etching adhesives. Dent Mater 25: 1484-1492.

Ye Q, Spencer P, Wang Y, Misra A (2007) Relationship of solvent to the photopolymerization process, properties, and structure in model dentin adhesives. J Biomed Mater Res A 80: 342-350.

Yiu CK, King NM, Pashley DH, et al., Tay FR (2004) Effect of resin hydrophilicity and water storage on resin strength. Biomaterials 25: 5789-5796.

Yiu CK, King NM, Suh BI, et al., Tay FR (2005a) Incompatibility of oxalate desensitizers with acidic, fluoride-containing total-etch adhesives. J Dent Res 84: 730-735.

Yiu CK, Pashley EL, Hiraishi N, et al., Tay FR (2005b) Solvent and water retention in dental adhesive blends after evaporation. Biomaterials 26: 6863-6872.

Zhang W, Yang W, Wu S, et al., Li Y (2014) Effects of acid etching and adhesive treatments on host-derived cysteine cathepsin activity in dentin. J Adhes Dent 16: 415-420.

9 用于黏结纤维桩的黏固剂材料的选择

克斯廷·比特（Kerstin Bitter）

摘 要

如何实现根管系统内可靠而有效的黏结，这是一个具有重要意义的问题。目前对于根管内恰当的黏结策略的选择仍然是有争论的，大量的研究数据也显示出了有争议的结果。

在根管桩道制备后，牙本质壁上覆盖了厚厚的玷污层，其中包含了牙本质碎屑、残留的封闭剂和牙胶，这些都会影响根管牙本质的黏结，这也向我们强调了改建玷污层的重要性。从这方面来说，黏结策略的选择对纤维桩的黏结是至关重要的。因此，我们为读者呈现了针对不同种类的纤维桩黏结材料的研究，并对其中取得的数据加以分析。

此外，根管桩道制备后清理和冲洗的方法，以及它们对不同黏结策略的黏结强度的影响也是重要的临床问题，对于这些问题，我们也将从理论和实践的角度去进行总结。

9.1 简介

纤维桩的弹性模量接近牙本质，因而被认为具有良好的生物力学性能。研究显示，富含水分的牙本质，其弹性模量为 18～25 GPa（Kinney et al. 2003），主要取决于该部位的牙本质及其牙本质小管的数量和方向，这些都会造成均质性结构向异质性结构的转变（Bar-On Daniel Wagner 2012）。虽然黏结性的纤维桩可能不像牙本质那样复杂，然而比起那些更硬的材料，例如金属桩，其机械性能还是更接近于牙本质。因此，应用纤维桩可以降低治疗失败的风险(Fernandes et al. 2003)。但是，即使存在这种假设，最近的一项前瞻性的临床研究结果显示，在 7 年的观察期内，纤维桩和金属桩在成功率方面没有显著性差异(Sterzenbach et al. 2012a)。

纤维桩治疗失败的原因更多是由于桩钉的脱落和折断，而牙根折断导致的失败相对比较少见(Naumann et al. 2012)。因此，对于根管治疗后的患牙保留，纤维桩黏结的步骤是很重要的影响因素。由于根管内的高 C 因素(黏结面积/非黏结面积)，黏结变得十分复杂(Tay et al. 2005)。此外，根管内可见度差，根管牙本质不规则结构(继发性牙本质和牙骨质)的湿度难以控制，根尖部根管内壁的牙本质小管数量减少，这些因素都会阻碍根管内的黏结(Mjor et al. 2001)。另外，一些其他的因素，诸如桩道的清洁程度、根充封闭剂的选择、桩钉植入前的根管冲洗，以及桩钉与根管内壁的贴合程度，都会影响纤维桩在根管内的固位。这些内容将会在本章节加以详述。

9.2　影响纤维桩黏结强度和固位的因素

9.2.1　预备后桩道的清洁程度

来自不同研究的结果显示，桩道预备后的根管内残留的封闭剂和牙胶往往会阻碍纤维桩与根管内壁的黏结(Serafino et al. 2004；Perdigao et al. 2007a)。图 9-1 显示的是在体视显微镜下，桩道预备后不同根管的清洁程度。这 4 张图像分别显示了干净的桩道(图 9-1a)，桩道内有封闭剂残留(图 9-1b、c)，桩道内有封闭剂和牙胶残留(图 9-1d)。

有研究分析了诸如氧化铝颗粒喷砂或者黏有浮石的旋转毛刷等的一些清洁方法的清洁效率及其对纤维桩固位效果的影响(Bitter et al. 2012)。结果显示，没有证据证实应用这些机械方法能够明显提高根管内的清洁程度。究其原因，喷砂设备由于在口腔内入路的受限，因此妨碍其在根管内的清洁作用。不过，在扫描电镜下的确能观察到喷砂处理后根管内壁的牙本质表面出现的变化(图 9-2b)。此外，扫描电镜结果显示，封闭剂层位于根管内玷污层的最表层(图 9-2a)，说明黏结前的根管清洁对于取得最理想的根管内黏结至关重要。

9 用于黏结纤维桩的黏固剂材料的选择

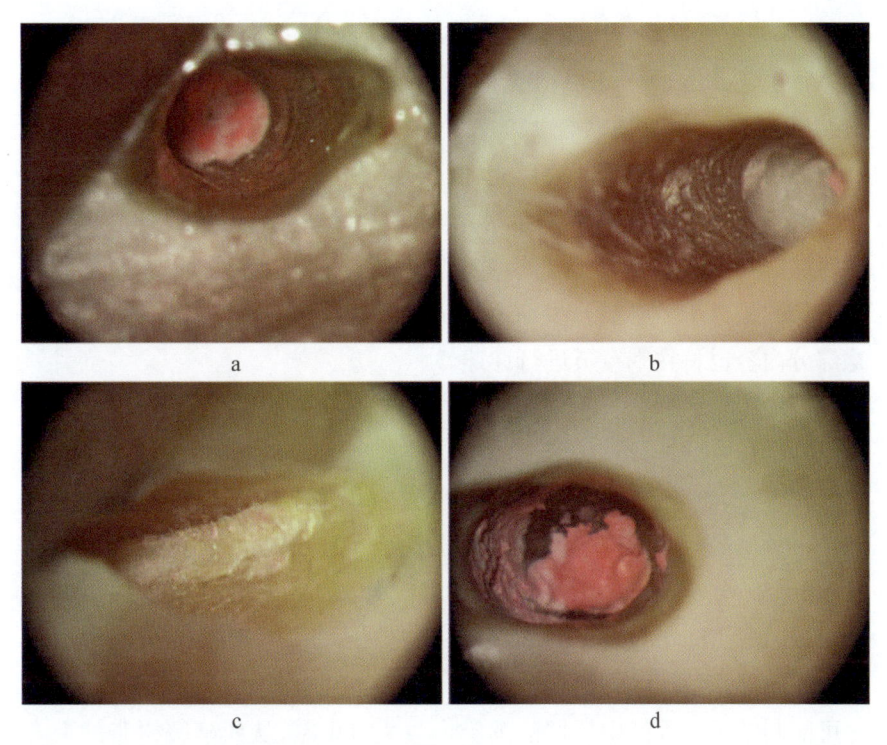

图 9-1 a.桩道预备及根管冲洗后干净的桩道；b.小块残留物；c.大块封闭剂残留物；d.暴露的大块封闭剂和牙胶残留物。

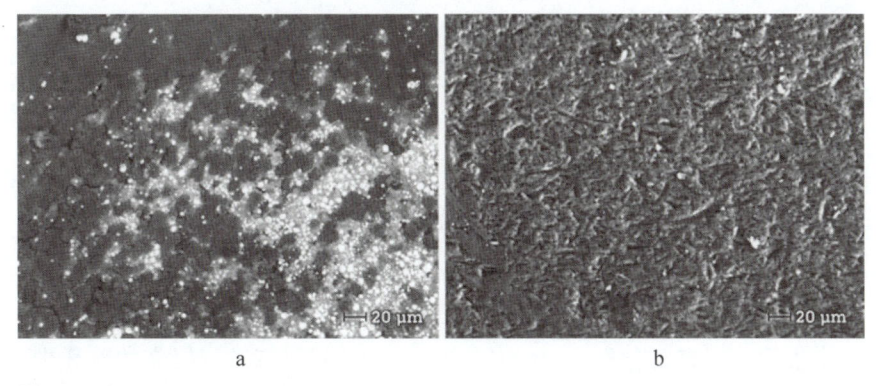

图 9-2 a.根管内牙本质的 SEM 显示，玷污层表面的封闭剂覆盖了牙本质小管开口；b.SEM 显示喷砂后的沟槽状结构。

同一项研究的结果还显示（Bitter et al. 2012），使用黏有浮石的旋转毛刷进行根管内清洁，会使得纤维桩的固位力显著降低；因此，不推荐这种不配合进一步冲洗操作的清洁措施（Bitter et al. 2012）。在另一项研究中,声波根管刷联合应用17%的EDTA可以有效地清除根管内壁附着的玷污层(Salman et al. 2010)。该结果得到了一项体外研究的支持,实验结果显示,在根管内联合17%EDTA的超声冲洗,能获得令人满意的清理效果和牙本质小管开放程度(Coniglio et al. 2008)。

在根管充填和桩道预备后,根管内壁上总是被残留的牙胶、封闭剂、玷污层以及牙本质碎屑所覆盖。因此,对根管内进行清洁,以获得更为清晰可见的桩道十分必要。手用器械机械清洁应该与冲洗操作联合应用,这部分内容也将在本章节进行详述。

9.2.2 根管充填的封闭剂的选择

图9-1显示的是残留的封闭剂,这有可能会阻碍根管内桩钉的黏结。大量体外实验研究比较了不同根管封闭剂对桩钉固位力的影响(Demiryurek et al. 2010；Aleisa et al. 2012；Vano et al. 2012；AlEisa et al. 2013；Mesquita et al. 2013)。其中一项研究发现,相较于环氧树脂类的封闭剂,丁香油类的封闭剂会降低纤维桩与黏结树脂之间的固位力,这可能归结于丁香油中残留的酚类会收集自由基,从而延缓树脂的聚合作用(Mayer et al. 1997)。然而,另一些研究则认为,封闭剂的化学结构并不会影响纤维桩与黏结树脂之间的固位力(Hagge et al. 2002；Kurtz et al. 2003),也不会影响碳素纤维桩的黏结界面(Mannocci et al. 2001)。尽管如此,在未进行根管充填的对照组中,纤维桩的固位力显示出了明显的增高,这说明残余的封闭剂很可能会阻碍根管内的黏结效果(Boone et al. 2001；Hagge et al. 2002)。

另一个因素是含有丁香油成分的材料的留置时间,这些材料在被去除之前会持续与根管壁牙本质接触;而长期的接触会降低黏结力(Hagge et al. 2002)。鉴于此原因,在根管充填后,应该立即将丁香油类的封闭剂完全去除。还有研究显示,在使用含丁香油的封闭剂进行根充的患牙中,如果将桩道预备的时间推迟至24个小时甚至是更长的7天后,纤维桩能获得的黏结强度要远高于根充后即刻预备组(Vano et al. 2012)。这种差异并未出现在应用环氧树脂类封闭剂进行根管充填的患牙(Vano et al. 2012)。作者推测,封闭剂固化完全后再行桩道预备,会使其造成的根管内"污染"降至最低。在所有的参考文献中,除了用管道水冲洗外,都没有提到其他冲洗策略；因此，鉴于最终冲洗能提高桩道的清洁程度，它也应该能减少根管内不同种类封闭剂对黏结效果的影响。

综上所述，尽管文献中表明了丁香油类的封闭剂存在阻碍黏结的可能，但封闭剂的种类对根管内的黏结强度和固位力的影响仍存在争议。已有报道称，这一问题可通过根管内壁的彻底清洁来解决（Schwartz and Robbins 2004）；而且，保证根管内壁不被任何种类的封闭剂"污染"也有助于整个黏结操作。

9.2.3 桩道预备后的最终冲洗

玷污层是在桩道预备过程中形成的，由残留在根管内的牙本质碎屑、牙胶和封闭剂组成。而且，玷污层会因为车针钻磨所导致的摩擦产热而被压紧（Khalighinejad et al. 2014）。除了前文所述的机械清理手段以外，很多化学制剂，如次氯酸钠（NaOCl）、乙二胺四乙酸（EDTA）、氯己定、乙醇以及它们的混合物，亦有一些研究比较了它们去除玷污层的能力，但同时也评价了其对纤维桩黏结强度的影响（Carvalho et al. 2009；Lindblad et al. 2010.2012；Cecchin et al. 2011；Bitter et al. 2014a；Khalighinejad et al. 2014）。次氯酸钠和EDTA是被广泛认可和使用的根管冲洗剂，长期而高浓度的应用可能会导致根管牙本质的机械性能的下降，比如挠曲强度、弹性模量和微硬度的降低（Tang et al. 2010）。这些牙本质结构上的变化会影响其本身与黏结剂的黏结强度（Dogan Buzoglu et al. 2007）。因此，桩道预备后的冲洗及其对不同黏结策略的黏结力的影响是值得探讨的问题，尤其是目前不同厂商对于应用次氯酸钠的看法相左，有些建议应用，有些则完全不建议。出于这种考虑，有学者设计了体外实验，桩道预备后分别用5种不同冲洗方法进行处理，而纤维桩与根管内壁牙本质之间采取了3种不同的黏结策略，以此来研究不同冲洗方法对黏结强度的影响（Bitter et al. 2013）。研究中以蒸馏水冲洗作为对照组，实验组则包括1%和5.25%浓度次氯酸钠的超声冲洗以及18%EDTA分别联合5.25%次氯酸钠及2%氯己定的冲洗。纤维桩的黏结采取3种不同的黏结策略，分别是自酸蚀-黏结系统、酸蚀-冲洗-黏结系统，以及自黏结树脂水门汀系统。冲洗系统对黏结强度的影响会因为黏结策略的不同而改变。对酸蚀-冲洗-黏结系统来说，相较于对照组，联合应用

EDTA 和 5.25%次氯酸钠的冲洗方法会造成数值上明显低于平均黏结强度，而应用 1%次氯酸钠的超声冲洗则获得了最高的黏结强度。这些结果来源于对黏结界面的分析，采用激光共聚焦显微镜（CLSM），在双重荧光模式下可以显示黏结剂渗透入高度脱矿的根管牙本质内的深度情况（图 9-3a-c）。虽然 18%EDTA 联合 5.25%次氯酸钠的应用能在玷污层去除方面达到令人满意的效果，但是其在导致深层牙本质的化学结构的变化方面，尤其是在联合应用磷酸的情况下，牙本质会出现过度脱矿，反而造成黏结效果不够理想。因此，该冲洗方法不能用于酸蚀-冲洗-黏结系统中。

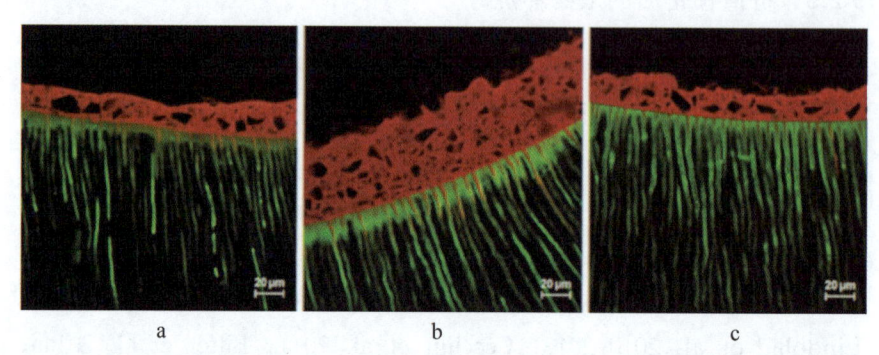

图 9-3　a. 用 NaCl 冲洗桩道后；b. 用 18%EDTA 和 5.25%NaOCl 冲洗桩道后；c. 用 1%NaOCl 冲洗桩道后。应用酸蚀-冲洗-黏结系统 XPBond 联合 Core X Flow 流体树脂（DENTSPLY DeTrey）在 CLSM 下形成的显微影像。和对照组 a 相比较，b 显示，红色标记的树脂渗入牙本质小管，而在绿色标记的黏结剂层形成了漏斗状的树脂突，这种情况明显增多。c 显示，形成了混合层，树脂材料渗入牙本质小管形成连续的树脂突。

在研究的自酸蚀-黏结系统中，不同的冲洗方法并未造成数值上的明显差异，这一结果也得到了其他研究的支持（Zhang et al. 2008；Fawzi et al. 2010）。该结果同样也来源于 CLSM 显示下的玷污层的有效去除和黏结剂渗透深度的分析（图 9-4a-c）；然而，这些并不能增强黏结效果。

对于自黏结树脂水门汀，相较于对照组，联合应用 18%EDTA 和 5.25%次氯酸钠去除玷污层会显著提高黏结强度（Bitter et al. 2013）。在 CLSM 上可看到（图 9-5a-c），黏结树脂渗透入牙本质小管内的深度明显增加。因此，不同的黏结策略需要特定的冲洗方法相匹配；然而，在每一分组中 1%次氯酸钠的超声冲洗总是能获得较好的黏结效果。因此，不管选用哪种黏结策略，均推荐 1%次氯酸钠的超声冲洗应用于桩道预备后的玷污层去除。

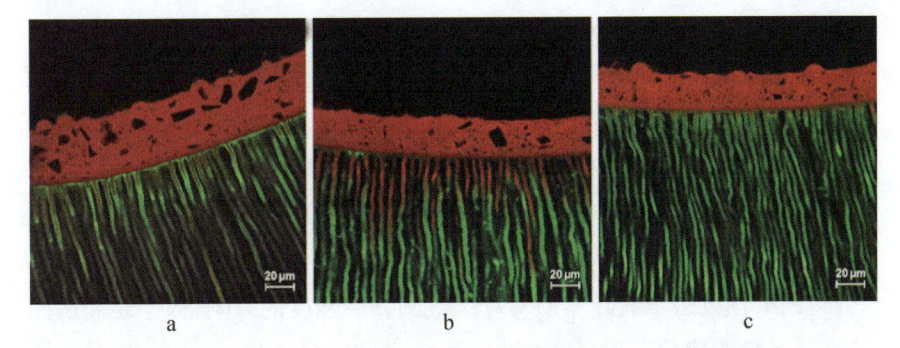

图 9-4 自酸蚀-黏结系统 AdheSE DC(绿色标记),联合 Multicore Flow 流体树脂(红色标记)(Ivoclar Vivodent)应用的图像,在所有分组中都观察到了薄而连续的混合层形成
a. 对照组;b. 用 18%EDTA 和 5.25%NaOCl 冲洗桩道去除玷污层后,树脂渗入牙本质小管的量显著增加;c. 用 1%NaOCl 冲洗桩道后,树脂更容易渗入牙本质小管。

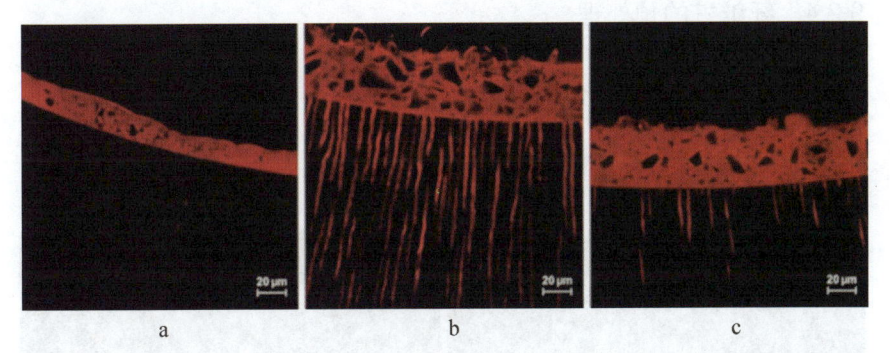

图 9-5 自黏结树脂水门汀 SmartCem2(DENTSPLY DeTrey)的 CLSM 图像
a. 对照组,没有树脂突形成;b. 用 18%EDTA 和 5.25%NaOCl 冲洗桩道后,树脂渗入牙本质小管增多;c. 用 1%NaOCl 冲洗后,树脂突形成相对 b 组较少。

包括黏结强度测试在内,对于牙髓治疗后的纤维桩修复的寿命,根管黏结的耐久性也是很重要的一个因素,该部分内容已经在第 8 章详述了。对于防止树脂-牙本质黏结剂的降解,一个策略是先在已脱矿的胶原蛋白基质上应用金属基质蛋白酶(MMP)的抑制剂,在进行牙本质黏结,详细内容可参见第 8 章。对于最终冲洗而言,氯己定作为非特异性的 MMP 抑制剂在黏结前使用,在黏结即刻和长期观察中都对桩钉的黏结强度没有不良影响(Lindblad et al. 2010, 2012;Cecchin et al. 2011)。然而,另有研究发现,氯己定冲洗后经温度循环处理和储存的样本,其根管牙本质与桩钉的黏结强度有明显的降低;同样的结果也出现在用热机械负荷处理的实验组中(Cecchin et al. 2014)。

之前在第 8 章阐述的乙醇湿黏结技术的简化流程，是在黏结前用 99% 的乙醇处理根管。无论是酸蚀-冲洗-黏结系统，还是自黏结树脂水门汀系统，这种处理都可以有效地防止热机械负荷(Cecchin et al. 2014)和温度循环实验下根中及根尖段的黏结强度的下降(Bitter et al. 2014a)。对此，研究者提出了假设，他们认为根管系统深处的湿度控制不足，可以通过应用乙醇置换水分，从而使得胶原蛋白基质获得疏水性来补偿这一点。然而，乙醇预处理根管牙本质对纤维桩的黏结强度的影响，似乎还和所用的黏结系统的成分有关(Carvalho et al. 2009；Cecchin et al. 2011)。因此，虽然从现有的结果来看，乙醇预处理根管牙本质是有前途的，但距离能够纳入临床治疗指南，尚需更多的研究来支持。

9.2.4 纤维桩的预处理

图 9-6 显示的是扫描电镜(SEM)下，黏结性纤维桩失败的两种情况，即根管牙本质与黏结剂界面的黏结失败(a)，以及纤维桩与黏结剂界面的黏结失败(b)。

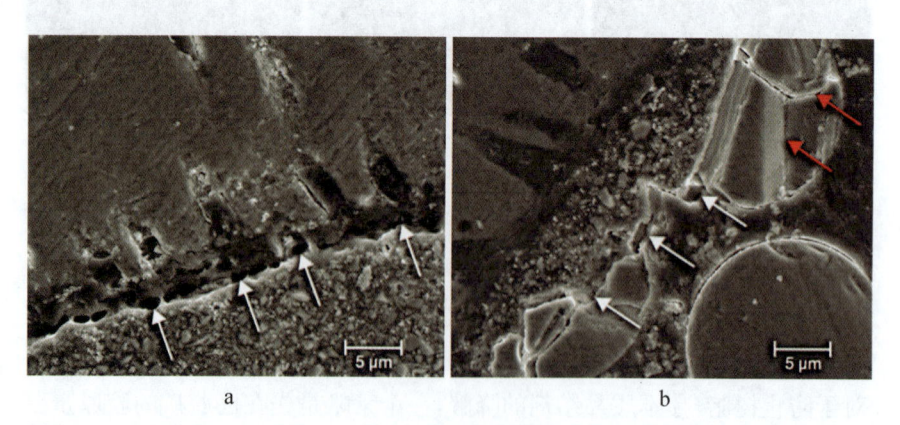

图 9-6　a. 根管牙本质与黏结水门汀之间的黏结失败的 SEM 图像(箭头所示)；b. 纤维桩与黏结水门汀之间的黏结失败的 SEM 图像(白箭头所示)；可见纤维桩结构破坏(红箭头所示)。

因此，桩钉表面与根管内壁牙本质表面的可靠黏结，是建立持久耐用的牙髓治疗后修复体的必要因素。尽管有研究表明，更多的黏结失败出现在根管内壁牙本质与黏结剂之间的界面上(Rasmick et al. 2010)，学者们还是提出了多种纤维桩的预处理流程，来提高其与黏结剂界面的黏结强度。

现有的纤维桩都是由单向纤维(玻璃或者石英)包埋在树脂基质内形

成的。厂商所用的树脂基质也不尽相同,包括了环氧树脂,甲基丙烯酸树脂,或者专用树脂(Zicari et al. 2012a)。不同的玻璃纤维桩在挠曲性能和微观形态学上各不相同,挠曲性能可能与树脂基质的机械性能、纤维和树脂基质的界面结合相关(Zicari et al. 2013)。而且,在微观形态学、表面结构和组成成分上的差异,也会影响预处理流程对纤维桩黏结强度的作用。为了提高桩钉与黏结剂的黏结强度,学者们针对纤维桩的化学及微机械预处理流程进行了研究。目前对桩钉表面进行微机械预处理的最常用的方法主要是喷砂和Cojet系统(3M ESPE公司)。喷砂处理的目的是为了去除树脂表层,将深层的玻璃纤维暴露,以求得可能的化学反应。另外,也可以使得表面粗糙。文献中的数据显示,喷砂处理能够提高纤维桩的黏结力(Balbosh 和 Kern 2006);另一些研究则认为,不管是不是使用硅烷偶联,喷砂处理对于纤维桩的黏结强度的作用依赖于桩的类型和黏结剂(Magni et al. 2007;Radovic et al. 2007)。而且,还有研究指出,喷砂处理会造成桩表面的不良改变,使得树脂基质和纤维之间的界面受到破坏,这都会导致纤维桩在加载负荷后的表面断裂(Soares et al. 2008)。因此,喷砂处理对于纤维桩长期稳定性的弱化作用不能排除。Cojet系统则是利用覆硅的氧化铝颗粒,对纤维桩表面进行摩擦化学包被,使其硅烷化(Zicari et al. 2012a)。同样,这一技术也存在着争议(Bitter et al. 2006;Zicari et al. 2012a),而且纤维桩的类型和黏结剂的种类也对其有很大影响,对纤维桩体的损害也能被观察到(图9-7a、b)。

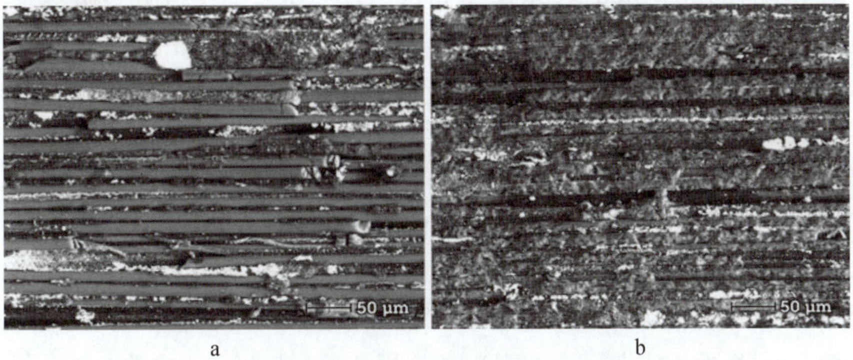

图9-7 二甲基丙烯酸酯基质的纤维桩(FRC Postec, Ivoclar Vivadent)的表面
a. 未处理;b. Cojet系统(3M ESPE)处理后。可见纤维桩表面有破坏。

在临床操作中,桩表面的硅烷偶联是最常用的化学预处理手段。然而,这一方法也出现了矛盾的结果(Goracci et al. 2005；Perdigao et al. 2006；Bitter et al. 2007；Zicari et al. 2012a)。硅烷化预处理的主要作用是提高表面的可湿性,在树脂及黏结剂的填料颗粒和纤维之间建立交联结构(Zicari et al. 2012a)。

这种预处理方法似乎高度依赖于纤维桩表面的成分及微观形态学特征(也即是在桩表面暴露的纤维和填料颗粒),同时也有赖于黏结树脂的组成成分。此外,有学者推断,材料之间正常的相互反应受到了水解弱化的阻碍,这种现象也随之影响了黏结树脂和硅烷化的桩钉之间产生的界面(Machado et al. 2015)。疏水性的树脂黏结剂应用在硅烷预处理的桩钉上会弱化水解作用,从而增强纤维桩的固位力(Machado et al. 2015)。

进一步的联合应用化学和微机械预处理手段,包括硅烷偶联前的氢氟酸处理(Monticelli et al. 2008a；Schmage et al. 2009a),可使得黏结剂依赖的纤维桩黏结强度提升。然而,已证实氢氟酸对桩表面的作用是时间依赖的,并且受到桩组成成分(树脂基质和纤维的种类)的影响。至于氢氟酸的应用时间,有报道称这项技术会对玻璃纤维造成实质性的损伤,从而影响桩钉的完整性(Valandro et al. 2006)。

其他的纤维桩预处理方法,例如过氧化氢浸泡(Vano et al. 2006),或者乙醇钠的应用(Monticelli et al. 2006a),都是通过溶解桩表面的环氧树脂或甲基丙烯酸树脂基质,使得纤维无损伤的暴露,从而达到提升黏结强度的目的。用10%过氧化氢侵蚀桩表面20分钟,能增加黏结剂和纤维桩之间的黏结强度(Monticelli et al. 2006b);但这似乎并不适用于临床。

近来,有报道称,发现了表面聚多巴胺的功能化能够在不破坏纤维桩表面的前提下,提高黏结剂与纤维桩之间的黏结力(Chen et al. 2014)。有必要进行更进一步的研究来评估这种表面改性是否也能对黏结的长期稳定起作用。

为了简化治疗流程,市场上常见的商品化的桩表面往往会预先被覆材料(图9-8)。有些桩用氢氟酸酸蚀,并用气化的二氧化硅颗粒被覆,浸泡的方式硅烷化,随后用可渗透入桩钉表面的 MMA 包被;有些则是用摩擦化学结合的方式进行硅烷偶联,随后用 25 μm 厚度的聚合物包被。仅有少数的研究比较了预被覆桩和普通桩在黏结强度方面的差异,发现差

9 用于黏结纤维桩的黏固剂材料的选择

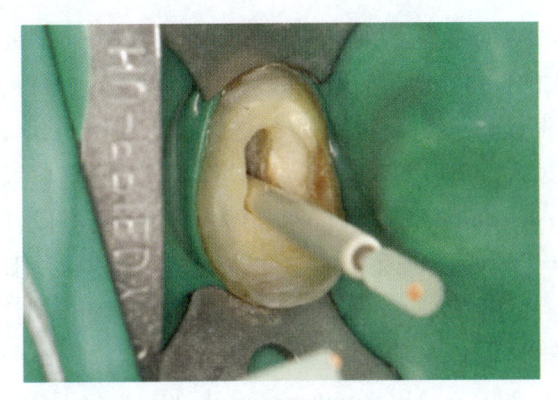

图9-8 临床上预包被纤维桩(Komet)试尖

别并不明显。对自黏结树脂水门汀 RelyX Unicem 而言,预被覆桩并不能提升黏结强度(Mazzitelli et al. 2012a;Schmage et al. 2012)。

需要注意的是,虽然有大量的关于纤维桩的预处理手段的研究,但在临床上其实更多见的治疗失败是发生在牙本质和黏结剂之间的界面上(Rasimick et al. 2010)。尽管如此,桩钉和黏结剂之间的理想黏结还是应该达到的。遗憾的是,由于桩表面的微观形态学和使用的黏结树脂基质的不同,导致不同预处理技术对黏结强度的影响也不同,因此很难取得通用的指导意见。一些侵入性的预处理技术,例如喷砂、Cojet 系统和氢氟酸处理可能会损伤桩钉,从而破坏桩钉的完整性,应尽可能避免。提高桩表面的可湿性,加强黏结树脂和纤维桩树脂基质的相容性是获得理想纤维桩黏结强度的重要手段。

9.2.5 桩的贴合度及树脂水门汀层的厚度

当氧化锌类的非黏结性水门汀用于根管桩的黏固时,桩钉与根管壁最大程度的贴合对提高桩钉固位性和抗折性是十分必要的(Sorensen 和 Engelman 1990)。而对于黏结性的纤维桩来说,形态完全与根管壁相贴合则并非必要(Perdigao et al. 2007a;Krastl et al. 2011);而且,对于一个横截面非圆形的根管而言,除非进行了"侵入性"的桩道预备,否则也很难获得均一的水门汀层厚度。而这种侵入恰恰是应该避免的,因为这会使得天然根管的牙本质基质缺失,根管立体形态也被破坏,而这些因素对维持牙齿的硬度至关重要(Lang et al. 2006)。根管毗邻的管内牙本质对维持牙齿的抗折性起了主要的作用，因此，要尽可能保留结构健康的管内牙本质(Kishen et al. 2004)。

直径较大的桩钉能够相应承担更大的咀嚼压力。较细的桩钉则容易折断，特别是根管和桩钉的直径不一致的时候(Lazari et al. 2013)。另一方面，将桩钉插入桩道后，伴随着黏结强度的显著下降，C因素也会出现明显的升高(Aksornmuang et al. 2011)。就树脂水门汀层厚度而言，厚者相较薄者产生较低的C因素，但这一差别并不大，厚度差距在100 μm，收缩仅有细微的变化(Alster et al. 1992)。因此，树脂水门汀厚度的小变化并不会对纤维桩抵抗脱出的黏结力产生影响(Perez et al. 2006；Perdigao et al. 2007a；Aksornmuang et al. 2011)，也不会对抗折性能产生显著影响(Buettel et al. 2009)，这些研究提示，黏结性纤维桩对根管的完美贴合并非必须。一项最近的有限元分析显示，越薄的水门汀层，受到的应力集中越强(Lazari et al. 2013)。但也有研究发现，树脂水门汀层的厚度并不会对其表面受到的应力集中产生影响(Spazzin et al. 2009)。而弹性模量比水门汀层厚度对应力集中的作用更大。还有研究者发现，过大的桩道预备会导致过小的脱出力(Egilmez et al. 2013；D'Arcangelo et al. 2007；Schmage et al. 2009b)。尽管如此，对黏结强度的作用，还会受树脂黏结剂的种类和如何定义"过大"的桩道预备影响。

综上所述，牙本质基质的缺失和立体形态的改变很可能会影响根管治疗后的牙齿的抗折性，应当尽可能避免"侵入性"的桩道预备。另外，在日常临床工作中，为了方便纤维桩的插入而进行的额外的桩道预备也需要重新考虑，而且形态上纤维桩的要求首先是与冠方修复体相匹配以求得固位力，其次桩道也需要制备得稍许宽大以利于桩钉的插入。完美与根管贴合的桩钉，虽然可使得水门汀层的厚度最薄，但并非必要。此外，也并不强求在每一个临床病例都进行常规的桩道预备，也可以有一些替代的桩道预备方法，比如应用超声工作尖(Rengo et al. 2014)或者圆钻(Bitter et al. 2012)，当然，选择贴合现有根管的桩钉也可以纳入考虑范围。

9.3 纤维桩黏结的黏结剂和系统

9.3.1 针对根管内黏结系统的选择：酸蚀-冲洗 vs 自酸蚀

除了上述影响根管内纤维桩黏结强度的因素，还有一些影响黏结的因素需要进行考虑,这些因素包括牙本质的脱水程度、根管内的湿度控制困难和视野受限等(Zicari et al. 2008)。根管内牙本质的黏结与冠部牙本质的黏结流程上大致接近,但黏结强度会普遍降低。"多步骤"的树脂基质的水门汀常采用的是"酸蚀-冲洗"和"自酸蚀"策略(Zicari et al. 2012b)。相对于手用器械,使用诸如桩道钻之类的机动器械预备的根管内会产生更厚的玷污层(Czonstkowsky et al. 1990)。基于根管内的黏结界面的形态学分析指出,磷酸由于其能有效去除厚而致密的玷污层,在根管内可能更有优势(Bitter et al. 2004)。当然,"自酸蚀"通常宣称比"酸蚀-冲洗"更为方便,技术敏感性也更低(Van Meerbeek et al. 2011)。由于根管内的复杂环境,这些因素可能更有作用,尤其是在湿度控制的方面。有研究者对两种策略加以双重聚合的手段进行根管内黏结,采用CLSM进行黏结界面的形态学分析(Bitter et al. 2014b)。正如预期,黏结界面的分析显示,"酸蚀-冲洗"黏结系统产生的混合层要厚于"自酸蚀"黏结系统(Bitter et al. 2014b)(图9-9a、b)。然而,自酸蚀黏结系统中也能观察到连续的薄层混合层和连接紧密的界面,显示使用自酸蚀黏结系统也能产生有效的玷污层改性。这些黏结系统中均含有共引发剂,例如苯亚磺酸钠。引发剂-催化剂系统会启动与之配套的双固化树脂基质黏结剂的黏结作用,并加速其聚合(Arrais et al. 2009)。因此,理论上不同类纤维桩内的光传导差异并不会影响不同黏结系统的黏结效果。

  关于这两种黏结策略在根管内的黏结效果,不同的研究显示出不同的结果。其中的两项研究认为上述两种黏结策略没有显著差异(Mazzoni et al. 2009;Bitter et al. 2014b),而一些研究则报道了"酸蚀-冲洗"系统的黏结强度低于"自酸蚀"系统(Zicari et al. 2008;Bitter et al. 2009a)。还有一些研究却得到了相反的结果,认为"自酸蚀"系统的黏结强度要低于"酸蚀-冲洗"或"自黏结"系统(Radovic et al. 2008)。这些争论提示,相较于黏结策略,根管内的黏结强度似乎更依赖于材料本身的性质。最新的一篇关于根管内黏结强度的综述提及,应用常规的树脂水门汀,无论采用哪种黏结策略,在黏结强度的数值上均没有明显差异(Sarkis-Onofre et al. 2013)。其他的一些相似研究则给出了许多不同的结论。

  黏结剂和牙本质之间的化学反应也许会进一步影响根管内的黏结效果和封闭性能(Van Meerbeek et al. 2011),而下方未被包裹进混合层的区

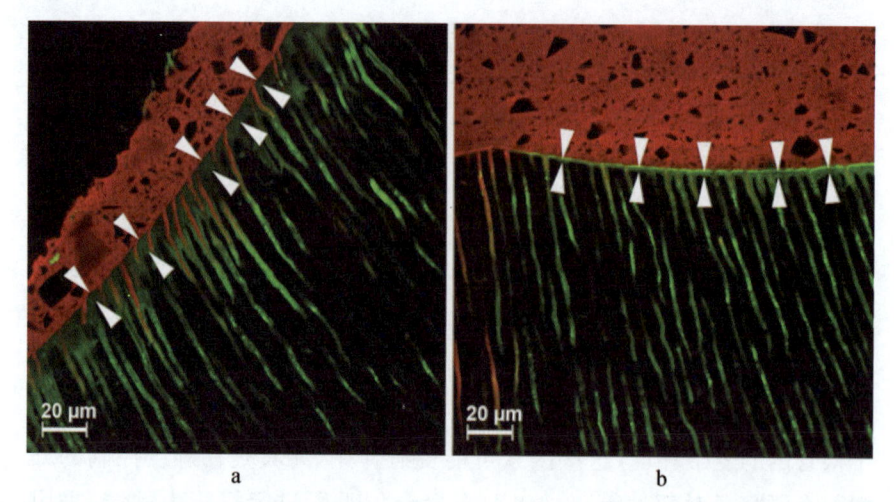

图9-9 在 CLSM 图像上测量形成混合层的厚度(箭头所示)
a. 酸蚀-冲洗-黏结系统 XP Bond 联合 Core X Flow 流体树脂(DENTSPLY DeTrey)处理组；b. 自酸蚀黏结系统 Futurabond DC 联合 Rebilda DC(VOCO GmbH)处理组。

域则可能会影响黏结的远期效果(Pashley et al. 2011)，类似的因素还包括聚合收缩的程度及产生的应力(Zicari et al. 2008)。这些因素很大程度依赖于所使用的材料本身，再一次证实材料本身的影响强于黏结方法的影响。

9.3.2 自黏结树脂水门汀对纤维桩的黏结效果

自黏结树脂水门汀是用来黏结牙齿基质的，在设计上摒弃了单独使用的黏结剂和酸蚀剂。可分为两种：一种由甲基丙烯酸酯单体组成，另一种由酸官能化的甲基丙烯酸酯单体组成。酸官能化的单体主要包含碳酸或者磷酸基团，行使牙齿基质脱矿和促进矿物盐(主要是钙盐)稳定形成的功能(Ferracane et al. 2011)，这在第8章中已做了详细阐述。这种简化的黏结方法技术敏感度低，对于根管这种黏结难度很大的部位似乎有着令人满意的效果(Zicari et al. 2012b)。首款商业化的自黏结树脂水门汀是 RelyX Unicem(3M ESPE 公司)。因此，绝大多数的文献中都选择了这款产品用于纤维桩黏结强度研究(Sarkis-Onofre et al. 2013)。在磷酸化甲基丙烯酸酯、填料和羟磷灰石进行中和反应时会产生水，而制造商宣称该产品有高度抗潮性(Zicari et al. 2012b)。关于玷污层去除和树脂突形成方面的相互关系，有实验进行了研究(Al-Assaf et al. 2007)，并有图像为证(图9-10、图9-11)(Bitter et al. 2009b)。

9　用于黏结纤维桩的黏固剂材料的选择　　199

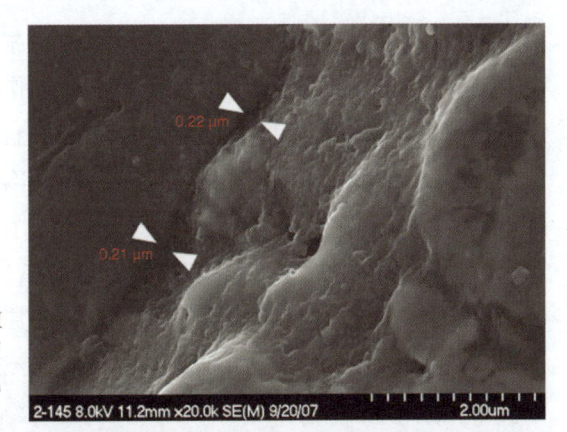

图 9-10　Rely-X Unicem(3M ESPE)和根管牙本质黏结界面的 SEM 图像。箭头所示，形成了 0.2 μm 厚的菲薄混合层。

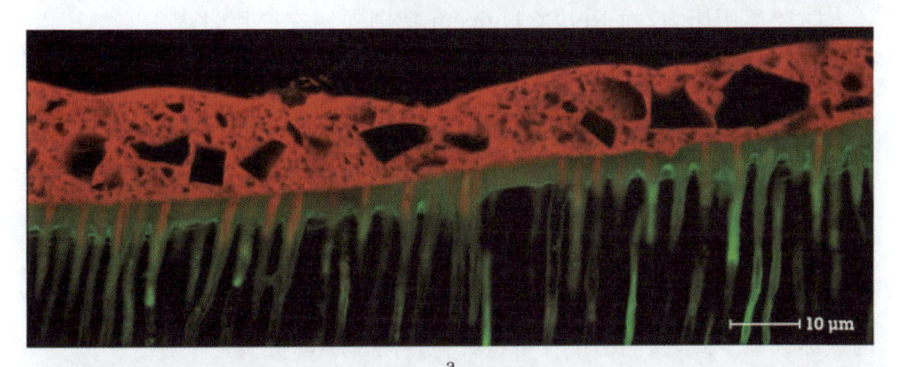

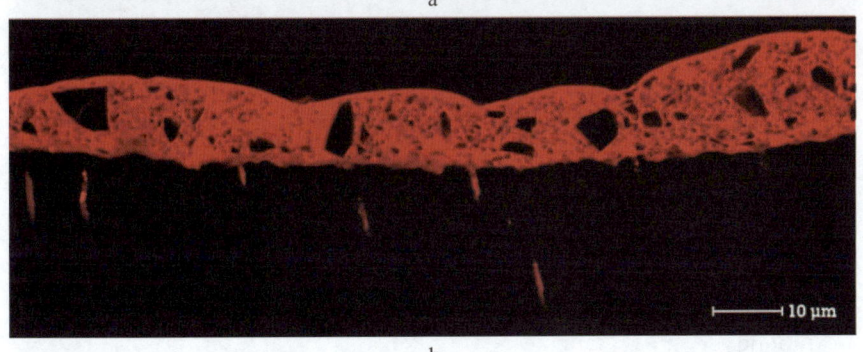

图 9-11　CLSM 图像显示
a. 应用酸蚀-冲洗-黏结系统 XP Bond 联合 Core X Flow 流体树脂(DENTSPLY DeTrey)进行根管黏结后，可获得良好的混合层及足量的树脂突；b. 应用自黏结树脂水门汀 SmartCem2(DENTSPLY DeTrey)进行根管黏结，无混合层形成，仅有零星树脂突进入牙本质小管。

　　自黏结树脂水门汀和羟磷灰石中的钙有良好的化学反应，这在文献中已有描述(Monticelli et al. 2008b)。该结果得到了最近的一项研究证实,自黏结树脂水门汀能显著提高纤维桩在根管内的黏结强度(Sarkis-Onofre et al. 2013),这说明这种简单而已操作的黏结方法在根管内的黏结中是有优势的。和多步法的黏结树脂相比,自黏结树脂也显现出了更少的微渗漏(Bitter et al. 2011)。此外,应用自黏结树脂 RelyX Unicem 对纤维桩和钛钉进行黏结,也显示出良好的临床操作性。有研究推测,自黏结树脂水门汀的高黏结强度可能是和其较低的聚合收缩应力有关(Frrassetto et al. 2012; Sarkis-Onofre et al. 2013)尽管其机械性能和黏结效果的品牌差异还是很大(Frrassetto et al. 2012; Mazzitelli et al. 2012b)。另一个使自黏结树脂 RelyX Unicem 具有良好黏结效果的原因可能是,桩钉插入时要运用压力,而 RelyX Unicem 特别强调在使用过程中需加压以利于水门汀与根管壁紧密贴合,从而获得较高的黏结强度(De Munck et al. 2004)。因此,我们可以得出结论,应用自黏结树脂水门汀作为纤维桩的黏结材料是可靠且恰当的选择,操作便利。近来,有研究指出,将自黏结树脂水门汀作为桩核,会对冠方的玻璃陶瓷全冠产生不良的破坏作用(Sterzenbach et al. 2014)。这种情况往往出现在长期浸泡在水环境中,学者推断是因为自黏结树脂水门汀吸水膨胀使得裂隙产生,从而导致冠的破坏。基于此,我们不推荐将这种材料用于堆砌桩核。

9.3.3 桩-核系统

纤维桩的临床优势是可以将桩与根管的黏结以及冠核的堆砌两个步骤合二为一,缩短了操作时间,简化了流程。因此,各个厂商都有相应的桩-核系统推荐使用(Bitter et al. 2014b)。这种二合一方式被描述为间接一体化结构(Tay 和 Psahley 2007)。然而,之前也有研究指出,冠核由于含有更高比例的填料,可能对黏结性的纤维桩产生不良的作用(Ferrari et al. 2009)。

桩-核系统可配合之前所说的多种黏结方式,比如"自酸蚀"或者"酸蚀-冲洗"黏结系统。而对黏结性纤维桩所涉及的冠核材料的测试数据,依据厂商和所用黏结系统的不同而存在很大差异(Mazzoni et al. 2009; Schmage et al. 2009a; Schmage et al. 2009b; Rodig et al. 2010; Bitter et al. 2014b)。但针对同一个桩-核材料,用不同的黏结方法黏结,研究结果显示,"自酸蚀"组和"酸蚀-冲洗"组并无显著差异(Bitter et al. 2014b)。

但是有一些学者则得出了不同的观点,这些研究对常规的树脂水门汀(自黏结或者多步法树脂水门汀)和桩-核材料进行了比较,结果显示,不管是使用"酸蚀-冲洗"黏结系统(Mazzoni et al. 2009)还是"自酸蚀"黏结系统(Rodig et al. 2010),相较于树脂水门汀而言,纤维桩对桩-核材料的黏结更为理想。另一项研究分别对桩-核及常规的树脂水门汀这两种材料和经过摩擦化学处理过的纤维桩进行黏结,数据显示未见明显不同(Schmage et al. 2012)。同一个研究团队对未经处理的纤维桩(Schmage et al. 2009a)和完全匹配的纤维桩(Schmage et al. 2009b)进行拉应力的测试,结果显示,这两种桩与冠核材料及树脂水门汀材料之间的拉应力没有显著差异,而在不同的冠核材料之间却存在差别。

目前仅有一项临床实验研究了桩黏结和冠核堆砌时使用相同或者不同材料对临床效果的影响(Juloski et al. 2014)。4年的随访结果显示,黏结性材料的种类并不会影响根管治疗后患牙的失败率。但是,对于是否在桩-核黏结中应用同一种材料,在制订相关的临床指南前,还应该进行进一步的体内和体外研究来确定其远期的临床效果。尽管如此,这些材料目前看来还是具有相当大的应用前景的。

9.4 结论

根管内的黏结对牙医来说迄今仍是一种挑战,尤其因为桩黏结的高C因素、根管内的视野受限,而根管内牙本质本身的物理特性使得其也较难作为黏结面。此外,经过了根管充填和桩道预备后的根管壁上总是会被残留的牙胶和封闭剂、玷污层和牙本质碎屑所包被,从而妨碍了根管内的黏结。因此,在高倍放大下清洁桩道使其清晰可见是不可缺少的步骤,而彻底清洁根管内壁防止其被封闭剂污染也大大有利于根管内的黏结。

对桩道用手用器械或者根管锉进行机械清洁,应该联合1%次氯酸钠的超声冲洗,随之用蒸馏水冲净。无论哪种黏结策略,这种最终冲洗方案都可以有效减少桩道内的玷污层。为了提升纤维桩的远期黏结效果,取得良好的修复成效,可以使用99%的乙醇溶液进行进一步的冲洗。然而,乙醇的预处理效果和黏结系统中的树脂成分息息相关,因此最终的指南出台还需要更多相关的研究支持。

为了提高纤维桩的黏结强度，学者测试了多种针对纤维桩表面的预处理方法。这些方法的效果很大程度依赖于桩表面的微观形态学、牙本质基质的成分，以及所用黏结树脂的种类。一些"侵入性"的预处理手段，例如喷砂、Cojet、氢氟酸，可能会破坏纤维桩的结构，影响其完整性，因此不推荐使用。增加桩表面的可湿性，提高黏结树脂和桩的相容性，似乎对理想的纤维桩黏结有着重要的作用。

"侵入性"的桩道预备方法会引起牙本质基质的缺失和天然根管的立体形态的改变，从而造成根管治疗后患牙的折断，因此应该尽量避免。与根管壁完美贴合的桩会产生很薄的树脂水门汀层，并不是十分必要的；而且，一些研究还报道了和根管过于贴合的桩修复反而容易出现问题。对于纤维桩黏结中使用的策略，不同的研究给出了不同的结果。这些研究的结果大不相同，但对于根管内黏结使用"自酸蚀"还是"酸蚀-冲洗"黏结系统会产生更高的黏结强度，所有研究的观点都是一致的，即这两种方式无明显差别，其结果的差异更多来源于黏结树脂本身而非方法的不同。有证据显示，对于纤维桩的黏结，自黏结系统更为可靠。另外，同时在桩的黏结和冠核的堆砌中使用同种树脂材料会简化临床操作，实验室研究也认为这是一种有应用前景的方式，但最终的意见还未统一。

黏结性纤维桩的水门汀层有着不均质的外观，这点常见于文献的表述（Perdigao et al. 2007b；Sterzenbach et al. 2012b）。然而，在水门汀层中空泡的存在会对黏结造成何种影响，这点尚有争议。根管专用的应用助剂能减少水门汀层中空泡的发生率（Watzke et al. 2008；Watzke et al. 2009），因此可推荐使用。

9.5　总结

临床中，在纤维桩的黏结中可参考以下几点：

- 高 C 因素，视野受限，残留的牙胶和封闭剂，以及玷污层都对根管内黏结提出挑战
- 清洁的根管内牙本质表面对黏结最为有益
- 无论何种黏结策略，在桩钉就位前的最终冲洗方案，推荐联合 1% 次氯酸钠和超声冲洗

- 99％的乙醇冲洗可以提升远期黏结效果
- 针对纤维桩的"侵入性"预处理，例如喷砂、Cojet 系统和氢氟酸，应避免使用
- 增加纤维桩表面可湿性，增强树脂水门汀和桩钉基质的相容性，对桩的黏结非常重要
- 应避免"侵入性"的桩道预备
- 尽可能保留完好的牙齿结构，对根管治疗后的患牙远期生存率至关重要
- 桩不需要完全和根管内壁贴合，较厚的树脂水门汀层并不一定会减弱纤维桩的固位力和修复体的稳定性
- 应用自黏结树脂水门体进行桩的黏结，更为可靠
- 根管专用的应用助剂能减少水门汀层中空泡的发生率

（顾申生 译）

参考文献

Aksornmuang J, Nakajima M, Senawongse P, Tagami J (2011) Effects of C-factor and resin volume on the bonding to root canal with and without fibre post insertion. J Dent 39: 422–429.

Al-Assaf K, Chakmakchi M, Palaghias G, Karanika-Kouma A, Eliades G (2007) Interfacial characteristics of adhesive luting resins and composites with dentine. Dent Mater 23: 829–839.

Aleisa K, Alghabban R, Alwazzan K, Morgano SM (2012) Effect of three endodontic sealers on the bond strength of prefabricated fiber posts luted with three resin cements. J Prosthet Dent 107: 322–326.

AlEisa K, Al-Dwairi ZN, Lynch E, Lynch CD (2013) In vitro evaluation of the effect of different endodontic sealers on retentive strength of fiber posts. Oper Dent 38: 539–544.

Alster D, Feilzer AJ, De Gee AJ, Mol A, Davidson CL (1992) The dependence of shrinkage stress reduction on porosity concentration in thin resin layers. J Dent Res 71: 1619–1622.

Arrais CA, Giannini M, Rueggeberg FA, Pashley DH (2007) Microtensile bond strength of dualpolymerizing cementing systems to dentin using different polymerizing modes. J Prosthet Dent 97: 99–106.

Arrais CA, Giannini M, Rueggeberg FA (2009) Effect of sodium sulfinate salts on the polymerization characteristics of dual-cured resin cement systems exposed to attenuated light-activation. J Dent 37: 219–227.

Balbosh A, Kern M (2006) Effect of surface treatment on retention of glass-fiber endodontic posts. J Prosthet Dent 95: 218–223.

Bar-On B, Daniel Wagner H (2012) Enamel and dentin as multi-scale bio-composites. J Mech Behav Biomed Mater 12: 174–183.

Bitter K, Paris S, Martus P, Schartner R, Kielbassa AM (2004) A Confocal Laser Scanning Microscope investigation of different dental adhesives bonded to root canal dentine. Int

Endod J 37: 840-848.

Bitter K, Meyer-Lueckel H, Priehn K, Martus P, Kielbassa AM (2006) Bond strengths of resin cements to fiber-reinforced composite posts. Am J Dent 19: 138-142.

Bitter K, Noetzel J, Neumann K, Kielbassa AM (2007) Effect of silanization on bond strengths of fiber posts to various resin cements. Quintessence Int 38: 121-128.

Bitter K, Paris S, Mueller J, Neumann K, Kielbassa AM (2009a) Correlation of scanning electron and confocal laser scanning microscopic analyses for visualization of dentin/adhesive interfaces in the root canal. J Adhes Dent 11: 7-14.

Bitter K, Paris S, Pfuertner C, Neumann K, Kielbassa AM (2009b) Morphological and bond strength evaluation of different resin cements to root dentin. Eur J Oral Sci 117: 326-333.

Bitter K, Perdigao J, Hartwig C, Neumann K, Kielbassa AM (2011) Nanoleakage of luting agents for bonding fiber posts after thermomechanical fatigue. J Adhes Dent 13: 61-69.

Bitter K, Eirich W, Neumann K, Weiger R, Krastl G (2012) Effect of cleaning method, luting agent and preparation procedure on the retention of fibre posts. Int Endod J 45: 1116-1126.

Bitter K, Hambarayan A, Neumann K, Blunck U, Sterzenbach G (2013) Various irrigation protocols for final rinse after post space preparation to improve bond strengths of fiber posts inside the root canal. Eur J Oral Sci 121: 349-354.

Bitter K, Aschendorff L, Neumann K, Blunck U, Sterzenbach G (2014a) Do chlorhexidine and ethanol improve bond strength and durability of adhesion of fiber posts inside the root canal? Clin Oral Investig 18: 927-934.

Bitter K, Glaser C, Neumann K, Blunck U, Frankenberger R (2014b) Analysis of resin-dentin interface morphology and bond strength evaluation of core materials for one stage postendodontic restorations. PLoS ONE 9, e86294.

Boone KJ, Murchison DF, Schindler WG, Walker WA 3rd (2001) Post retention: the effect of sequence of post-space preparation, cementation time, and different sealers. J Endod 27: 768-771.

Buettel L, Krastl G, Lorch H, Naumann M, Zitzmann NU, Weiger R (2009) Influence of post fit and post length on fracture resistance. Int Endod J 42: 47-53.

Carvalho CA, Cantoro A, Mazzoni A, Goracci C, Breschi L, Ferrari M (2009) Effect of ethanol application on post-luting to intraradicular dentine. Int Endod J 42: 129-135.

Cecchin D, de Almeida JF, Gomes BP, Zaia AA, Ferraz CC (2011) Infl uence of chlorhexidine and ethanol on the bond strength and durability of the adhesion of the fiber posts to root dentin using a total etching adhesive system. J Endod 37: 1310-1315.

Cecchin D, Giacomin M, Farina AP, Bhering CL, Mesquita MF, Ferraz CC (2014) Effect of chlorhexidine and ethanol on push-out bond strength of fiber posts under cyclic loading. J Adhes Dent 16: 87-92.

Chen Q, Cai Q, Li Y, Wei XY, Huang Z, Wang XZ (2014) Effect on push-out bond strength of glass-fiber posts functionalized with polydopamine using different adhesives. J Adhes Dent 16: 177-184.

Coniglio I, Carvalho CA, Magni E, Cantoro A, Ferrari M (2008) Post space debridement in ovalshaped canals: the use of a new ultrasonic tip with oval section. J Endod 34: 752-755.

Czonstkowsky M, Wilson EG, Holstein FA (1990) The smear layer in endodontics. Dent Clin North Am 34: 13-25.

D'Arcangelo C, Cinelli M, De Angelis F, D'Amario M (2007) The effect of resin cement film thickness on the pullout strength of a fiber-reinforced post system. J Prosthet Dent 98: 193-198.

De Munck J, Vargas M, Van Landuyt K, Hikita K, Lambrechts P, Van Meerbeek B (2004) Bonding of an auto-adhesive luting material to enamel and dentin. Dent Mater 20: 963-971.

Demiryurek EO, Kulunk S, Yuksel G, Sarac D, Bulucu B (2010) Effects of three canal sealers on bond strength of a fiber post. J Endod 36: 497-501.

Dogan Buzoglu H, Calt S, Gumusderelioglu M (2007) Evaluation of the surface free energy on root canal dentine walls treated with chelating agents and NaOCl. Int Endod J 40: 18-24.

Egilmez F, Ergun G, Cekic-Nagas I, Vallittu PK, Lassila LV (2013) Influence of cement thickness on the bond strength of tooth-colored posts to root dentin after thermal cycling. Acta Odontol Scand 71: 175-182.

Fawzi EM, Elkassas DW, Ghoneim AG (2010) Bonding strategies to pulp chamber dentin treated with different endodontic irrigants: microshear bond strength testing and SEM analysis. J Adhes Dent 12: 63-70.

Fernandes AS, Shetty S, Coutinho I (2003) Factors determining post selection: a literature review. J Prosthet Dent 90: 556-562.

Ferracane JL, Stansbury JW, Burke FJ (2011) Self-adhesive resin cements - chemistry, properties and clinical considerations. J Oral Rehabil 38: 295-314.

Ferrari M, Carvalho CA, Goracci C, Antoniolli F, Mazzoni A, Mazzotti G, Cadenaro M, Breschi L (2009) Influence of luting material filler content on post cementation. J Dent Res 88: 951-956.

Frassetto A, Navarra CO, Marchesi G, Turco G, Di Lenarda R, Breschi L, Ferracane JL, Cadenaro M (2012) Kinetics of polymerization and contraction stress development in self-adhesive resin cements. Dent Mater 28: 1032-1039.

Goracci C, Raffaelli O, Monticelli F, Balleri B, Bertelli E, Ferrari M (2005) The adhesion between prefabricated FRC posts and composite resin cores: microtensile bond strength with and without post-silanization. Dent Mater 21: 437-444.

Goracci C, Corciolani G, Vichi A, Ferrari M (2008) Light-transmitting ability of marketed fiber posts. J Dent Res 87: 1122-1126.

Hagge MS, Wong RD, Lindemuth JS (2002) Effect of three root canal sealers on the retentive strength of endodontic posts luted with a resin cement. Int Endod J 35: 372-378.

Juloski J, Fadda GM, Monticelli F, Fajo-Pascual M, Goracci C, Ferrari M (2014) Four-year survival of endodontically treated premolars restored with fiber posts. J Dent Res 93: 52S-58S.

Khalighinejad N, Feiz A, Faghihian R, Swift EJ Jr (2014) Effect of dentin conditioning on bond strength of fiber posts and dentin morphology: a review. Am J Dent 27: 3-6.

Kinney JH, Marshall SJ, Marshall GW (2003) The mechanical properties of human dentin: a critical review and re-evaluation of the dental literature. Crit Rev Oral Biol Med 14: 13-29.

Kishen A, Kumar GV, Chen NN (2004) Stress-strain response in human dentine: rethinking fracture predilection in postcore restored teeth. Dental Traumatology 20: 90-100.

Krastl G, Gugger J, Deyhle H, Zitzmann NU, Weiger R, Muller B (2011) Impact of adhesive surface and volume of luting resin on fracture resistance of root filled teeth. Int Endod J 44: 432-439.

Kurtz JS, Perdigao J, Geraldeli S, Hodges JS, Bowles WR (2003) Bond strengths of tooth-colored posts, effect of sealer, dentin adhesive, and root region. Am J Dent 16: 31A-36A.

Lang H, Korkmaz Y, Schneider K, Raab WH (2006) Impact of endodontic treatments on the rigidity of the root. J Dent Res 85: 364-368.

Lazari PC, Oliveira RC, Anchieta RB, Almeida EO, Freitas Junior AC, Kina S, Rocha EP (2013) Stress distribution on dentin-cement-post interface varying root canal and glass fiber post diameters. A three-dimensional finite element analysis based on micro-CT data. Journal of applied oral science : revista FOB 21: 511-517.

Lindblad RM, Lassila LV, Salo V, Vallittu PK, Tjaderhane L (2010) Effect of chlorhexidine on initial adhesion of fiber-reinforced post to root canal. J Dent 38: 796-801.

Lindblad RM, Lassila LV, Salo V, Vallittu PK, Tjaderhane L (2012) One year effect of chlorhexidine on bonding of fibre-reinforced composite root canal post to dentine. J Dent 40: 718-722.

Machado FW, Bossardi M, Ramos Tdos S, Valente LL, Munchow EA, Piva E (2015)

Application of resin adhesive on the surface of a silanized glass fiber-reinforced post and its effect on the retention to root dentin. J Endod 41: 106-110.

Magni E, Mazzitelli C, Papacchini F, Radovic I, Goracci C, Coniglio I, Ferrari M (2007) Adhesion between fiber posts and resin luting agents: a microtensile bond strength test and an SEM investigation following different treatments of the post surface. J Adhes Dent 9: 195-202.

Mannocci F, Ferrari M, Watson TF (2001) Mikroleakage of endodontically treated teeth restored with fibre posts and composite cores after cyclic loading: a confocal microscopic study. J Prosthet Dent 85: 284-291.

Mayer T, Pioch T, Duschner H, Staehle HJ (1997) Dentinal adhesion and histomorphology of two dentinal bonding agents under the influence of eugenol. Quintessence Int 28: 57-62.

Mazzitelli C, Papacchini F, Monticelli F, Toledano M, Ferrari M (2012a) Effects of post surface treatments on the bond strength of self-adhesive cements. Am J Dent 25: 159-164.

Mazzitelli C, Monticelli F, Toledano M, Ferrari M, Osorio R (2012b) Effect of thermal cycling on the bond strength of self-adhesive cements to fiber posts. Clin Oral Investig 16: 909-915.

Mazzoni A, Marchesi G, Cadenaro M, Mazzotti G, Di Lenarda R, Ferrari M, Breschi L (2009) Push-out stress for fibre posts luted using different adhesive strategies. Eur J Oral Sci 117: 447-453.

Mesquita GC, Verissimo C, Raposo LH, Santos-Filho PC, Mota AS, Soares CJ (2013) Can the cure time of endodontic sealers affect bond strength to root dentin? Braz Dent J 24: 340-343.

Mjör IA, Smith MR, Ferrari M, Mannocci F (2001) The structure of dentine in the apical region of human teeth. Int Endod J 34: 346-353.

Monticelli F, Osorio R, Toledano M, Goracci C, Tay FR, Ferrari M (2006) Improving the quality of the quartz fiber postcore bond using sodium ethoxide etching and combined silane/adhesive coupling. J Endod 32: 447-451.

Monticelli F, Toledano M, Tay FR, Sadek FT, Goracci C, Ferrari M (2006) A simple etching technique for improving the retention of fiber posts to resin composites. J Endod 32: 44-47.

Monticelli F, Osorio R, Sadek FT, Radovic I, Toledano M, Ferrari M (2008a) Surface treatments for improving bond strength to prefabricated fiber posts: a literature review. Oper Dent 33: 346-355.

Monticelli F, Osorio R, Mazzitelli C, Ferrari M, Toledano M (2008b) Limited decalcification/diffusion of self-adhesive cements into dentin. J Dent Res 87: 974-979.

Naumann M, Koelpin M, Beuer F, Meyer-Lueckel H (2012) 10-year survival evaluation for glassfiber- supported postendodontic restoration: a prospective observational clinical study. J Endod 38: 432-435.

Pashley DH, Tay FR, Breschi L, Tjaderhane L, Carvalho RM, Carrilho M, Tezvergil-Mutluay A (2011) State of the art etch-and-rinse adhesives. Dent Mater 27: 1-16.

Perdigao J, Gomes G, Lee IK (2006) The effect of silane on the bond strengths of fiber posts. Dent Mater 22: 752-758.

Perdigao J, Gomes G, Augusto V (2007a) The effect of dowel space on the bond strengths of fiber posts. J Prosthodont 16: 154-164.

Perdigao J, Monteiro P, Gomes G, Santos V (2007b) Restoring teeth with prefabricated fiber-reinforced resin posts. Pract Proced Aesthet Dent 19: 359-364.

Perez BE, Barbosa SH, Melo RM, Zamboni SC, Ozcan M, Valandro LF, Bottino MA (2006) Does the thickness of the resin cement affect the bond strength of a fiber post to the root dentin? Int J Prosthodont 19: 606-609.

Radovic I, Monticelli F, Goracci C, Cury AH, Coniglio I, Vulicevic ZR, Garcia-Godoy F, Ferrari M (2007) The effect of sandblasting on adhesion of a dual-cured resin composite to methacrylic fiber posts: microtensile bond strength and SEM evaluation. J Dent 35: 496 - 502.

Radovic I, Mazzitelli C, ChieffiN, Ferrari M (2008) Evaluation of the adhesion of fiber posts cemented using different adhesive approaches. Eur J Oral Sci 116: 557 - 563.

Rasimick BJ, Wan J, Musikant BL, Deutsch AS (2010) A review of failure modes in teeth restored with adhesively luted endodontic dowels. J Prosthodont 19: 639 - 646.

Rengo C, Spagnuolo G, Ametrano G, Juloski J, Rengo S, Ferrari M (2014) Micro-computerized tomographic analysis of premolars restored with oval and circular posts. Clin Oral Investig 18: 571 - 578.

Rodig T, Nusime AK, Konietschke F, Attin T (2010) Effects of different luting agents on bond strengths of fiber-reinforced composite posts to root canal dentin. J Adhes Dent 12: 197 - 205.

Salman MI, Baumann MA, Hellmich M, Roggendorf MJ, Termaat S (2010) SEM evaluation of root canal debridement with Sonicare CanalBrush irrigation. Int Endod J 43: 363 - 369.

Sarkis-Onofre R, Skupien J, Cenci M, de Moraes R, Pereira-Cenci T (2013) The role of resin cement on bond strength of glass-fiber posts (GFPs) luted into root canals: a systematic review and meta-analysis of in vitro studies. Oper Dent Schmage P, Cakir FY, Nergiz I, Pfeiffer P (2009a) Effect of surface conditioning on the retentive bond strengths of fiber reinforced composite posts. J Prosthet Dent 102: 368 - 377.

Schmage P, Pfeiffer P, Pinto E, Platzer U, Nergiz I (2009b) Influence of oversized dowel space preparation on the bond strengths of FRC posts. Oper Dent 34: 93 - 101.

Schmage P, Nergiz I, Markopoulou S, Pfeiffer P (2012) Resistance against pull-out force of prefabricated coated FRC posts. J Adhes Dent 14: 175 - 182.

Schwartz RS, Robbins JW (2004) Post placement and restoration of endodontically treated teeth: a literature review. J Endod 30: 289 - 301.

Serafi no C, Gallina G, Cumbo E, Ferrari M (2004) Surface debris of canal walls after post space preparation in endodontically treated teeth: a scanning electron microscopic study. Oral Surg Oral Med Oral Pathol Oral Radiol Endod 97: 381 - 387.

Soares CJ, Santana FR, Pereira JC, Araujo TS, Menezes MS (2008) Influence of airborne-particle abrasion on mechanical properties and bond strength of carbon/epoxy and glass/bis-GMA fiberreinforced resin posts. J Prosthet Dent 99: 444 - 454.

Sorensen JA, Engelman MJ (1990) Effect of post adaptation on fracture resistance of endodontically treated teeth. J Prosthet Dent 64: 419 - 424.

Spazzin AO, Galafassi D, de Meira-Junior AD, Braz R, Garbin CA (2009) Influence of post and resin cement on stress distribution of maxillary central incisors restored with direct resin composite. Oper Dent 34: 223 - 229.

Sterzenbach G, Franke A, Naumann M (2012a) Rigid versus Flexible Dentine-like Endodontic Posts- Clinical Testing of a Biomechanical Concept: Seven-year Results of a Randomized Controlled Clinical Pilot Trial on Endodontically Treated Abutment Teeth with Severe Hard Tissue Loss. J Endod 38: 1557 - 1563.

Sterzenbach G, Karajouli G, Naumann M, Peroz I, Bitter K (2012b) Fiber post placement with core build-up materials or resin cements-An evaluation of different adhesive approaches. Acta Odontol Scand 70: 368 - 376.

Sterzenbach G, Karajouli G, Tunjan R, Spintig T, Bitter K, Naumann M (2014) Damage of lithium-disilicate all-ceramic restorations by an experimental self-adhesive resin cement used as core build-ups. Clin Oral Investig 19: 281 - 288.

Tang W, Wu Y, Smales RJ (2010) Identifying and reducing risks for potential fractures in endodontically treated teeth. J Endod 36: 609 - 617.

Tay FR, Pashley DH (2007) Monoblocks in root canals: a hypothetical or a tangible goal. J Endod 33: 391 - 398.

Tay FR, Loushine RJ, Lambrechts P, Weller RN, Pashley DH (2005) Geometric factors affecting dentin bonding in root canals: a theoretical modeling approach. J Endod 31: 584 - 589.

Valandro LF, Yoshiga S, de Melo RM, Galhano GA, Mallmann A, Marinho CP, Bottino MA (2006) Microtensile bond strength between a quartz fiber post and a resin cement: effect of post surface conditioning. J Adhes Dent 8: 105 - 111.

Van Meerbeek B, Yoshihara K, Yoshida Y, Mine A, De Munck J, Van Landuyt KL (2011) State of the art of self-etch adhesives. Dent Mater 27: 17 - 28.

Vano M, Goracci C, Monticelli F, Tognini F, Gabriele M, Tay FR, Ferrari M (2006) The adhesion between fibre posts and composite resin cores: the evaluation of microtensile bond strength following various surface chemical treatments to posts. Int Endod J 39: 31 - 39.

Vano M, Cury AH, Goracci C, Chieffi N, Gabriele M, Tay FR, Ferrari M (2008) Retention of fiber posts cemented at different time intervals in canals obturated using an epoxy resin sealer. J Dent 36: 801 - 807.

Vano M, Cury AH, Goracci C, ChieffiN, Gabriele M, Tay FR, Ferrari M (2012) The effect of immediate versus delayed cementation on the retention of different types of fiber post in canals obturated using a eugenol sealer. J Endod 32: 882 - 885.

Watzke R, Blunck U, Frankenberger R, Naumann M (2008) Interface homogeneity of adhesively luted glass fiber posts. Dent Mater 24: 1512 - 1517.

Watzke R, Frankenberger R, Naumann M (2009) Probability of interface imperfections within SEM cross-sections of adhesively luted GFP. Dent Mater 25: 1256 - 1263.

Zhang L, Huang L, Xiong Y, Fang M, Chen JH, Ferrari M (2008) Effect of post-space treatment on retention of fiber posts in different root regions using two self-etching systems. Eur J Oral Sci 116: 280 - 286.

Zicari F, Couthino E, De Munck J, Poitevin A, Scotti R, Naert I, Van Meerbeek B (2008) Bonding effectiveness and sealing ability of fiber-post bonding. Dent Mater 24: 967 - 977.

Zicari F, De Munck J, Scotti R, Naert I, Van Meerbeek B (2012a) Factors affecting the cement-post interface. Dent Mater 28: 287 - 297.

Zicari F, Van Meerbeek B, Scotti R, Naert I (2012b) Effect of fibre post length and adhesive strategy on fracture resistance of endodontically treated teeth after fatigue loading. J Dent 40: 312 - 321.

Zicari F, Coutinho E, Scotti R, Van Meerbeek B, Naert I (2013) Mechanical properties and micro-morphology of fiber posts. Dent Mater 29: e45 - e52.

临时修复体

10

乔奇·佩尔迪高(Jorge Perdigao)
乔治·戈梅斯(George Gomes)

摘　要

准备行部分或全覆盖修复体修复的患牙必须用临时修复体进行保护和加固，以帮助最终修复体重建形态和功能。临时性修复也能为患者的管理提供重要的工具，帮助医生了解治疗的效果和不足。因此，一个高质量的临时修复体对治疗的成功是十分重要的。本章将对现有的临时修复体的材料，及它们的优缺点进行详述。

10.1 简介

根据口腔修复学会(2005)对临时修复体的定义为："暂时修复体是一种固定/活动的齿科修复体或颌面部赝复体，在进行最终的修复之前的观察期设计以提升美学、稳定性和/或功能。这种修复体常被用来帮助医师确定最终修复体的有效性及其形态和功能——同义词——临时修复体，临时充填体。"

理想的临时修复对最终修复体的成功十分重要，对整个治疗的效果也起着决定性的作用(表 10 - 1)(Vahidi 1987；Gratton 和 Aquilino 2004)。除了寿命以外，对临时修复体的要求和期望，应该与之后的最终修复体完全相同。而且，由于临时修复体可能会使用较长一段时间，等到其他治疗(冠延长术等)完成后才进行最终修复。因此，其强度应该足以维持其结构的完整。在其他情况下，当需要对患牙的恢复情况或者牙髓活力进行延长观察时，也需要利用临时修复体占据缺损部位以防止移位。

表 10-1　临时修复体的用途

保护牙髓组织,稳定牙备后的基牙
保护患牙,远离龋损
提供舒适性和功能
提供缺牙的即刻修复
防止基牙移位
提升美观度
维持牙周健康
加强患者的居家口腔护理
当修复体去除后,通过获得可视的手术路径,来辅助牙周治疗
为牙周手术的敷料提供附着的支架
通过牙周治疗和评估,进行松牙固定
在正畸移动牙齿过程中提供支抗的固定
在进行最终修复前,辅助咬合调整
帮助评估面型改变、语言及咀嚼功能
在修复治疗计划中帮助确定有问题基牙的预后

临时修复体常被用作诊断工具,来测试可能在最终修复体上出现的美学、位置、形态、尺寸和咬合关系等方面的变化(Zinner et al. 1989；Wassell et al. 2002；Hammond et al. 2009)。临时修复体也是理想的检测牙备量是否足够的工具。因此,临时修复体对最终修复体而言就是起了蓝图的作用,可使医师在进行最终修复前就能够预见是否有理想的治疗效果(Fox et al. 1984；Luthardt et al. 2000)。此外,具有理想美学设计的临时修复体也能增进患者对临床医师技术的信任感。

10.2　材料

临时修复体的材料有多种选择。单组分的材料包括临时修复体专用的丙烯酸树脂、双丙烯酸(bis-acryl)基质的复合树脂、双酚 A-双甲基丙烯酸缩水甘油酯(bis-GMA)基质的复合树脂、预制的聚碳酸酯冠、金属冠、赛璐珞冠、树脂冠,以及复合树脂直接修复。丙烯酸树脂、bis-acryl 或

10 临时修复体

bis-GMA 自混合的复合树脂材料,预制的树脂冠也是比较适合作为临时修复体材料。

对于临时修复体材料的选择主要基于其机械、物理性能及生物相容性(Duke 1999)。这些材料可按照不同的方法进行分类,一些学者建议按照化学组成,将其分为甲基丙烯酸树脂和复合树脂。

用于前牙的临时修复体总是比那些后牙修复体有着更为复杂的美学要求(Sham et al. 2004)。这些美学要求随着近些年来患者对齿科美学的需求与日俱增而显得越来越重要。在前牙区的单个临时冠并不需要很高的抗压强度。另一方面,用于长桥的临时修复材料应该具有更大的张力,这点与用于单冠的材料截然不同(Koumjian 和 Nimmo,1990)。长期使用的临时修复材料则需要更耐用(Amet 和 Phinney,1995)。用于临时修复的材料要求在表 10-2 中已列出。

表 10-2 临时修复体的要求

生物学	保存活髓(完美封闭作用)
	对牙髓和其他组织无刺激
	低产热
	最少的单体存留
	维持牙周健康,促进组织再生
	具有正常生理凸度和外展隙
	不会妨碍常规的居家口腔清洁
物理/机械	形态稳定,无孔
	坚固耐用
	良好的边缘密合
	低传热
	理想的操作性能(自混合),固化时间短
	不用损伤牙齿即可方便取出
美学	良好的美学设计,牙色分层
	接近牙齿外形
	为美学设计提供诊断性治疗
	良好的抛光性,抗锈蚀

(续表)

功　能	提供和维持稳定的咬合关系
	有充分的邻面接触,防止印模取出后的移位
	为咬合建立提供诊断性治疗
	易于修理或重做
其　他	价格低廉
	无异味
	易于抗感染措施的实施

临时修复体常常通过两种途径制作：① 定制；② 预成形制作。这两种都可以通过临床直接法、技工加工间接法或者直接/间接联合法完成(Vahidi 1987)。虽然间接法需要增加技工加工的成本和制作时间,但定制仍被认为是目前最佳的临时修复体制作手段(Christensen, 1996)。

10.2.1　定制临时修复体的材料

定制能够提供临时修复体与基牙之间紧密的接触。最常用于临时修复体的材料包括：① 聚甲基丙烯酸甲酯(PMMA)树脂；② 聚甲基丙烯酸乙酯(PEMA)树脂；③ 双丙烯酸酯树脂；④ 氨基甲酸酯二甲基丙烯酸酯(UDMA)树脂；⑤ bis-GMA 树脂(Krug 1975；Liu et al. 1986；Vahidi 1987；Wassell et al. 2002；Strassler 2009)。其中,PMMA 和双丙烯酸酯树脂是最为常用的临时修复材料。

丙烯酸树脂是目前使用的最古老的材料。自固化的丙烯酸树脂制作临时修复体操作简便,易于充填入缺损,是一种简便和快捷的方法。它的缺点也很多,最重要的是聚合收缩明显,操作时间短,异味和明显的固化产热,这些都有可能会对牙髓造成损伤(Grajower et al. 1979；Michalakis et al. 2006；Chen et al. 2008)。残留的甲基丙烯酸酯单体也可能会诱发细胞毒性和过敏反应(Lee et al. 2002；Lai et al. 2004)。

丙烯酸树脂通常指的是两种不同的化学成分的材料,一种是 PEMA,另一种是 PMMA。其他一些丙烯酸材料也可用于临时修复,但本章涉及的主要是以上这两种。

10.2.1.1 聚甲基丙烯酸甲酯(PMMA)

PMMA 材料在 20 世纪 40 年代被引入作为临时修复体的直接和间接法所用到的材料(Kaiser 和 Cavazos 1985；Duke 1999；Burns et al. 2003；Christensen 2004)。自固化的 PMMA 树脂可调整粉液比例来获得不同的牙色。相对于其他甲基丙烯酸酯树脂，PMMA 临时修复体具有悠久的使用历史、廉价的费用、可接受的边缘适应性(Wang et al. 1989；Duke 1999；Christensen 2004)，以及较高的机械强度(Wang et al. 1989)。然而，PMMA 的抗磨性能较低，随着时间的推移，材料本身会产生磨损(Vallittu et al. 1994)。

用 PMMA 树脂很难实现理想的美学要求，并且也很费时。这种材料的颜色稳定性和表面质地都比较差，并具有多孔性(Luthardt et al. 2000；Bidra 和 Manzotti 2012)，这就是为何这种材料在美学表现上有问题的原因。一些学者建议可使用液体表面光亮剂，以阻止蛋白质的吸附，从而防止形成生物膜(Davidi et al. 2008)。也有学者建议用其他材料，例如聚碳酸酯冠和双丙烯酸酯树脂替代丙烯酸树脂(Bidra 和 Manzotti 2012)。

在 PMMA 聚合过程中的温度升高明显高于聚甲基丙烯酸乙酯、光固化的聚氨酯二甲基丙烯酸酯和双丙烯酸酯树脂(Lieu et al. 2001)。PMMA 树脂材料聚合造成的牙髓内的升温，可以五倍于热的液体正常产热引起的升温(Plant et al. 1974)。当应用直接法制作临时修复体时，不推荐使用 PMMA 树脂。然而，对于应用间接法制作临时修复体，基于出色的物理性能，PMMA 是很好的选择(Kaiser 和 Cavazos 1985)。一些常用的商品化的 PMMA 材料见表 10-3。

表 10-3 临时修复体的定制材料

材料	商品名	制造商
PMMA 树脂	Alike	GC 美国
	Trim Plus	Harry J. Bosworth
	Jet Set-4	Lang 齿科制造
	Unifast LC	GC 美国

(续表)

材 料	商 品 名	制 造 商
PEMA 树脂	Trim	Harry J. Bosworth
	Trim II	Harry J. Bosworth
	Snap	Parkell
	Splintline	Lang 齿科制造
UDMA 复合树脂	Revotek LC	GC 美国
Bis-GMA 复合树脂	Triad VLC Provisional Material	Dentsply
	TempSpan	Pentron Clinical
Bis-acryl 复合树脂	Access Crown	Centrix
	Cool Temp Natural	Coltene
	Integrity	Dentsply
	Luxatemp Solar	DMG 美国
	Protemp Plus/Prompt 4	3M ESPE
	Structur	VOCO
	Telio CS C & B	Ivoclar Vivadent
	Temphase	Kerr
	Ultra-Trim	Harry J. Bosworth

Bis-GMA　双酚 A-双甲基丙烯酸缩水甘油酯
PEMA　　聚甲基丙烯酸乙酯
PMMA　　聚甲基丙烯酸甲酯
UDMA　　氨基甲酸酯二甲基丙烯酸酯
Bis-acryl　双丙烯酸酯

10.2.1.2　聚甲基丙烯酸乙酯(PEMA)

PEMA 树脂是 20 世纪 60 年代引入作为临时修复材料,相较于 PMMA 树脂,有着各自的优缺点。有一项研究显示,与 PMMA 和双丙烯酸酯材料相比较,PEMA 具有更高的抗折性能(Osman 和 Owen 1993),被认为是一种可用于直接法制作短期使用的临时修复体的理想选择(Vahidi 1987; Christensen 1996)。一些常用的商品化的 PEMA 材料见表 10-3。

10.2.1.3　复合树脂

Bis-acryl　双丙烯酸酯

Bis-acryl 复合树脂的引入是为了克服甲基丙烯酸的缺点。有报道称,用于临时修复,bis-acryl 树脂比其他树脂材料更有优势(表 10-4)。

表 10-4 Bis-acry 复合树脂的优点*

与不含填料的丙烯酸树脂相比,含填料的丙烯酸复合树脂具有更硬,更能对抗食物性溶剂和咀嚼磨损的能力
应用快捷、简便
快速固化,在 60~75 秒后可从口腔中去除
有弹性,可行嵌体,易于去除
低弹性模量,可抵抗咀嚼力
聚合收缩最小
聚合时产热最少,不易对牙髓造成热损伤
X 线阻射
易于用流体树脂修补
良好的颜色稳定性和抗着色能力
混匀时仅有少量异味

* 引自 Hagge et al.(2002),Garcia 和 Aquilino(2004),Strassler(2009)
UDMA　氨基甲酸酯二甲基丙烯酸酯

　　Bis-acry 复合树脂是一种类似 bis-GMA 的疏水性材料,一般以双组分自混合输送系统应用于临床,易于使用,但较其他种类的定制临时材料昂贵。其具有较低的聚合收缩,良好的边缘密合和抗挠强度(Strassler et al. 2007)。固化后在表面虽然存在厚的阻聚氧化层使得其抗着色能力比甲基丙烯酸酯树脂弱,但容易用流体树脂修复(Hagge et al. 2002;Bohnenkamp 和 Garcia 2004)。Bis-acry 复合树脂材料比 PMMA 有着更强的微硬度和抗磨损能力(Diaz-Arnold et al. 1999;Strassler et al. 2007),PMMA 则更脆。Bis-acry 复合树脂可以用于树脂直接修复的抛光工作尖进行抛光,产生的表面质地取决于充填材料的颗粒大小(图 10-1)。

　　在咬合、形态、边缘精确度和修型方面,不管在前牙还是后牙,Bis-acry 复合树脂均显示出了较 PMMA 更优良的性能(Solow 1999;Young et al. 2001)。相较于在真空成型的聚丙烯酸印模,其在聚乙烯基硅氧烷印模中应用会显著降低髓腔内升高的温度(Castelnuovo 和 Tjan 1997)。表 10-3 列出了常用的 Bis-acry 复合树脂。

a   b

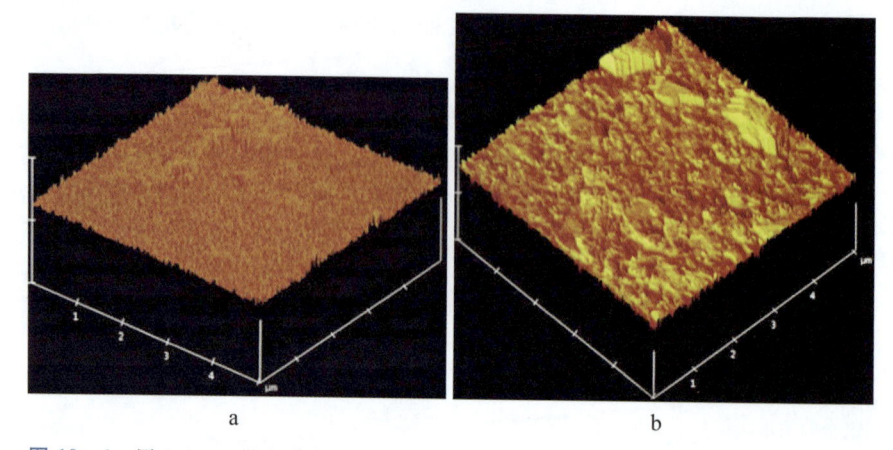

图 10-1　用 Sof-Lex 抛光碟(3M ESPE)抛光不同 bis-acryl 树脂后的原子力显微镜图像 (5 μm×5 μm)
a. Protemp Plus 或者 Protemp 4(3M ESPE);b. Structur(VOCO)。

这种材料现在是许多美国开业牙医和牙科医院行临时修复的首选。

UDMA　氨基甲酸酯二甲基丙烯酸酯

一类用于临时修复的光固化树脂材料,面世于 20 世纪 80 年代(Emtiaz 和 Tarnow 1988)。其中一些材料含有填料,例如二氧化硅颗粒,可有效提高聚合收缩等物理性能(passon 和 Goldfogel 1990)。光固化的 UDMA 树脂不会像 PMMA 一样残留单体,这也是其组织毒性较低的原因(Khan et al. 1988)。该材料比那些技工室制作的临时修复体和直接树脂修复体费用更少且省时(Haddix 1988)。此外,这类材料具有油灰状结构且可以被流体树脂修补,因而十分适用于口腔。不过,用于临时修复的 UDMA 树脂比 bis-acryl 和 PEMA 树脂的边缘密合性差(Tjan et al. 1997)。光固化的 UDMA 树脂比较脆,这使得其不能用于高强度的后牙修复(Prestipino 1989)。对于前牙修复,它们不像其他材料一样有较好的抗着色能力,且仅能用于有限几种色度。目前使用的 UDMA 树脂已在表 10-3 中列出。

Bis-GMA　双酚 A-双甲基丙烯酸缩水甘油酯

双重固化的临时修复树脂材料也是可用的(表 10-3)。TempSpan(Pentron Clinical)是其中一种,它以乙烯基聚硅氧烷膏剂的形式应用于口腔内(TempSpan Clear Matrix Material,Pentron Clinical)。与甲基丙烯酸酯相比,Bis-GMA 材料具有良好的边缘密合性、完美的抛光性、较低的聚合收缩和最小的放热反应,且可用流体树脂进行修补。和所有的

10 临时修复体

树脂基质的材料一样，Bis-GMA 比甲基丙烯酸酯基质的材料更为昂贵。

10.2.1.4 用于 CAD/CAM 的材料

现在可通过 CAD/CAM 技术将高密度的 PMMA 树脂块切磨成高度美观的临时修复体（表 10-5）。这些修复体可通过单/多单元的精密切磨，以获得更良好的强度。这种新技术有若干缺点，其中一项便是费用，因为在临床试戴前必须将模型送技工室进行加工。

表 10-5　用于 CAD/CAM 临时修复体制作的材料
（Guth et al. 2013；Keul et al. 2014）

商品名，制造商	成　分
artBloc Temp, Merz Dental	不含填料的 PMMA
Telio CAD, Ivoclar Vivodent	不含填料的 PMMA
Telio CAD for Zenotec, Wieland Dental	不含填料的 PMMA
Cercon base PMMA, Dentsply	不含填料的 PMMA
VITA CAD-Temp, VITA Zahnfabrik	含 14%微填料的 PMMA
Polycon ae, Straumann	高度交联的 PMMA（IPN，互穿聚合物网络）
New Outline, Anaxdent	不含填料的 PMMA
Quattro Disc eco PMMA, Goldquadrat	不含填料的 PMMA

近期有研究对 11 个 CAD/CAM 切磨的树脂进行分析，显示不同品牌的材料在透光率上差别很大，数值从 33.1%～54.5%（Guth et al. 2013）。另一项研究发现，CAD/CAM 树脂较常规固化树脂磨损率更低。然而，CAD/CAM 树脂显示出了比玻璃离子水门汀更高的磨损值，只有 Telio CAD（Ivoclar Vivodent）例外（Stawarczyk et al. 2013）。

10.2.2　用于预成型的临时修复材料

临时的预成冠通常是由牙齿外形的壳组成，成分往往是聚碳酸酯树脂、PMMA 树脂、赛璐珞和金属等。用丙烯酸酯树脂重衬，使得冠严密适合牙备后的牙齿，但通常需要对它们进行边缘修整和咬合调整。目前市场上有不同尺寸的商品化预成冠，适合不同解剖特点的牙齿。尽管如此，可用的尺寸和形态也是有限的。与定制的修复体相比，这种处理方法比较快捷，但疗效可能较差，会造成尺寸不合的临时修复（Christensen 1996）。"bead-brush"技术或者流体树脂可应用以缩小治疗差距(Hammond et al. 2009)。

10.2.2.1 赛璐珞冠

赛璐珞冠是由纤维醋酸酯构成的薄层外壳(Strassler 2009)。Crowns Forms(Dentsply)，Full Forms(Directa AB)和Odus Pella Transparent Crown Forms(Moore Co.)是其中的几种商品。它们在被修整以适合龈缘线之后，可以用丙烯酸树脂或复合树脂加以充填。

10.2.2.2 牙色树脂冠

聚碳酸酯树脂冠在口腔修复学中，对单冠的临时修复有着悠久的历史(Bidra 和 Manzotti 2012)。这种冠可通过超细纤维加强其结构强度，并提升美观性能。正如其他的预成冠一样，它和牙体的吻合度较差，必须用丙烯酸树脂加以重衬。最终的边缘修整和咬合调整可能会比较耗费时间(Gratton 和 Aquilino 2004)。聚碳酸酯树脂冠和PMMA材料相比，在很多方面，包括颜色稳定性、抗磨损性、硬度、美观性和机械强度，都有着优势(King et al. 1973；Bidra 和 Manzotti 2012)。牙科从业者往往将聚碳酸酯树脂冠作为模型，用丙烯酸树脂重衬制备后的基牙，来定制临时修复体。这其中，最常用的商品化聚碳酸酯树脂冠是由3M ESPE公司和Directa AB公司出品的。

PMMA树脂冠也是常用的牙色冠，例如GC Crowntek(GC America)。和聚碳酸酯树脂冠一样，它也可以用PMMA或者PEMA树脂重衬。

10.2.2.3 金属冠

铝 目前有两种铝冠，一种是铝壳冠(Miltex)，另一种是金阳极氧化冠(3M ESPE)。基于其较高的柔性和延展性，铝冠很容易与牙体贴合，但这一点同样也会导致较为快速的磨损，从而造成穿孔(Lui et al. 1986)。此外，铝金属有时也会产生一些异味。

锡 锡冠(Directa AB)的主要成分是锡，而Iso-Form冠(3M ESPE)的主要成分则是锡银。就像铝冠一样，锡冠拥有合适的延展性，能快速成型，而咬合面则被强化，使得其更能对抗磨损(Lui et al. 1986)。往往应用在后牙的短期临时修复中，并可作为牙色冠的模板。

不锈钢 不锈钢冠(不锈钢后牙永久冠，3M ESPE)一般用于长期的修复，但相对于其他两种金属冠，它的硬度较高，延展性也较差，因此很难成型。

金属冠由于其美观性能较差，一般均用于后牙修复。

10.2.2.4　Protemp™冠

Protemp™冠材料(3M ESPE)是一种预成的、可塑的 bis-GMA 复合树脂，可用于单个后牙和尖牙的临时冠修复(图10-2)。冠尺寸可选，可通过修剪调整至合适的高度。一旦冠就位并有邻间接触建立，便需要患者咬合以获得足够的咬合关系。然后按照咬合面、颊面、舌面的顺序，将冠进行光固化2~3秒。然后取出临时修复体，光固化1分钟，用金刚石车针修整外形，在黏结之前完成抛光。冠边缘可用流体树脂补偿。这种临时修复结合了复合树脂的优点(高抛光性、美观性、抗磨性、边缘贴合)和预成冠的优点(方便、易清理、不用模板)(Strassler 2009)。Protemp™冠的色度沿用通用的分类。

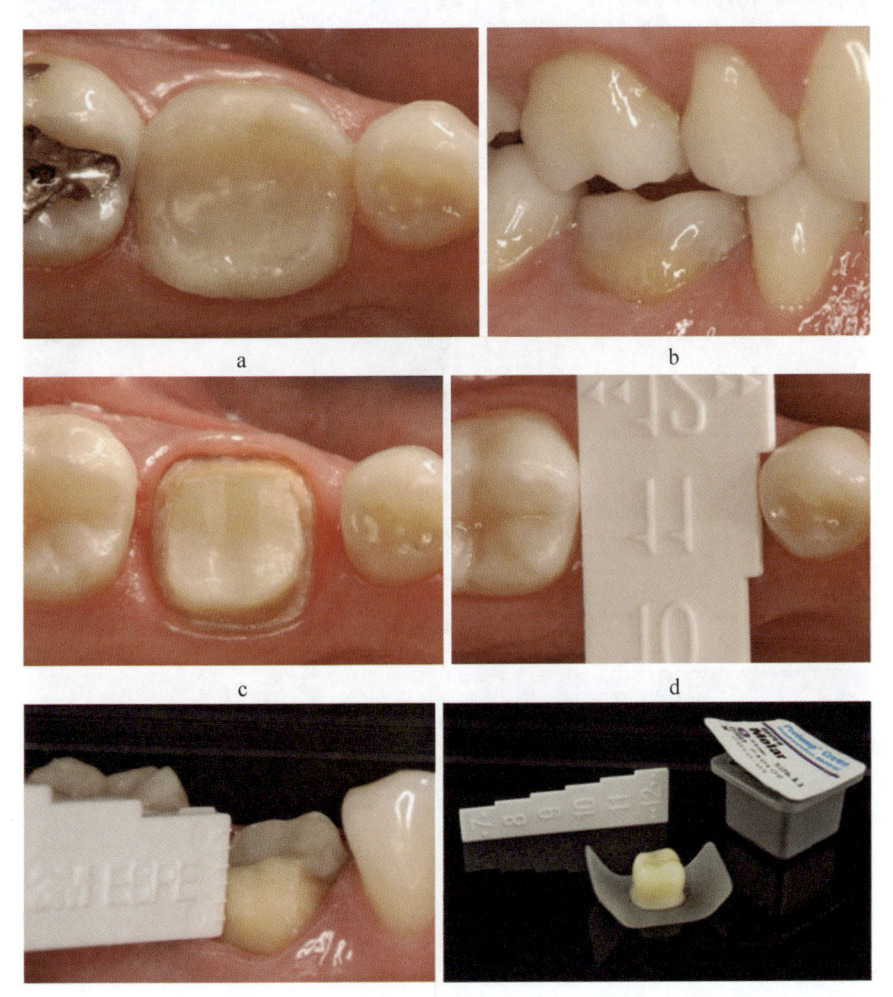

a

b

c

d

e

f

根管治疗后的牙体修复

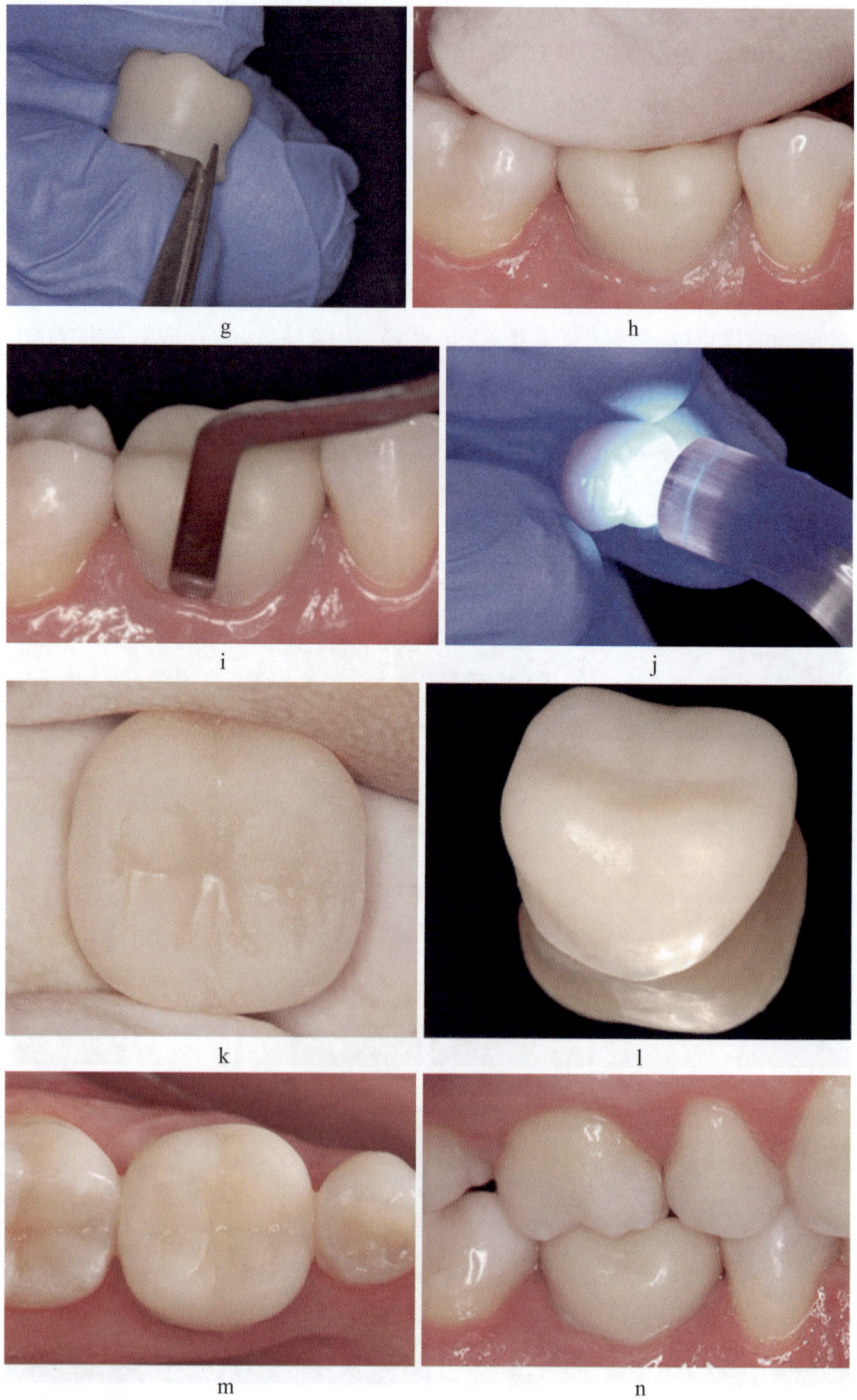

g

h

i

j

k

l

m

n

10 临时修复体

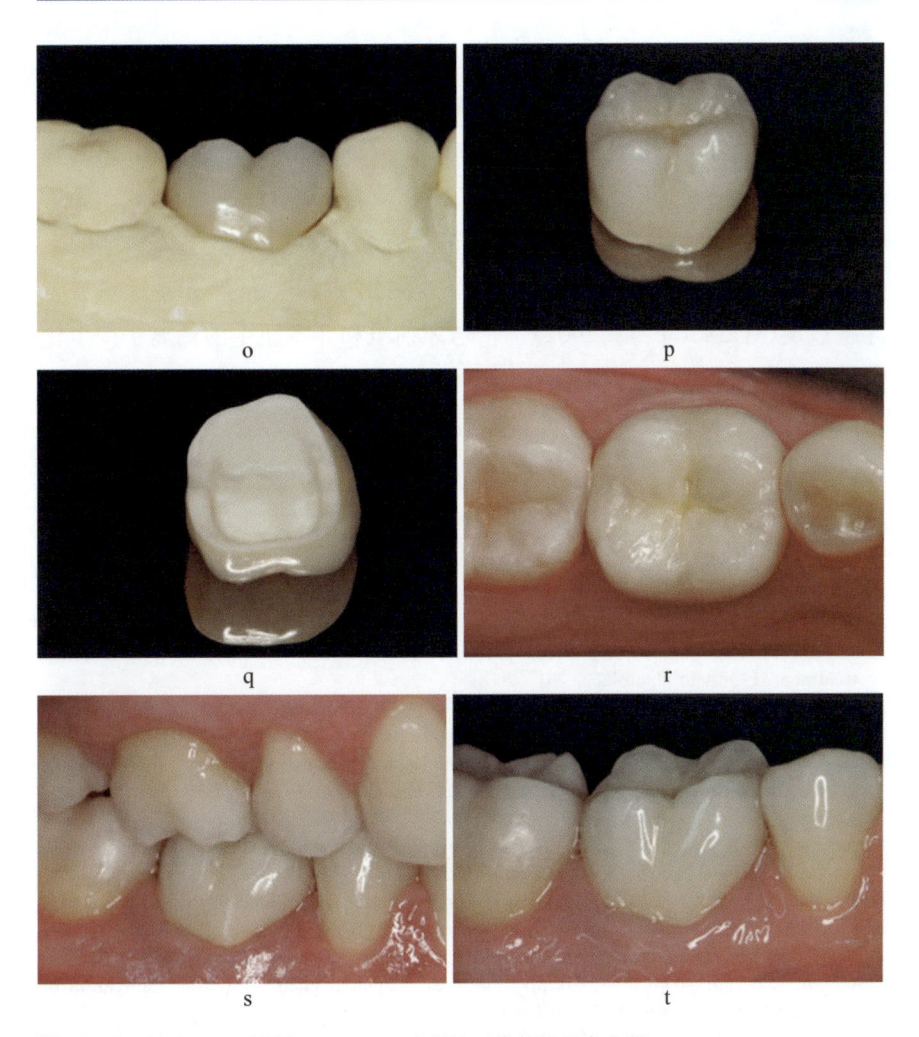

图 10-2 用 Protemp™ 冠(3M ESPE)进行临时修复的临床步骤
a. 根管治疗并树脂直接修复后的下颌第一磨牙术前图；b. 颊面观；c. 按照氧化锆冠的要求进行牙备；d. 用 Protemp 冠标尺测量近远中间隙；e. 冠高度测量；f. 选择匹配测量结果的冠；g. 用剪修整冠边缘；h. 冠在轻微润湿的牙体上就位；i. 嘱患者轻柔咬合。颊侧部分用树脂修补，颊侧光固化 3 秒；j. 将冠轻柔取下，在体外每个面都光固化 40 秒；k. 冠试戴，调整咬合；l. 用合金抛光针、Sof-Lex 抛光碟(3M ESPE)和 PoGo 抛光尖(Dentsply)等进行冠抛光；m. 取完印模后，用 Temp-Bond NE(Kerr 公司)进行冠黏结，去除多余的黏结剂；n. 临时修复体的颊面观；o、p. 技工加工中心进行氧化锆全冠的制作；q. 冠内壁组织面用氧化铝颗粒进行喷砂处理；r. 永久修复体用自黏结树脂水门汀进行黏结；s、t. 术后图。

10.2.3 临时黏结材料

既然临时修复体需要易于拆除，对黏结剂很重要的一点是能够提供良好的边缘封闭性,以防止活髓牙的牙髓激惹及根管治疗后牙齿的再感染。临时黏结材料应具备良好的机械性能、低溶解性及对牙齿的足够黏结力,以对抗细菌及其产物的渗透(Baldissara et al. 1998)。最常用的临时黏结材料包括:① 氢氧化钙水门汀;② 氧化锌丁香油水门汀;③ 无丁香油的氧化锌水门汀(Baldissara et al. 1998)。一般用于永久黏结的聚羧酸盐水门汀,在牙备不理想的情况下也可用于临时黏结,如基牙短或者牙备过度(Wassell et al. 2002)。它与牙釉质和牙本质中的钙离子产生化学结合,可提供更理想的封闭作用。

临时黏结材料的机械性能较差,以便于到期拆除。

(顾申生 译)

参考文献

Amet EM, Phinney TL (1995) Fixed provisional restorations for extended prosthodontic treatment. J Oral Implantol 21: 201–206.

Baldissara P, Comin G, Martone F, Scotti R (1998) Comparative study of the marginal microleak-age of six cements in fixed provisional crowns. J Prosthet Dent 180: 417–422.

Bidra AS, Manzotti A (2012) A direct technique for fabricating esthetic anterior fixed provisional restorations using polycarbonate veneers. Compend Contin Educ Dent 33(452–4): 456.

Bohnenkamp DM, Garcia LT (2004) Repair of bis-acryl provisional restorations using flowable composite resin. J Prosthet Dent 92: 500–502.

Burns DR, Beck DA, Nelson SK (2003) A review of selected dental literature on contemporary provisional fixed prosthodontic treatment: report of Committee on Research in Fixed Prosthodontics of the Academy of Fixed Prosthodontics. J Prosthet Dent 90: 474–497.

Castelnuovo J, Tjan AH (1997) Temperature rise in pulpal chamber during fabrication of provisional resinous crowns. J Prosthet Dent 78: 441–446.

Chen H-L, Lai Y-L, Chou I-C, Hu C-J, Lee S-Y (2008) Shear bond strength of provisional restoration materials repaired with light-cured resins. Oper Dent 33: 508–515.

Christensen GJ (1996) Provisional restorations for fixed prosthodontics. J Am Dent Assoc 127: 249–252.

Christensen GJ (2004) Making provisional restorations easy, predictable and economical. J Am Dent Assoc 135: 625–627.

Davidi MP, Beyth N, Weiss EI, Weiss EI, Eilat Y, Feuerstein O, Sterer N (2008) Effect of liquid-polish coating on in vitro biofilm accumulation on provisional restorations: Part 2. Quintessence Int 39: 45–49.

Diaz-Arnold AM, Dunne JT, Jones AH (1999) Microhardness of provisional fixed prosthodontic materials. J Prosthet Dent 82: 525–528.

Duke ES (1999) Provisional restorative materials: a technology update. Compend Contin Educ Dent 20: 497–500.

Emtiaz S, Tarnow DP (1988) Processed acrylic resin provisional restoration with lingual cast metal framework. J Prosthet Dent 79: 484–488.

Federick DR (1975) The provisional fixed partial denture. J Prosthet Dent 34: 520–526.

Fox CW, Abrams BL, Doukoudakis A (1984) Provisional restorations for altered occlusions. J Prosthet Dent 52: 567-572.

Grajower R, Shaharbani S, Kaufman E (1979) Temperature rise in pulp chamber during fabrication of temporary self-curing resin crowns. J Prosthet Dent 41: 535-540.

Gratton DG, Aquilino SA (2004) Interim restorations. Dent Clin North Am 48: 487-497.

Güth JF, Zuch T, Zwinge S, Engels J, Stimmelmayr M, Edelhoff D (2013) Optical properties of manually and CAD/CAM-fabricated polymers. Dent Mater J 32: 865-871.

Haddix JE (1988) A technique for visible light-cured provisional restorations. J Prosthet Dent 59: 512-514.

Hagge MS, Lindemuth JS, Jones AG (2002) Shear bond strength of bis-acryl composite provisional material repaired with flowable composite. J Esthet Restor Dent 14: 47-52.

Hammond BD, Cooper JR, Lazarchik DA (2009) Predictable repair of provisional restorations. J Esthet Restor Dent 21: 19-24; discussion 25.

Kaiser DA, Cavazos E (1985) Temporization techniques in fixed prosthodontics. Dent Clin North Am 29: 403-412.

Keul C, Müller-Hahl M, Eichberger M, Liebermann A, Roos M, Edelhoff D, Stawarczyk B (2014) Impact of different adhesives on work of adhesion between CAD/CAM polymers and resin composite cements. J Dent 42: 1105-1114.

Khan Z, Razavi R, von Fraunhofer JA (1988) The physical properties of a visible light-cured temporary fixed partial denture material. J Prosthet Dent 60: 543-545.

King CJ, Young FA, Cleveland JL (1973) Polycarbonate resin and its use in the matrix technique for temporary coverage. J Prosthet Dent 30: 789-794.

Koumjian JH, Nimmo A (1990) Evaluation of fracture resistance of resins used for provisional restorations. J Prosthet Dent 64: 654-657.

Krug RS (1975) Temporary resin crowns and bridges. Dent Clin North Am 19: 313-320.

Lai YL, Chen Y-T, Lee SY, Shieh T-M, Hung S-L (2004) Cytotoxic effects of dental resin liquids on primary gingival fibroblasts and periodontal ligament cells in vitro. J Oral Rehabil 31: 1165-1172.

Lee S-Y, Lai Y-L, Hsu T-S (2002) Influence of polymerization conditions on monomer elution and microhardness of autopolymerized polymethyl methacrylate resin. Eur J Oral Sci 110: 179-183.

Lieu C, Nguyen TM, Payant L (2001) In vitro comparison of peak polymerization temperatures of 5 provisional restoration resins. J Can Dent Assoc 67: 36-39.

Lui JL, Setcos JC, Phillips RW (1986) Temporary restorations: a review. Oper Dent 11: 103-110.

Luthardt RG, Stössel M, Hinz M, Vollandt R (2000) Clinical performance and periodontal out-come of temporary crowns and fixed partial dentures: a randomized clinical trial. J Prosthet Dent 83: 32-39.

Michalakis K, Pissiotis A, Hirayama H, Kang K, Kafantaris N (2006) Comparison of temperature increase in the pulp chamber during the polymerization of materials used for the direct fabrication of provisional restorations. J Prosthet Dent 96: 418-423.

Osman YI, Owen CP (1993) Flexural strength of provisional restorative materials. J Prosthet Dent 70: 94-96.

Passon C, Goldfogel M (1990) Direct technique for the fabrication of a visible light-curing resin provisional restoration. Quintessence Int 21: 699-703.

Plant CG, Jones DW, Darvell BW (1974) The heat evolved and temperatures attained during setting of restorative materials. Br Dent J 137: 233-238.

Prestipino V (1989) Visible light cured resins: a technique for provisional fixed restorations. Quintessence Int 20: 241-248.

Sham ASK, Chu FCS, Chai J, Chow TW (2004) Color stability of provisional prosthodontic materials. J Prosthet Dent 91: 447-452.

Solow RA (1999) Composite veneered acrylic resin provisional restorations for complete veneer crowns. J Prosthet Dent 82: 515-517.

Stawarczyk B, Özcan M, Trottmann A, Schmutz F, Roos M, Hämmerle C (2013) Two-body wear rate of CAD/CAM resin blocks and their enamel antagonists. J Prosthet Dent 109: 325-332.

Strassler HE, Anolik C, Frey C (2007) High-strength, aesthetic provisional restorations using a bis-acryl composite. Dent Today 26: 128-130, 3.

Strassler HE (2009) In-office provisional restorative materials for fixed prosthodontics: part 1-polymeric resin provisional materials. Inside Dent 5: 70-74.

The Academy of Prosthodontics (2005) The glossary of prosthodontic terms. J Prosthet Dent 94: 46.

Tjan AH, Castelnuovo J, Shiotsu G (1997) Marginal fidelity of crowns fabricated from six proprietary provisional materials. J Prosthet Dent 77: 482-485.

Tyas MJ, Burrow MF (2004) Adhesive restorative materials: a review. Aust Dent J 49: 112-121.

Vahidi F (1987) The provisional restoration. Dent Clin North Am 31: 363-381.

Vallittu PK, Lassila VP, Lappalainen R (1994) Wetting the repair surface with methyl methacrylate affects the transverse strength of repaired heat-polymerized resin. J Prosthet Dent 72: 639-643.

Wang RL, Moore BK, Goodacre CJ, Swartz ML, Andres CJ (1989) A comparison of resins for fabricating provisional fixed restorations. Int J Prosthodont 2: 173-184.

Wassell RW, St. George G, Ingledew RP, Steele JG (2002) Crowns and other extra-coronal restorations: provisional restorations. Br Dent J 192: 619-630.

Young HM, Smith CT, Morton D (2001) Comparative in vitro evaluation of two provisional restorative materials. J Prosthet Dent 85: 129-132.

Zinner ID, Trachtenberg DI, Miller RD (1989) Provisional restorations in fixed partial prosthodontics. Dent Clin North Am 33: 355-377.

铸造桩与核 11

沃克-金·西奥格(WookJin Seong)

摘 要

铸造桩、核(D&C)技术作为传统的修复方式已使用了相当长的一段时间,尽管近年来预制纤维桩技术在临床中运用得越来越多,但是仍旧有许多临床医师在一些病例中选择使用铸造桩核技术。一些体外和体内研究结果已经表明,预制纤维桩核技术较铸造桩核具有相似甚至更好的临床效果,但我们认为,在对这两种技术进行比较时,应考虑剩余牙体组织量,使用何种黏结技术以及研究人员的临床专业知识等。本章将重点介绍:① 铸造桩&核在流行的预制纤维桩和复合树脂核组合应用中的适应证。② 影响铸造桩&核长期成功的因素。③ 制造铸造桩&核及随后的全冠修复的两种不同的临床技术(直接和间接取模)及各自的顺序。④ 铸造桩&核的黏结以及全冠修复。

11.1 介绍

用桩来帮助牙冠固位的概念已经超过两个世纪。早在18世纪,皮埃尔·福查(Pierre Fauchard)使用木桩嵌入根管的空间中来保留牙冠(Prothero 1921)。此后又出现许多不同设计的桩作为牙冠的组成部分,但后来又消失了。随着对无髓牙修复兴趣的提高,桩冠分离逐渐替代了桩冠一体(Shillingburg 和 Kessler 1982)。即使在预制金属桩与银汞合金和复合树脂核芯材料的组合出现之后,一体式铸造桩&核仍作为根管治疗后牙体修复的标准做法。由于纤维柱无论对患者和临床医师的操作均较便利，以及复合树脂黏结技术的飞速发展，近年来，纤维桩和高强度复合树脂核心材料的组合已经得到了普遍应用，使其几乎取代了铸造桩&核的金标准。本章将对铸造桩&核的应用，以及目前流行的纤维桩和复合树脂核这两个体系进行讨论。

11.2　铸造桩 & 核的适应证

　　为了能够使用直接法制造以及黏结铸造桩&核，以及黏结铸造桩&核，在铸造桩&核的通路、根管口、髓室和临床牙冠的内部轴向壁均不应存在明显倒凹。如果计划在具有多个轴向壁并已经进行过牙髓处理的牙齿中放置铸造桩&核，则必须要去除原先不必要去除的牙体组织来为铸造桩&核创造合适的插入路径，如果铸造桩&核与牙体组织之间的间隙过大，则应当填充水门汀。在这两种情况下，铸造桩&核修复的整体强度都将受到影响。许多临床研究表明，剩余健康牙体结构的量对桩核修复体的保留有显著影响，提示我们应尽可能多的保留健康牙体组织以增强修复体的预后（Creugers 等人 2005；Ferrari 等 2007, 2012）。因此，当牙齿只具有有限量的牙体组织（例如一个或更少的侧壁具有或不具有理想的肩台）时，制造铸造桩&核不会使髓室或临床牙冠的内部轴向壁减少过多的牙体结构，才考虑使用铸造桩&核（如仅剩余一壁或更少的侧壁/具有或不具有理想的肩台时则不适合使用）。

　　为了比较预制纤维桩和铸造桩&核的研究结果，需要进一步的研究，对每个研究对象（预制纤维桩与铸造桩&核）的剩余牙体结构，应用的黏结技术方面和研究人员的临床专业知识等是否处于类似水平进行比较。有许多早期的预制金属桩研究被排除在外，因为自从性能较好的纤维桩自 1989 年引入临床以来，已基本上取代了预制金属柱。1993 年的一项 meta 分析和 2002 年的一篇系统综述（Heydecke 和 Peters 2002）中表明，铸造桩&核和预制纤维柱的比较没有随机对照试验（RCT）。2007 年科克伦（Cochrane）的综述和 2009 年西奥多普若（Theodosopoulou）和乔克利塔基斯（Chochlidakis）的系统综述（Theodosopoulou 和 Chochlidakis 2009）中都介绍了只有一项随机对照试验（RCT）比较了铸造桩&核和预制纤维柱。Cochrane 的综述指出，2000 年由法拉利等人发表的随机对照试验(2000)具有偏倚的高风险,并得出结论,需要有更多的随机对照试验(RCT)来确认纤维增强型桩和核系统是否优于铸造桩&核。

法拉利等人的随机对照试验包括200例患者的200颗经牙髓治疗的牙齿伴牙齿结构的严重丧失,临床治疗后4年评估了铸造桩&核和树脂桩系统(碳纤维柱)的临床疗效(Theodosopoulou和Chochlidakis 2009)。其中树脂桩有2%的失败率(全部是牙髓治疗失败),而铸造桩&核有14%的失败率(9%根折;2%冠脱落;3%牙髓治疗失效)。尽管作者指出,将200颗牙齿随机分为两组,但没有进一步描述研究人员的随机分组和结果评估是否采用盲法。此外,作者没有定义牙体结构严重丧失的纳入标准,并且没有量化随机分配前的200颗牙齿的剩余牙体结构。碳纤维柱使用的是多步骤酸蚀冲洗黏结技术和双固化树脂水门汀黏结技术,而铸造桩&核使用的是磷酸锌水门汀黏固技术。由于所有200例患者均在6个月内入选,多名临床医师可能已经进行了临床治疗,且没有对9个根折病例的铸造桩&核的长度和宽度进行进一步的描述,但作者推测,大量的根折可能是由于根管的不受控区域的应力集中,事实上铸造桩&核的固位是通过与根管壁的摩擦力而获得的。经验丰富的医师能够仔细制订计划并熟练进行根管预备和铸造桩&核的试戴,如果铸造桩能够被动匹配并且其长度尽可能长,且根尖部4~5 mm的密封能够保持,则这两个推测的原因都不会发生。

最近发表出版一些比较铸造桩&核和纤维桩的小规模短期随机对照试验(Ferrari等2000;Preethi和Kala 2008;Zicari等2011)。在1~3年随访期间,样本量范围从30~205个。这些研究均显示这两种修复方式的失败率都非常低,并得出结论,铸造桩&核和纤维桩显示了相似的临床表现。2014年发表的一篇经过3年随访的随机对照试验,对仅包括0~0.5 mm肩台高度的72颗牙齿,随机分配使用铸造桩&核或纤维桩(Zicari等2011)。纤维桩和铸造桩&核都采用树脂水门汀黏结,均由完成了12小时授课和培训的本科生和研究生进行操作。结果表明,3年内共有4个失败病例,纤维桩和铸造桩&核的保存率在统计学分析中无显著差异(分别为91.9%和97.1%)。其中两个纤维桩脱落,一个前磨牙纤维桩引起根折,一个磨牙铸造桩&核引起根折。

由于比较铸造桩&核和纤维桩的临床研究仍旧相对较少,其他临床研究要么集中在纤维桩或单独的铸造桩&核上进行回顾。一篇关于985个纤维柱的回顾性研究报告表明,在7～11年的治疗期间,其失败率为8%(Ferrari 等 2007)。其中牙髓治疗失效最多,为39例,其次为桩脱落,为21例,第三为冠脱落,有17例。这篇研究报道指出,这些机械性失败病例总是与缺少冠方牙体组织有关。换言之,当只保留了有限量的剩余的牙齿结构,如仅有一个或更少的侧壁和/或没有理想的肩台时,纤维桩系统发生失败的可能性较大。一项针对360例经牙髓治疗的前磨牙,进行的6年随机对照实验结果表明,在3种不同的剩余牙齿组织量的患牙中(一壁,仅有肩台,无肩台),使用两种不同类型的纤维桩,其成功率分别为29%～78%,(Ferrari 等 2012)。在这3种情况中,纤维桩的成功率明显低于具有足够牙体组织量(两至四壁)的情况。这3种情况中,失败的模式包括桩脱落、柱/核折断、牙冠脱落、牙髓治疗失败和根折。

一项为期5年的随机对照试验,由18名医师完成的319个铸造金属桩核修复体,报告在5年内的总体保持率为96%(Creugers 等 2005)。如果把在最小肩台高度的牙齿中使用铸造桩&核的病例分离出来统计,则在5年内58个病例中发生了3例失败(3次铸造桩&核脱落)(94.8%)。一些早期的铸造桩&核的临床研究显示出良好的成功率:96个桩91%超过6年(Sarkis-Onofre 等 2014),516个桩92%超过4.8年(Bergman 等 1989),456个桩85%超过6年(Mentink 等 1993),27个桩100%超过10年(Torbjömer 等人,1995)。

比较铸造桩和纤维桩之间的抗折裂性的meta分析发现,有13个体外研究表明铸造桩组显示出比纤维桩组更高的抗折裂性(Ellner 等 2003)。但是铸造桩&核的断裂模式往往是灾难性的破坏,如根部中1/3斜向或横向折裂或垂直折裂,而纤维桩失败则多是可修复的,如牙根的颈1/3或树脂核心的折断。研究假设纤维桩与牙根牙本质之间有相似的弹性模量,纤维桩和牙根牙本质之间的厚树脂水门汀作为应力吸收层,与坚硬的、合适的铸造桩相比可能降低了根折的风险。尽管铸造桩的断裂模式可能是灾难性的,但是在体外研究中看到,当根管预备和桩长/宽度比受到良好的控制时,用铸造桩系统修复的抗断裂能力显著高于纤维桩。

综上所述,研究表明,保留健康的牙齿结构对于经牙髓治疗过的牙体修复的长期成功是至关重要的,因此不鼓励为了制造出铸造桩&核而去除健康的牙体结构来消除倒凹。因此,仅当存在一壁或更少的牙体组织,具有/不具有理想的肩台时,才考虑使用铸造桩&核,因为铸造桩&核不会减少髓室和/或临床牙冠内轴壁的牙体组织。

如许多临床研究所示,仅余留一个侧壁或更少,带有/不带肩台的牙齿,无论使用预制纤维桩还是铸造桩&核,其长期修复成功率并不高。因此,对于根管治疗后牙齿的修复,临床医生应该进行铸造桩&核治疗,通过仔细设计治疗计划和熟练操作,将铸造桩&核治疗作为尝试修复的最终选择。如果铸造桩&核失败,应选择拔牙和种植或固定、活动义齿修复,以取代治疗失败的牙齿。由于铸造桩&核是受损牙齿冠修复的最后选择,整个过程的目标是要建立牙根-水门汀-铸造桩&核-水门汀-牙冠之间最强的连接,最大程度上使修复牙齿可以维持的时间更久,避免所修复牙齿灾难性失败模式的可能。

11.3 影响铸造桩&核长期成功的因素

铸造桩&核的失败方式包括牙髓治疗失败、根折、桩脱落(有/无牙结构折断),以及冠脱落(Creugers 等 2005)。没有关于发生桩断裂、桩核连接部断裂及核断裂报道,因为铸造桩&核通常是一整块合金铸造的。基于这几种失败方式,以下因素被认为是铸造桩&核修复牙髓治疗牙齿长期预后的决定因素。

11.3.1 保留健康的牙体结构

有许多体外和体内研究显示,无论是铸造桩&核还是预制纤维桩,保留牙齿结构都是桩核修复长期成功的决定性因素。一项 319 个铸造金属桩的随机对照试验,进行了为期 5 年的随访后得出结论,"剩余牙本质高度"这一因素对桩和核修复体的保存有显著影响("实质牙本质高度"为 98%±2%,"最小牙本质高度"为 93%±3%)(Creugers 等 2005)。

近来,将实验室测试与 3-D 有限元分析相结合的体外研究报道显示,无论是桩系统,铸造桩&核,或预制纤维桩,存在 2 mm 肩台(相对于无肩台),对牙髓治疗后的牙齿均显示良好的应力分布并显著提高抗断裂性(Zhou and Wang 2013;Santos-Filho 等 2010)。因此,当使用铸造桩&核来支撑全冠时,不要去除不必要去除的牙体组织,保留尽可能多的健康牙体组织非常重要。

11.3.2 铸造桩 & 核的长度

由于水门汀和铸造桩之间没有化学结合,影响机械固位的粗糙度和表面积是确保铸造桩固位的关键因素。研究已经证明使用更长而不是较厚的铸造桩确实可以提高固位力(Verissimo 等 2014)。体外研究测试具有 3 种不同长度(9 mm、12 mm、15 mm)和顶端直径(0.5 mm、0.9 mm、1.1 mm)的喷砂锥形金属桩的固位强度时发现,固位强度随长度以及桩的直径按比例增加(Shillingburg 等 1970)。除了喷砂之外,使用手持式金刚砂旋转器械对牙本质壁进行粗糙化,并且使用树脂黏结剂,可显著增加桩的固位力,差异有统计学意义(Nergiz 等 2002)。由于保持足够的牙根牙本质厚度,对于防止铸造桩&核的根折发生非常重要,因此增加铸造桩长度以及桩和牙本质壁的粗糙化,是最大限度使桩固位的最有效和最安全的方式。

据悉,相比较长的根管桩,较短的桩被认为会增加根折的发生率(图11-1)。对下颌前磨牙模型的有限元分析研究报道,铸造桩&核的桩尖端区域承受最大的剪切应力,并随着桩长度从 4 mm(90 MPa)增加到 10 mm(30 MPa)而下降(Balbosh 等 2005)。作者得出结论,在以纤维桩和复合树脂核心恢复牙齿结构时,颈部区域的黏结完整性对于修复是否成功起关键作用,而对于铸造桩&核,桩与牙根牙本质的黏结对于修复体长期保存是必不可少的。另外一项体外研究结合实验室测试与三维有限元分析发现,长 7 mm 的长铸造桩(相对于 12 mm 长的桩)显示了明显较

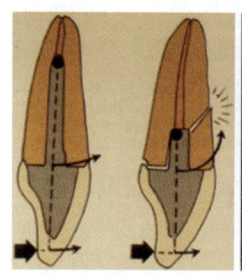

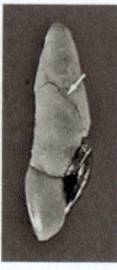

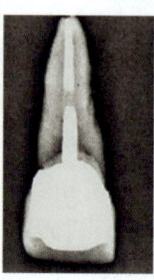

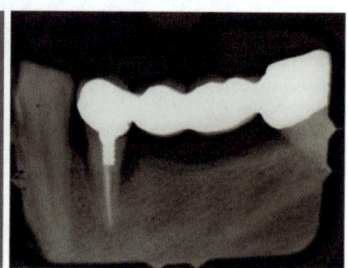

图 11-1 在弯曲时,短桩可以引起应力集中在牙根牙本质的侧方,从而容易引起根折。桩长度越长,力分布在牙根长度上越均匀,因此出现根折的机会较少

11 铸造桩与核

低的抗断裂值,并产生较高的牙折率(Zhou 和 Wang 2013)。作者进一步得出结论,当使用铸造桩&核时,桩应尽可能地长,而纤维桩的生物力学性能对桩的长度不太敏感。

11.3.3 根管预备过程中操作者的临床专业知识

(a)如果根管预备偏离牙体中心,牙钻的切割边缘可能会在牙本质的轴向壁上形成台阶。形成台阶的根部牙本质壁会更薄,并且应力会集中在台阶部位,当使用铸造桩&核时,可能会增加的根折的概率。

(b)根管预备过短可能会导致铸造桩过短,反过来也可能增加脱落和根折的机会。

(c)根管预备过宽可能会导致余留的牙根牙本质壁过薄,也可能增加根折的机会。

(d)根管预备过长或不适当的去除牙胶尖可能会破坏 4~5 mm 的根尖封闭。如第 1 章所示。根尖封闭不全会导致牙髓治疗失败。

11.3.4 铸造桩 & 核和冠的黏固／黏结技术

铸造桩&核与根部牙本质不充分黏结或使用机械性能弱的封闭水门汀可增加桩的脱落以及根折的可能性。全冠与铸造桩&核/牙齿边缘的不充分黏结或使用机械性能弱的水门汀可能会增加冠脱落的机会(Heintze 2010;Kainose 等 2014)。

11.4 预制铸造桩 & 核的临床过程和后续的全冠修复

一旦选定了铸造桩&核,经过仔细的临床和影像学检查,后续就可以选择预制纤维桩核心的叠加,为牙髓治疗后的牙齿进行最后的全冠恢复。铸造桩&核和牙冠治疗的临床顺序如图 11-2 所示。

对铸造桩&核而言,除非牙体牙髓科医师已经预备好根管空间,否则在开始进行根管预备之前首先应进行牙冠预备(图 11-3)。经过理想的牙冠预备后,使用 X 线片确定理想的桩长度。理想的桩长度应是最长可能的长度,保留 4~5 mm 根尖段牙胶尖封闭,而桩宽度不应该超过牙根直径的 1/3。除非牙体牙髓科医师已经完成根管预备,否则应使用加热的垂直充填器(♯5-7,♯9-11)或 System B (SybronEndo)进一步去除牙胶尖。如果没有这些器械可用,可使用适当尺寸的 Gates-Glidden 钻和 Peeso 钻来去除牙胶尖并预备根管空间(图 11-4)。在完成根管预备之前,应拍摄治疗中 X 线片,以确保根管预备保持中心,并保留足够的根尖封闭。使用适当尺寸的 Peeso 钻,小心完成根管预备。理想情况下,在预备的根管轴壁上不应有牙胶尖、台阶或严重的倒凹出现,以实现铸造桩&核与牙根牙本质壁的最大黏结,并减少负荷较重时根折的风险。

第一次就诊
— 治疗前 X 线片
— 冠的预备
— 根管的预备
— 治疗中 X 线片
— 根管预备的完成
选择 1
— 使用 EZ 桩直接制作铸造桩&核模型
— 临时冠与 EZ 桩的制作和黏固
选择 2
— 预备后根管使用根管桩钉取印模
— 临时冠与 EZ 桩的制作和黏固

第二次就诊
— 铸造桩&核的黏固
— 在铸造桩&核上精细冠预备
— 冠制作的最终印模
— 临时冠制作和黏固

第三次就诊
— 冠黏固

图 11-2 铸造桩&核和冠治疗的临床过程

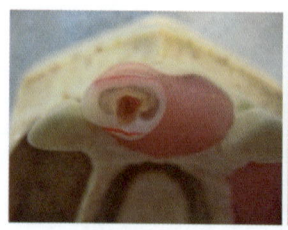

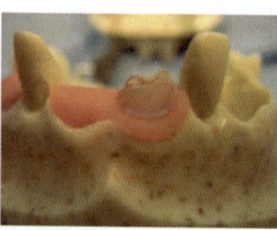

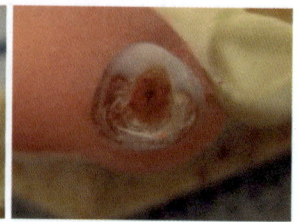

图 11-3 在根管预备之前,如果牙髓病学医生尚未预备根管空间,须进行理想的根管预备

11 铸造桩与核

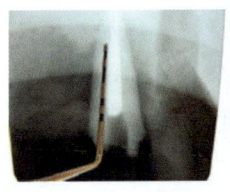

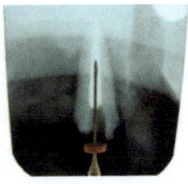

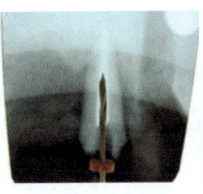

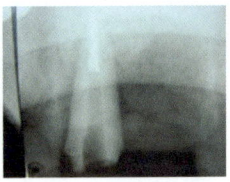

图 11-4 理想的桩长度由 X 线片确定。使用加热的根管垂直充填器(#5~7，#9~11)/System B 或 Gates-Glidden 钻或 Peeso 钻进行牙胶尖清除和根管预备，如果牙髓病学医师没有预备好根管空间。在完成根管预备之前，强烈建议拍摄治疗中 X 线片

11.4.1 应用 EZ 桩和自固化树脂的直接模型技术

从患者口中直接进行模型制作，用于经牙髓治疗的单根单个牙齿的铸造桩&核修复。直接模型可以在患者的口中完成，之后送到技工室进行铸造。同样的技术也可以用来制作直接修复和间接印模制备技术的临时修复体。铸造桩&核直接模型中的桩是使用 EZ 桩系统制成的(白色复合塑料根管桩；Merritt EZ Cast Post Inc.)(Leong 等 2009)。将白色热塑性塑料棒加热至颜色清晰呈熔化状态为止。将塑性复合塑料根管桩放置到已经预备好的根管中，待材料冷却到白色的固体化合物状态，将白色复合塑料根管桩从根管内取出(图 11-5)。如果取出的白色复合桩有空隙或长度短于到根管口的距离，则需要再加入额外的部分熔融化合物，然后将桩放回根管空间以形成完美的桩的形状。完成了铸造桩&核直接模型的桩的部分，直接法的核的部分是用自固化丙烯酸树脂制造的(Pattern Resin LS,GC America Inc.)。

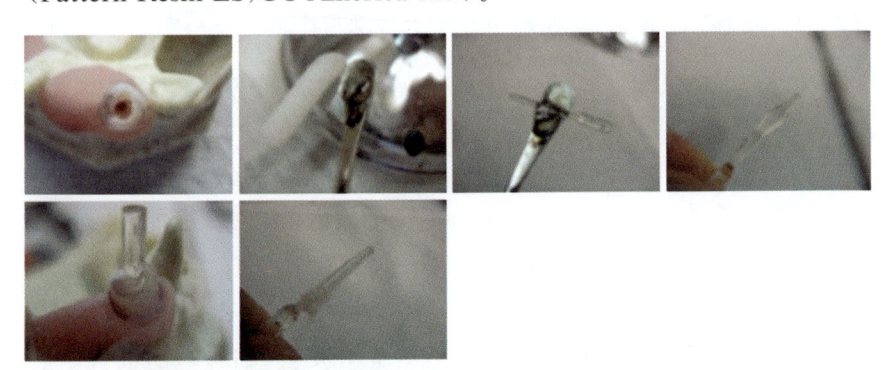

图 11-5 直接法制作铸造桩&核使用 EZ 桩系统(白色热塑性复合塑料根管桩)。白色的复合材料一旦加热将变成透明色。取用融化的化合物与塑料根管桩一起放入预备好的根管。一旦颜色变白后硬固，将白色复合物与塑料根管桩从根管内取出

当根管桩完全贴合患者的根管,用紫貂刷将模型树脂聚合物和单体环刷在塑料根管桩的周围。必须小心不要将树脂单体或聚合物滴落在患者的软组织上。当足够的自凝树脂包围在根管桩周围并硬化,则可对直接模型的核部分用金刚砂钻原位制备。如果在预备过程中直接桩&核模型不稳固,可使用牙周探针将模型保持在适当的位置。直接模型的核部分应与剩余的牙颈部连续,不应留下额外的溢出物。拆下完整的直接桩&核模型,以确保核部分与桩紧密相连。按照制备指南进行预备,以确保获得理想的核形状。当核部分的制作完成,达到理想的解剖形态,桩核的直接模型是通过其被动贴合进入根管空间的。为了减小由铸造桩&核引起的牙根折裂的概率,最终的铸造桩&核应被动地放置,而不与牙根牙本质的轴向壁发生摩擦。将直接桩&核模型的白色化合物或红自凝丙烯酸树脂的倒凹用热蜡刀和/或金刚砂钻削磨,直到获得直接模型与根管空间的绝对被动贴合(图11-6)。

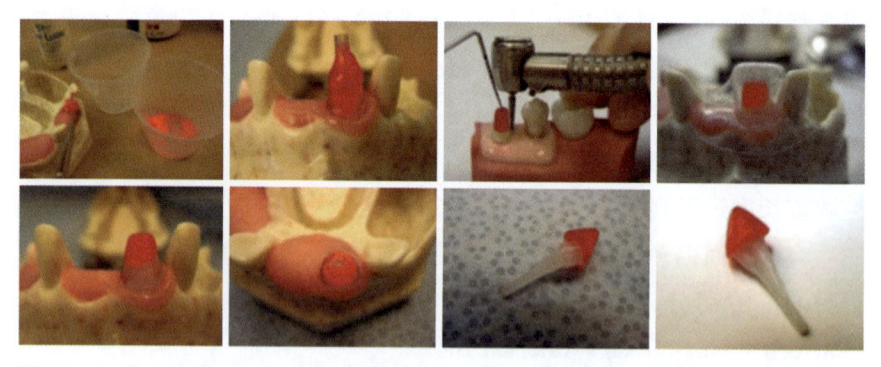

图11-6 铸造桩&核模型的核部分是在患者的口腔采用自固化丙烯酸树脂(模型树脂)和紫貂刷加在塑料根管桩的周围。安置后,直接铸造桩&核模型用一个牙周探针按住,核部分预备作理想基牙。真空外形制备指南可用于确认核部分的理想制备。消除EZ桩模型来源的任何倒凹,直接铸造桩&核模型应该无缝过渡到剩余的牙齿结构并与根管被动贴合

将桩&核的直接模型放置在一个拉链袋内,避免放错地方。另一个EZ桩是使用相同方法来制造单件临时冠和EZ桩。当桩的部分完成,塑料根管桩的柄部采用加热的#7蜡刀处理成钉头状。确保含有塑料钉头的白色塑料桩钉在患者口腔内充分安置,临时冠的油灰基质不影响钉头。将临时修复材料应用于油灰基质中,并将该基质固定在牙齿上。硬固后,单件EZ桩临时冠从根管空间取出。这时我们应检查

11　铸造桩与核

临时冠,以确保临时冠和白色复合桩之间的交界处是坚强和无缝的。在这种特殊情况下,EZ 桩的倒凹连接是我们所希望的,以获得临时冠的辅助固位。这种冠的黏固使用临时水门汀,水门汀仅限用于冠缘,而不是在 EZ 桩周围,以便于在以后的就诊中从根管空间除去水门汀(图 11-7)。咬合应该精心调整,而后患者结束本次治疗。直接桩＆核模型送到技工室进行铸造。

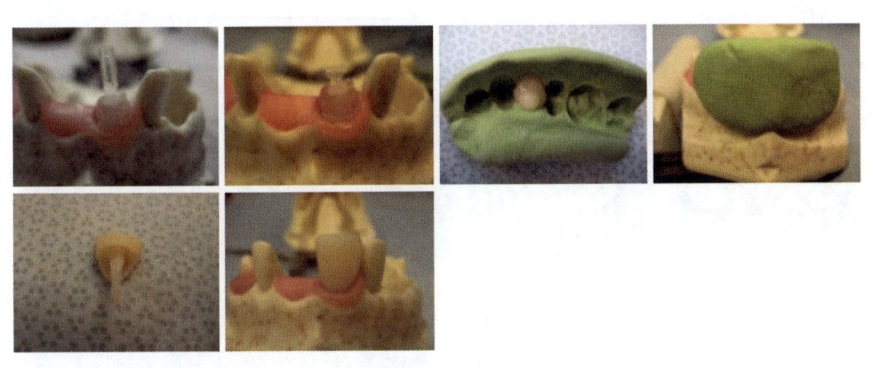

图 11-7　用相同方法另外制作 1 个 EZ 桩模型的临时冠。与通过增加 GC 模型树脂来制作直接模型的核部分不同,桩钉的头部是用加热的 ♯7 蜡刀去按压塑料根管桩形成。临时修复材料应用到油灰基质中,而这种基质被覆盖在牙齿上。硬固后,将单件临时冠-EZ 桩从根管空间取出。在此病例中,余留 EZ 桩的倒凹连接是为了临时冠的辅助固位。临时冠-EZ 桩用的临时水门汀黏固

11.4.2　间接印模技术

在预备后的根管中应用这种印模技术是多颗牙齿铸造桩＆核或在多根管的单颗磨牙中制作多个铸造桩＆核的适应证。在患者口腔内为多颗牙齿制作直接桩＆核模型并不能有效地利用时间。此外,如果患者怀孕或对自固化丙烯酸树脂过敏,间接印模技术也是其适应证,间接印模技术还适用于单个铸造桩＆核制作。

在多个牙或多根牙上完成牙冠的预备和根管的预备后,可在根管空间试用不同尺寸的塑料根管桩,根管桩应松弛地贴合根管而没有牵拉感,并切成适当长度。使用加热的 ♯7 蜡刀,制作钉头作为印模过程中的一个附加固位。钉头的位置应该包含在理想的核轮廓内,使印模托盘不妨碍塑料桩。每个根管应该有一个正确的尺寸和长度的塑料根管桩。所有的根管桩涂有聚乙烯基硅氧烷(PVS)印模胶。将适当尺寸的排龈线放置

在预备的牙齿颈缘,清洁根管并用纸尖干燥。将 PVS 轻体印模材料的窄针头深置于根管空间内,挤出 PVS 印模材料,注射器针尖后退。一旦根管充满了 PVS 印模材料,将涂布黏结剂的塑料根管桩穿过 PVS 材料推入根管。更多的 PVS 印模材料应用在牙齿的边缘,并将盛有单体 PVS 印模材料的托盘安放到患者的口中。一旦印模材料凝固,取出托盘,并且对根管空间和牙冠边缘的印模进行仔细评估(图 11-8)。去除牙齿颈缘周围的排龈线。

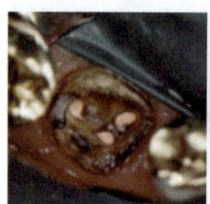

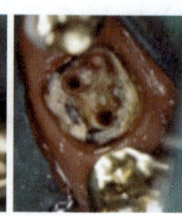

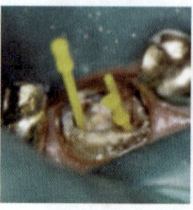

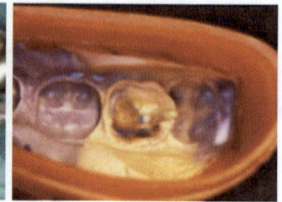

图 11-8　间接印模技术

使用相同的 EZ 桩技术,制作临时修复体并用临时水门汀黏固。如果需要,多个临时修复体连接成夹板,方便医生并获得更好的固位。精心调整咬合后让患者返回。最终的 PVS 印模将送技工室进行铸造桩&核的制作。图 11-9 显示了两件键和键槽铸造桩&核制作技工室程序。间接印模技术用在多颗牙齿的多个铸造桩&核上,如图 11-10 所示。一旦铸造桩&核准备黏固,自黏结双固化树脂水门汀可用于将铸造桩&核黏结到牙根的牙本质壁上。在 6~10 分钟的凝固时间后,可进行已黏结的铸造桩&核和牙齿边缘的最终牙冠预备,然后制作全冠的最终 PVS 印模。临时冠制作并用临时水门汀黏固。一旦牙冠准备好黏固,自黏结双固化树脂水门汀可用于将全冠黏结到铸造桩&核和牙齿边缘。仔细调整咬合。

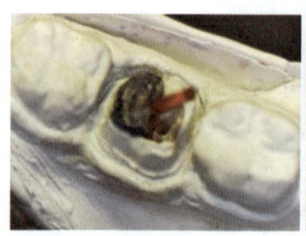

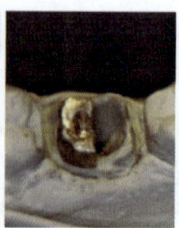

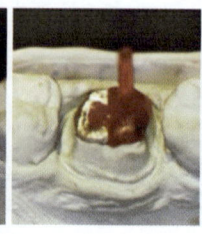

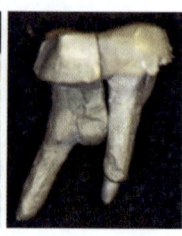

图 11-9　使用铸石间接印模技术制作的两片铸造桩&核的实验室程序

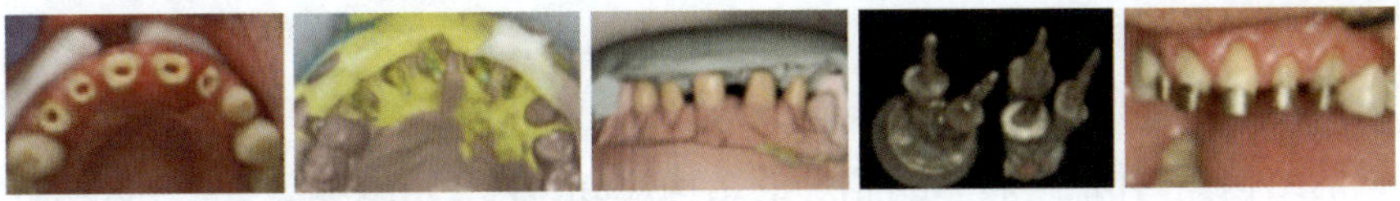

图 11-10　采用间接印模技术的多个铸造桩&核治疗过程(Dr. John Keyes 提供)

11.5　黏固/黏结铸造桩 & 核以及全冠修复体

铸造桩&核的脱落和牙冠的脱落是根管治疗后牙齿修复失败的常见原因。选择合适的黏固/黏结材料是铸造桩&核降低脱落和根折的非常重要的措施。当使用树脂水门汀封闭时,用 50 μm 氧化铝颗粒对铸造桩&核喷砂已被证明能增加铸造桩&核的固位(Rosenstiel 等 1977)。使用手持金刚砂旋转切削工具在粗糙的牙根牙本质壁(196D.644.090;Erlangen Post System;Brasseler)内旋转 3 次,并使用树脂黏结水门汀,统计学显示显著提高根管桩的固位(nergiz 等 2002)。在一项体外对铸造桩&核使用不同的水门汀的黏结效果的研究中发现,双固化树脂水门汀(838 N)的抗折强度明显高于树脂改性玻璃离子水门汀(613 N)和磷酸锌水门汀(643 N)(Young 等 1985)。

近期的两个有限元分析研究认为,较高的应力集中在铸造桩&核的尖端和铸造桩-牙本质壁的界面,而纤维桩和树脂堆集病例中应力集中在颈部黏结区(balbosh 等 2005;Santos-Filho 等 2014)。作者进一步得出结论：铸造桩的黏结对铸造桩&核修复的牙齿的保留至关重要。因此,在铸造桩&核与牙本质壁之间获得最长时间的绝对被动贴合是非常重要的,而喷砂后的铸造桩&核应采用自黏结双固化树脂水门汀黏结到粗糙化了的牙根牙本质上。当铸造桩&核用自黏结树脂水门汀黏结,抗折强度高于纤维桩组(Zhou and Wang 2013;Santos-Filho 等 2014)。这些结果与 meta 分析研究结论相一致,结合 13 项体外研究,结果表明铸造桩比纤维桩具有更高的抗断裂能力(Ellner 等 2003)。

一项 91 例 3 年以上的随机对照试验,比较了不同弹性模量钛桩和纤维桩的自黏结树脂水门汀黏结的临床效果(Naumann 等 2007)。结果显示,3 年期间均无失败病例。钛的弹性模量约为 110 GPa,高于金的弹性模量,此临床结果间接支持使用金合金铸造桩&核时使用自黏树脂水门汀。

有限元研究发现,健康的牙齿结构趋于通过釉质转移负荷,围绕在牙齿中心,进入牙根的牙本质,表明应力将会更加集中在具有较高的弹性模量的结构上,并最终转移到相邻的结构(Santos-Filho等2014)。这就解释了为什么加载冠的应力集中在比纤维桩和复合树脂核芯的弹性模量更高的铸造桩&核上。为了减少对铸造桩&核应力集中和向牙根部牙本质传递负荷,在铸造桩&核的铸石模型上制作牙冠时保留足够的无效腔,当硬的牙冠和铸造桩&核之间使用复合树脂水门汀时,就能提供足够的水门汀空间。同时冠边缘之间应具有对牙齿边缘的紧密接触,无论是牙釉质还是牙根牙本质。随着这种紧密的适应,更多的应力转移会发生在牙冠到牙齿边缘,而不是转移到铸造桩&核上并随之传到牙根的牙本质壁上,从而使牙冠和铸造桩&核连接稳固,引导更好的应力分布,推荐使用双固化复合树脂水门汀,如自黏结树脂水门汀。同类型的自粘树脂水门汀可用于将铸造桩&核黏结于牙根的牙本质壁上,也可用于将牙冠黏结于铸造桩&核/牙齿边缘上。

体外研究表明,金属冠较烤瓷冠、铸造桩&核较纤维桩,2 mm较1 mm或0 mm的肩台,有着显著更高的抗断裂性(Santos-Filho等2014)。作者认为,无论使用的是铸造桩还是纤维桩,高弹性模量的氧化铝强化陶瓷冠增加了系统的硬度,从而影响了应力分布。铸造桩&核系统的抗断裂抗力范围从724 N～1 026(Santos-Filho等2014),高于人的上颌和下颌第一磨牙之间产生的最大咬紧力。如果患者有磨牙症或紧咬牙,对铸造桩&核修复的后牙应进行仔细地咬合调整,以增加修复的长期成功率。

11.6 总结

研究表明,尽可能多的保留健康牙齿结构,是根管治疗后牙齿修复长期成功的最重要因素,因此不主张磨除健康的牙齿结构只是为了消除倒凹来制作铸造桩&核。当只有一个壁或更少/有或没有理想的肩台时,应考虑铸造桩&核,这样就不需要再从髓腔和/或临床牙冠的内轴壁处减少牙体组织了。

许多临床研究表明,无论使用哪种类型的桩(纤维桩或铸造桩),仅余一壁或更少/有或无肩台的牙齿,长期修复成功率都不高。因此,对于根管治疗后牙齿的修复，临床医师应该将铸造桩&核治疗作为最后的尝试。如果铸造桩&核失败，应选择拔牙和种植或固定、活动义齿修复，以取代治疗失败的牙齿。由于铸造桩&核的修复是受损牙齿最后的选择，整个过程的目标是要建立牙根-水门汀-铸造桩&核-水门汀-牙冠之间最强的连接，为的是修复牙齿可以维持时间最久，直到它失败而不再担心修复牙齿的失败模式。

当根管治疗后的牙齿出现牙齿结构受损时，预制纤维桩更趋于机械性失败，包括桩脱落，桩核断裂和冠脱落。铸造桩&核可以消除纤维桩与核修复之间的至少一个弱连接，因此桩核的断裂或冠的脱落率可降低。另一方面，铸造桩&核失败造成根折的原因主要是由于短桩的存在和牙根的牙本质和铸造桩&核之间不同的弹性模量。而使用纤维桩时，桩的长度对根折率并没有显著影响，但是使用铸造桩&核时则有明显影响，短的铸造桩与根折相关性更大。因此，临床医师的专业知识、在根管预备中获得理想的桩的长度和保持最多的牙根牙本质，以及去除牙根牙本质轴向壁的薄壁弱尖，对减少根折的失败率是非常重要的，特别是当使用不同弹性模量的铸造桩&核时。

获得理想的根管预备桩的空间，同时保持最多的牙齿结构，建议使用完全被动贴合模式的喷砂铸造桩&核，用自黏结双固化树脂水门汀黏固，能提供最大程度的固位和强度。桩尽可能长，并保持4～5 mm根尖密封，用复合树脂水门汀封闭被动贴合的铸造桩和牙根之间的牙本质空隙，铸造桩&核-树脂水门汀-牙根系统可成为一个坚固的结构，能够使0.2 mm厚的牙周韧带及周围骨组织承担大部分咬合负荷。铸造桩&核没有薄弱的交界处，而预制纤维桩和核之间存在薄弱的交界。因此，铸造桩&核交界处和铸造核的变形可能小于纤维桩与核系统的变形。在经根管治疗且剩余牙齿结构有限的牙齿上，结合应用具有长桩的被动贴合适应的单件铸造桩&核与复合树脂水门汀黏结的铸造桩&核的技术，可以降低铸造桩&核失败率、根折、铸造桩&核脱落，以及牙冠脱落。

完全被动法制作的全冠可以进一步用自黏结双固化树脂水门汀与铸造桩&核部分进行黏固，以提供牙冠的最大固位力以及牙冠-树脂水门汀-铸造核/牙齿边缘之间的最大强度。通过实现最强最坚固的牙根-树脂水门汀-铸造桩&核-树脂水门汀-牙冠系统，铸造桩&核修复根管治疗后的牙齿可能类似于最初牙齿的工作模式,牙周膜可发挥减震机制功能,从而减少根折的发生率、提高长期成功率。

即使在对比铸造桩&核和预制纤维桩核修复系统的有效性和优势研究中,有一些研究结果有冲突,经过精心设计和熟练操作制作的铸造桩&核,可能在余留牙齿结构有限的根管治疗后的牙齿中,仍是比预制纤维桩和核更为优先的选择。铸造桩&核作为修复治疗的最后选择,适用于那些希望尽可能长时间的保存患牙,且当铸造桩&核失败时也愿意接受拔牙和牙种植或固定义齿治疗的患者。

(孙喆 译)

参考文献

Baibosh A, Ludwig K, Kern M (2005) Comparison of titanium dowel retention using four different luting agents. J Prosthet Dent 94: 227–233.

Bergman B, Lundquist P, Sjögren U, Sundquist G (1989) Restorative and endodontic results after treatment with cast posts and cores. J Prosthet Dent 61: 10–15.

Bolla M, Muller-Bolla M, Borg C, Lupi-Pegurier L, Laplanche O, Leforestier E (2007) Root canal posts for the restoration of root filled teeth. Cochrane Database Syst Rev CD004623. http: //www.ncbi.nlm.nih.gov/pubmed/17253516.

Creugers NH, Mentink AG, Kayser AF (1993) An analysis of durability data on post and core restorations. J Dent 21: 281–284.

Creugers NH, Mentink AG, Fokkinga WA, Kreulen CM (2005) 5–year follow-up of a prospective clinical study on various types of core restorations. Int J Prosthodont 18: 34–39.

Ellner S, Bergendal T, Bergman B (2003) Four post-and-core combinations as abutments for fixed single crowns: a prospective up to 10–year study. Int J Prosthodont 16: 249–254.

Ferrari M, Vichi A, Garcia-Godoy F (2000) Clinical evaluation of fiber-reinforced epoxy resin posts and cast post and cores. Am J Dent 13: 15B–18B.

Ferrari M, Cagidiaco MC, Goracci C, Vichi A, Mason PN, Radovic I, Tay F (2007) Long-term retrospective study of the clinical performance of fiber posts. Am J Dent 20: 287–291.

Ferrari M, Vichi A, Fadda GM, et al., Goracci C (2012) A randomized controlled trial of endodontically treated and restored premolars. J Dent Res 91: 725–785.

Heintze SD (2010) Crown pull-off test (crown retention test) to evaluate the bonding effectiveness of luting agents. Dent Mater 26: 193–206.

Heydecke G, Peters MC (2002) The restoration of endodonticaily treated, single-rooted teeth with cast or direct posts and cores: a systematic review. J Prosthet Dent 87: 380–386.

Kainose K, Nakajima M, Foxton R, et al., Tagami J (2014) Stress distribution in root filled teeth restored with various post and core techniques: effect of post length and crown height. Int Endod J. doi: 10.1111/iej.12397 [Epub ahead of print].

Leong EW, Choon Tan KB, Nicholls JI, Chua EK, Wong KM, Neo JC (2009) The effect of preparation height and luting agent on the resistance form of cemented cast crowns under load fatigue. J Prosthet Dent 102: 155–164.

Mentink AGB, Meeuwissen R, Kfiyser AF, Mulder J (1993) Survival rate and failure characteristics of the all metal post and core restoration. J Oral Rehabil 20: 455–461.

Naumann M, Sterzenbac G, Alexandra F, Dietrich T (2007) Randomized controlled clinical pilot trial of titanium vs. glass fiber prefabricated posts: preliminary results after up to 3 years. Int J Prosthodont 20: 499-503.

Nergiz I, Schmage P, Ozcan M, Platzer U (2002) Effect of length and diameter of tapered posts on the retention. J Oral Rehabil 29: 28-34.

Preethi G, Kala M (2008) Clinical evaluation of carbon fiber reinforced carbon endodontic post, glass fiber reinforced post with cast post and core: a one year comparative clinical study. J Conserv Dent 1 I: 162-167.

Prothero JH (1921) Prosthetic dentistry. Medico-Dental Publishers, Chicago, pp. 1153-1174.

Rosenstiel SF, Land MF, Holloway JA (1977) Custom-cast post fabrication with a thermoplastic material. J Prosthet Dent 77: 209-211.

Santos-Filho PC, Verfssimo C, Soares PV, et al., Marcondes Martins LR (2014) Influence of ferrule, post system, and length on biomechanical behavior of endodontically treated anterior teeth. J Endod 40: 119-123.

Sarkis-Onofre R, Jacinto Rde C, Boscato N, et al., Pereira-Cenci T (2014) Cast metal vs. glass fiber posts: a randomized controlled trial with up to 3 years of follow up. J Dent 42: 582-587.

Shillingburg HT, Kessler JC (1982) Restoration of the endodontically treated tooth. Quintessence Publishing Co., Inc, Chicago, pp. 13-44.

Shillingburg HT, Fisher DW, Dewhirst RB (1970) Restoration of the endodontically treated posterior teeth. J Prosthet Dent 24: 401-409.

Theodosopoulou JN, Chochlidakis KM (2009) Systematic review of dowel (post) and core materials and systems. J Prosthodont 18: 464-472.

Torbjörner A, Karlsson S, Odman PA (1995) Survival rate and failure characteristics for two post designs. J Prosthet Dent 73: 439-444.

Verfssimo C, Simamoto Jfinior PC, Soares CJ, et al., Santos-Filho PCF (2014) Effect of the crown, post, and remaining coronal dentin on the biomechanical behavior of endodontically treated maxillary central incisors. J Prosthet Dent 111: 234-246.

Young HM, Shen C, Maryniuk GA (1985) Retention of cast posts relative to cement selection. Quintessence Int 16: 357-360.

Zhou L, Wang Q (2013) Comparison of fracture resistance between cast posts and fiber posts: a meta-analysis of literature. J Endod 39: 11-15.

Zicari F, van Meerbeek B, Debels E, et al., Naert I (2011) An up to 3-year controlled clinical trial comparing the outcome of glass fiber posts and composite cores with gold alloy-based posts and cores for the restoration of endodontically treated teeth. Int J Prosthodont 24: 363-372.

临床过程 12

乔治·戈梅斯(George Gomes)
乔奇·佩尔迪高(Jorge Perdigão)

摘 要

本章用图阐述了两例上颌中切牙分别用自黏结水门汀与纤维桩黏固,复合树脂堆塑和烤瓷氧化锆冠的一步一步地治疗过程。两个视频还将演示以黏结技术用材料和器械在根管中黏固纤维桩。

下面是使用自黏结黏固技术或常规黏固技术一步一步黏结纤维桩治疗方案。

12.1 自黏结黏固技术

材料

Ⅰ.纤维桩

Ⅱ.自酸蚀树脂水门汀

Ⅲ.双固化树脂核芯

1. 用(蒸馏)水冲洗根管并用纸尖干燥。
2. 将伸长的尖端插入根管内,并在根尖区域开始注射自黏结水门汀。
3. 立即将桩插入根管,保持桩上轻柔的垂直压力为5~10秒。
4. 用小毛刷清除桩周围多余的水门汀;光固化40秒。
5. 用低速圆钻暴露牙本质的新鲜面,以免过量的自黏结树脂水门汀扩散到冠部牙本质。用30%~40%的磷酸酸蚀暴露的牙本质和牙釉质15秒,冲洗10秒,然后空气轻轻吹干。

6. 应用牙本质黏结剂作用 20 秒,空气轻轻吹干,以蒸发溶剂,按各自的制造商推荐的操作流程,光固化 20 秒。

7. 根据牙体制备的大小,树脂核芯堆塑材料可以徒手或使用成型片。如果一个明显的赛璐珞冠形状需要塑造核芯的形状,则选择相应的尺寸。用剪刀修整赛璐珞冠的外形,调整成型片对应牙齿结构。

8. 注入复合材料,从不同方向光固化 40 秒。

12.2 传统黏固技术

材料

Ⅰ. 纤维桩

Ⅱ. 黏结系统

Ⅲ. 双固化复合树脂水门汀

Ⅳ. 双固化复合材料核芯

1. 酸蚀-冲洗技术是首选,用 30%～40% 的磷酸酸蚀根管壁和预备的冠方 15 秒。如果需要,用纸尖将酸蚀剂涂布在全部根管壁上。

2. 冲洗 10 秒;以纸尖干燥根管。

3. 用小头小毛刷将牙本质黏结剂送入根管,并在根管内反复旋转刷几次;涂黏结剂于牙齿冠方作用 20 秒。

4. 用纸尖将黏结剂溶剂从根管中吸出,直至纸尖从根管中返回呈干燥状态。在冠方上,轻轻用空气吹干黏合剂以蒸发溶剂。按各自的制造商推荐的流程光固化 20 秒。

5. 刷去桩表面残留的黏结剂,空气吹干 5 秒,光固化 10 秒。

6. 将双固化树脂水门汀注入根管,从根尖区开始。

7. 立即将桩插入根管,保持轻微垂直压力 5～10 秒。

8. 光固化复合材料 40 秒。

9. 根据制备的大小,树脂核芯堆塑材料可以徒手或使用成型片。如果一个明显的赛璐珞冠形状需要塑造核芯的形状,则选择相应的尺寸。用剪刀修整赛璐珞冠的外形,调整成型片对应牙齿结构。

10. 注入复合材料,从不同方向光固化 40 秒。

12 临床过程

临床病例,纤维桩、复合材料堆塑和烤瓷氧化锆全冠的两例修复体

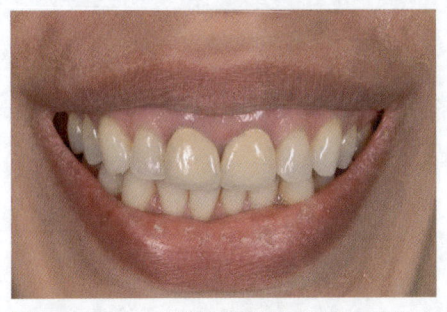

图 12 - 1　24 岁的女性患者,主诉为美学上的缺陷"所有的时候我都不敢笑。"有上颌中切牙外伤史,曾行根管治疗和金属烤瓷冠修复。患者的既往病史无特殊情况。

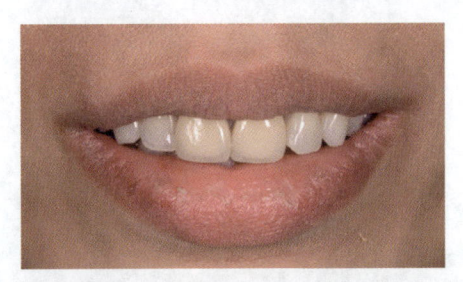

图 12 - 2

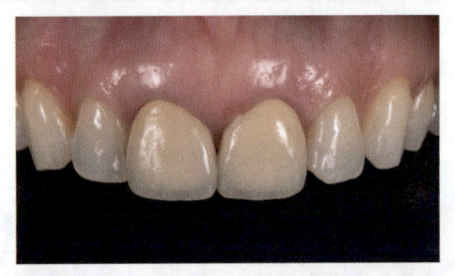

图 12 - 3

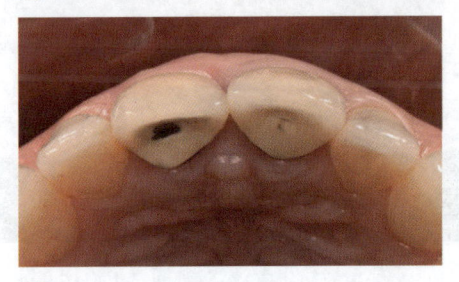

图 12 - 4
图 12 - 2、12 - 3、12 - 4　美学缺陷牙冠的基本情况观察

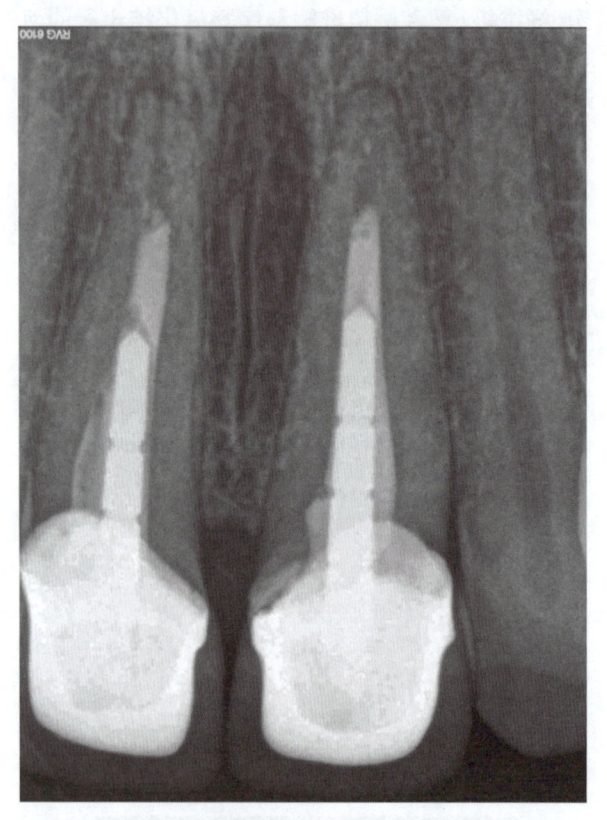

图 12-5 上颌中切牙-根尖片的基本条件显示扩大了的根管内有预制金属桩,以及根管治疗有缺陷。

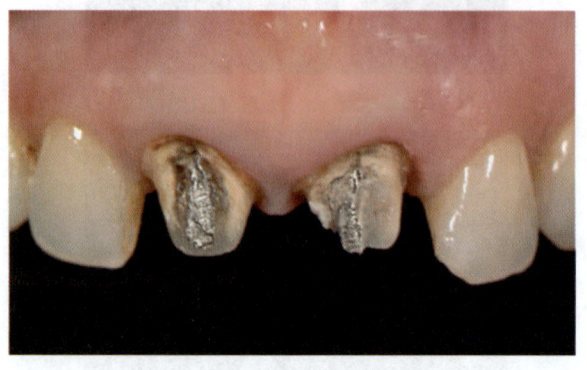

图 12-6 上蜡型后给患者观察,她同意了治疗方案。现有的金属烤瓷冠和各自的黏结剂被拆除。

12 临床过程

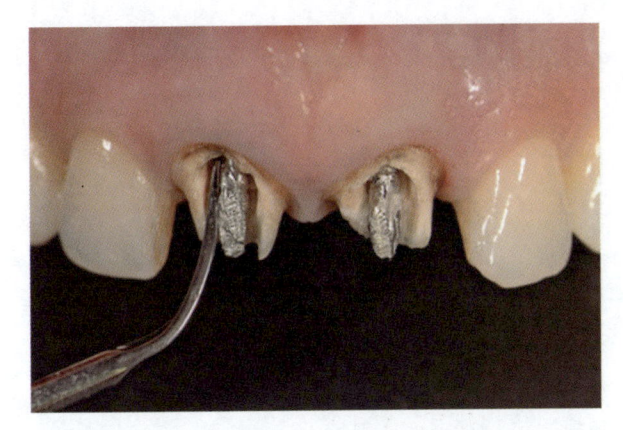

247

图 12-7 预制金属桩用超声波装置和高速手机的小金刚砂车针去除

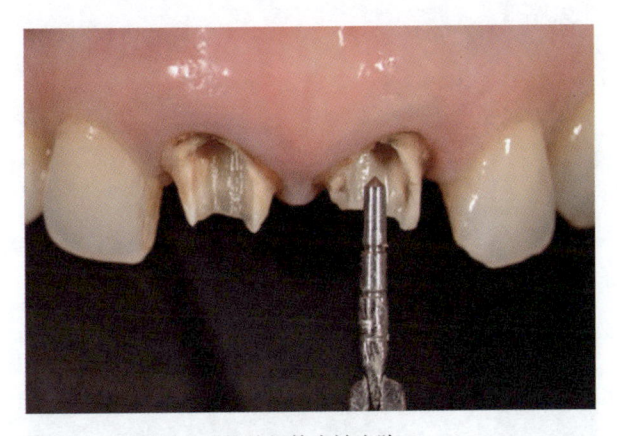

图 12-8 预制金属桩从根管内被去除

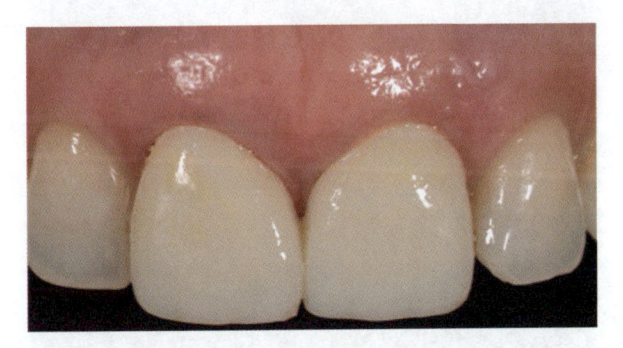

图 12-9 定制的预成临时修复体用双丙烯酸复合树脂制作（Protemp Plus/4，3M ESPE）

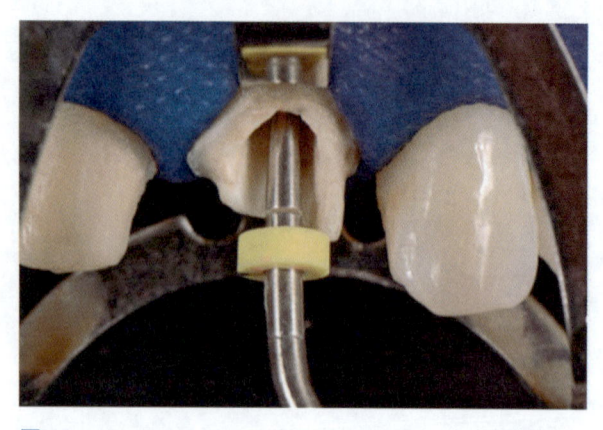

图 12‑10 根管再治疗后,牙胶尖用 System B 的热源（Sybronendo）去除直至先前在根尖片确定的根管长度。然后,剩余的牙胶尖用手用垂直充填器压紧,保留至少 5 mm 的根尖封闭。

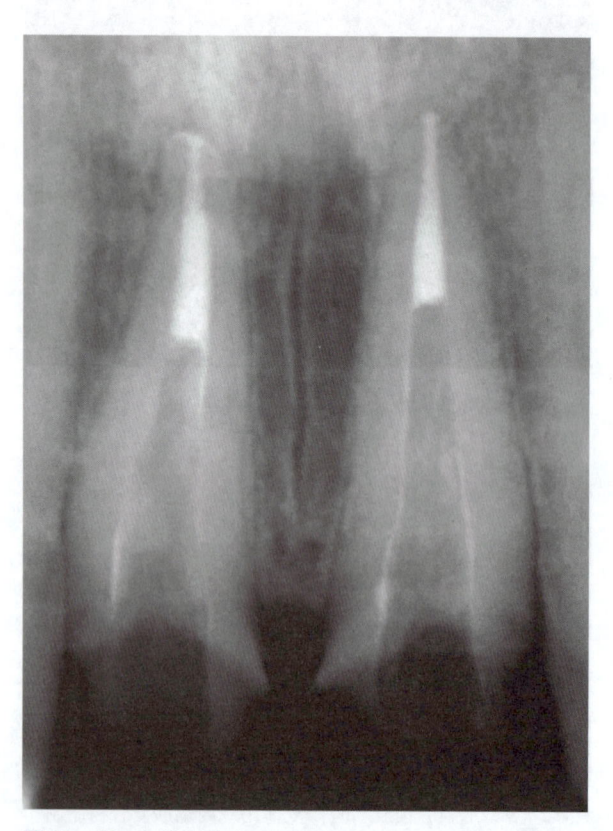

图 12‑11 根管再治疗后的根尖片

12 临床过程

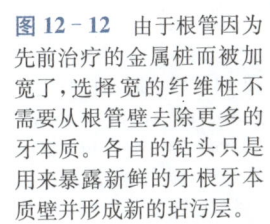

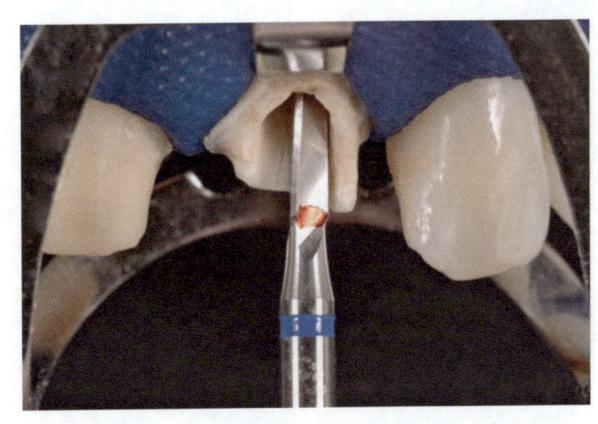

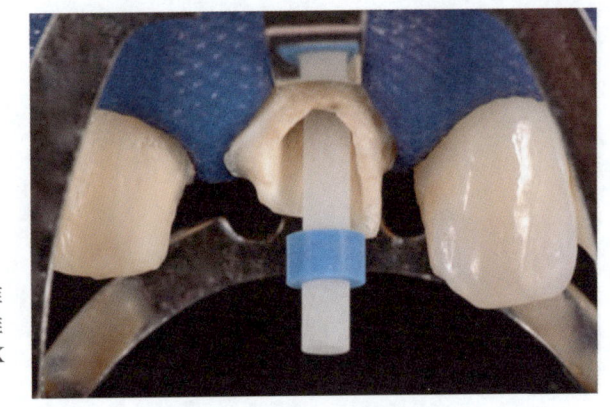

图 12‑12　由于根管因为先前治疗的金属桩而被加宽了,选择宽的纤维桩不需要从根管壁去除更多的牙本质。各自的钻头只是用来暴露新鲜的牙根牙本质壁并形成新的玷污层。

图 12‑13　各自试用双锥度纤维桩(#3 RelyX 纤维桩,3M ESPE),并拍摄 X 线片检查是否适应根管。

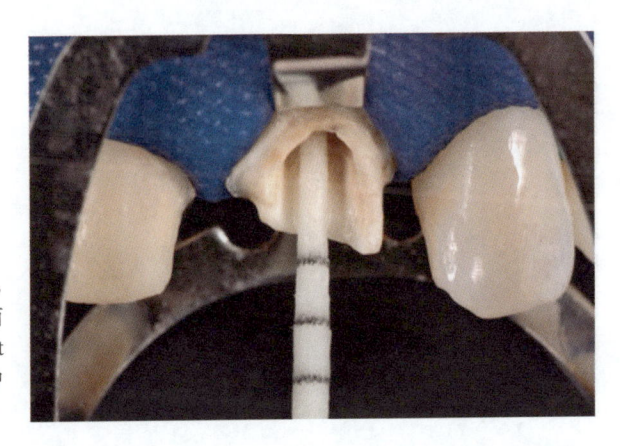

图 12‑14　根管用 2.5% NaOCl 冲洗,纸尖干燥。而后,95% 乙醇用 Monoject (Covidien)冲洗注射器冲洗根管,以纸尖干燥根管。

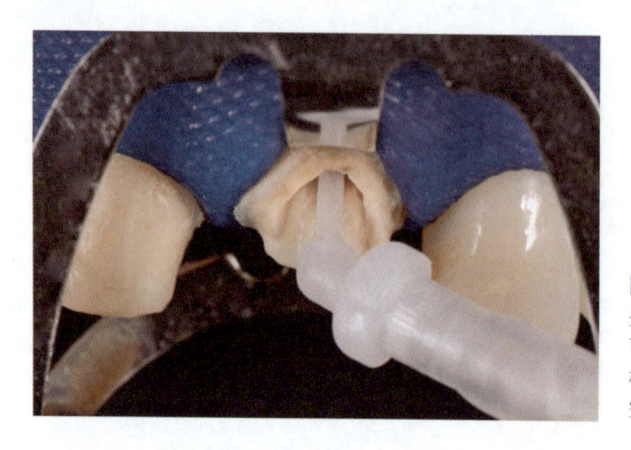

图 12-15 用加长的注射头将自黏结水门汀 RelyX Unicem 2（3M ESPE）注入根管内，从桩的根尖部分空间开始。

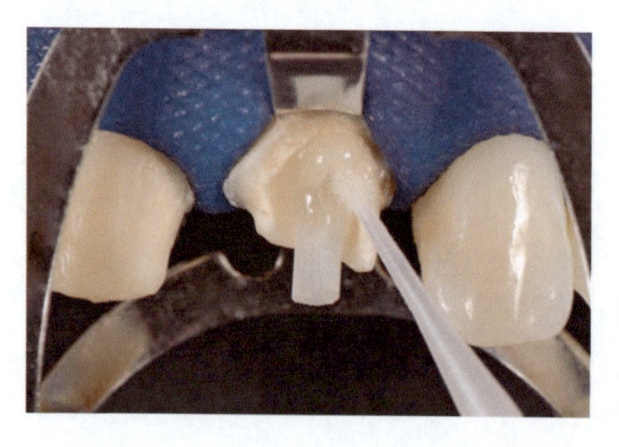

图 12-16 多余的水门汀用一次性刷子去除，避免堵塞桩周围区域的复合堆塑材料的固位肩领。

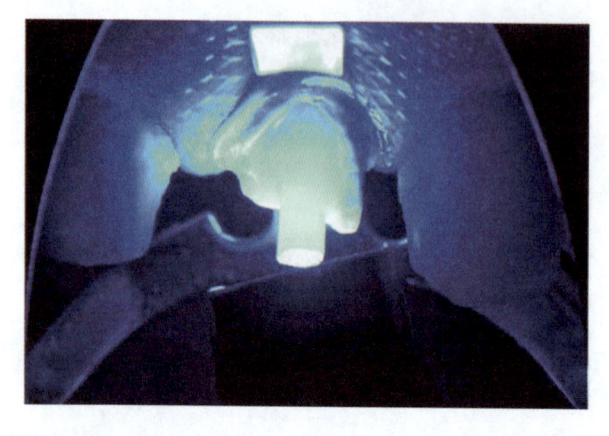

图 12-17 暴露的自黏结水门汀光固化 40 秒

12 临床过程

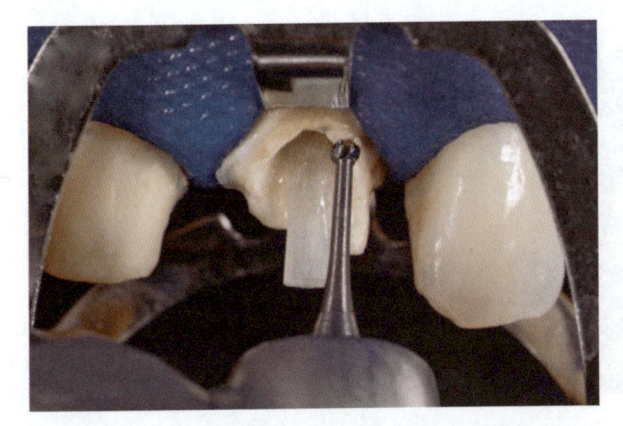

图 12-18 用低速圆钻暴露新鲜牙本质表面,去除残留水门汀碎屑并形成新的玷污层。

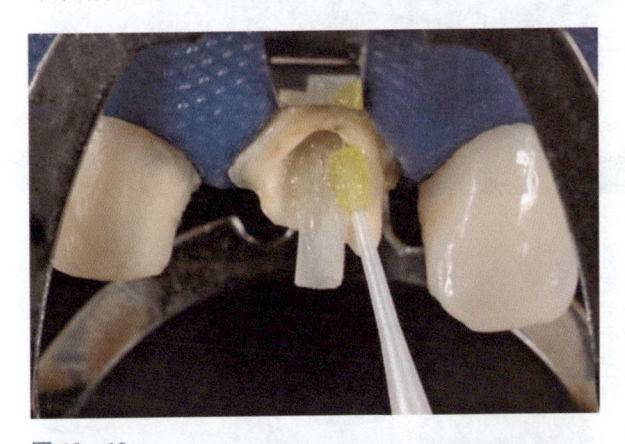

图 12-19

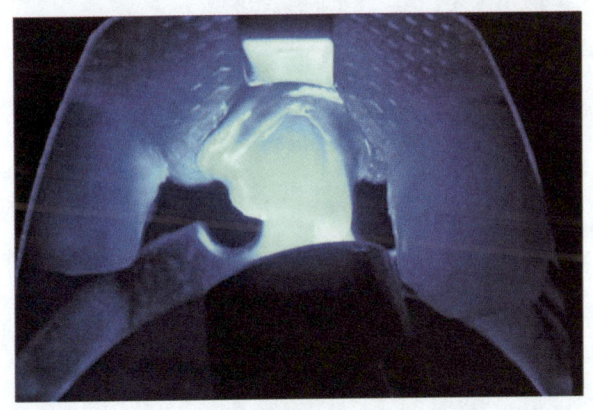

图 12-20
图 12-19、12-20 用34%磷酸酸蚀15秒后,冲洗10秒,再用空气轻轻吹干,涂布牙本质黏结剂,用空气轻轻吹干以蒸发溶剂,光固化20秒。

根管治疗后的牙体修复

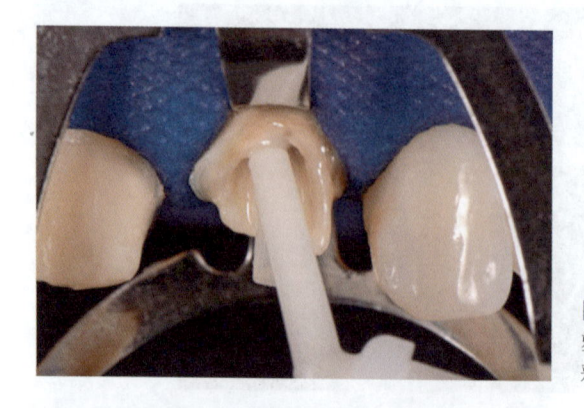

图 12-21　注入双固化复合堆塑材料（Paracore，Coltene），从颊侧和舌侧分别光固化 40 秒。

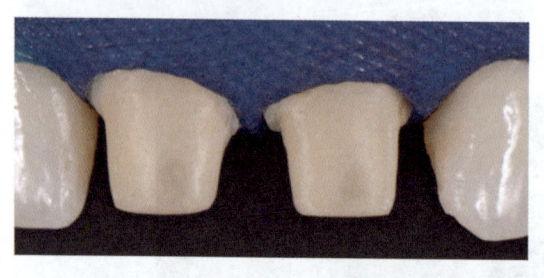

图 12-22　15 分钟后预备完成

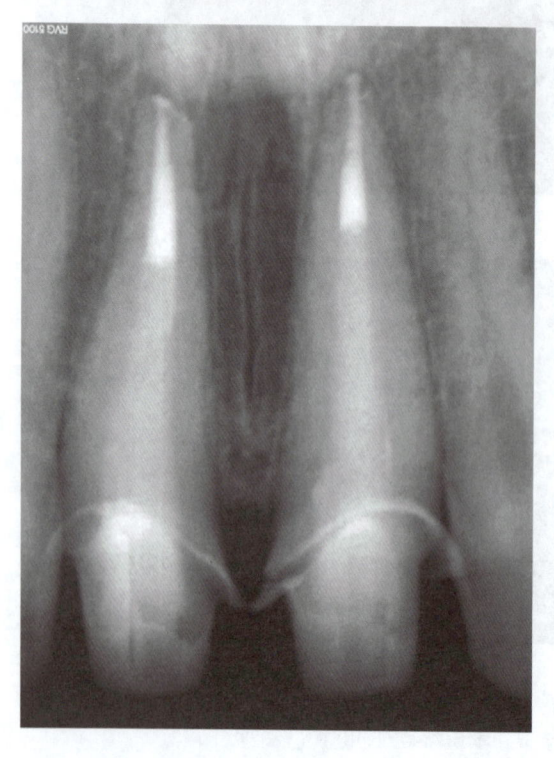

图 12-23　根尖片显示桩黏固在根管内，以及核心堆塑完成

12　临床过程

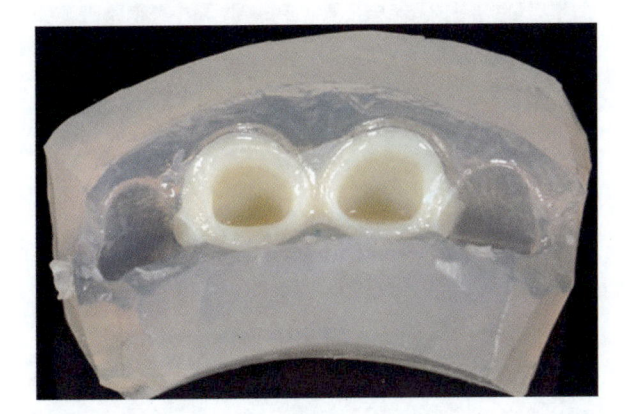

图 12-24

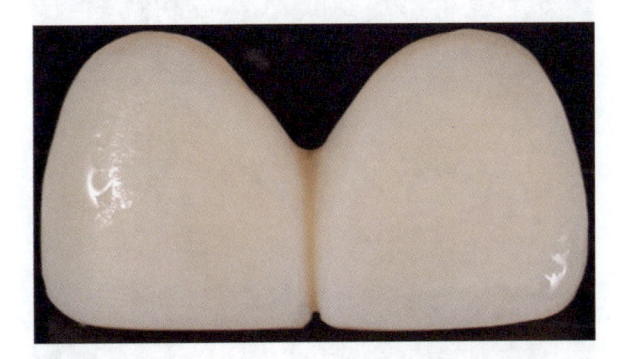

图 12-25

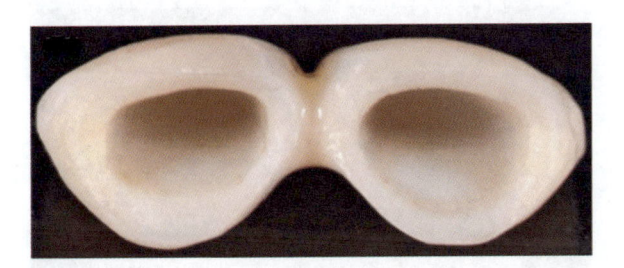

图 12-26
图 12-24、12-25、12-26　新定做的临时修复体使用聚硅氧烷基质填充双丙烯复合树脂制作（Protemp Plus/4,3M ESPE）。聚乙烯硅氧烷模板复制了术前的蜡型,作为最终修复的蓝图。根据患者的建议作了调整。临时修复体用砂纸盘和橡胶抛光头抛光。

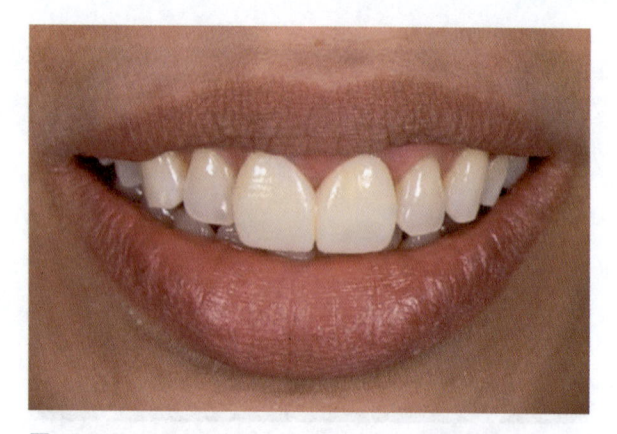

图 12-27

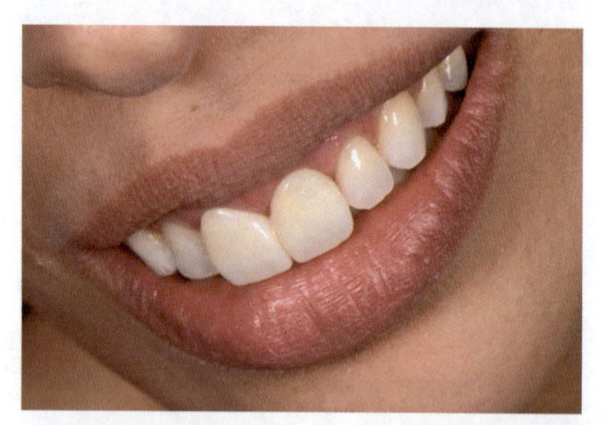

图 12-28

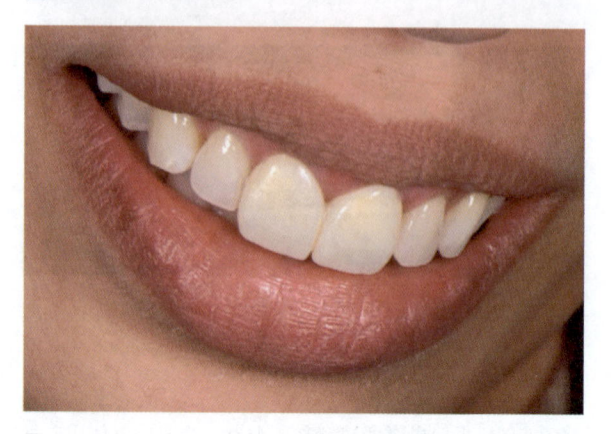

图 12-29
图 12-27、12-28、12-29　在最终修复体制作之前,以临时修复体的自然的外观作为蓝图,测试了美学、外形和咬合的变化。

12　临床过程

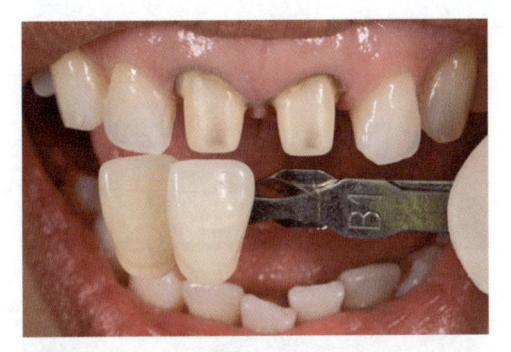

图 12-30　比色的记录和比色图的绘制

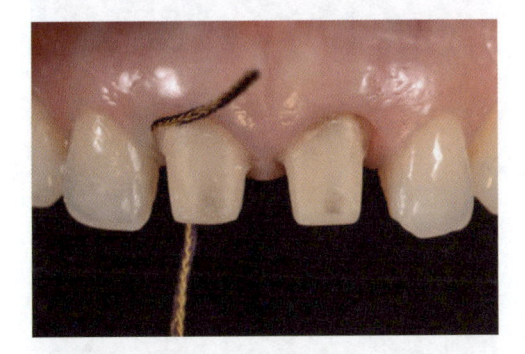

图 12-31

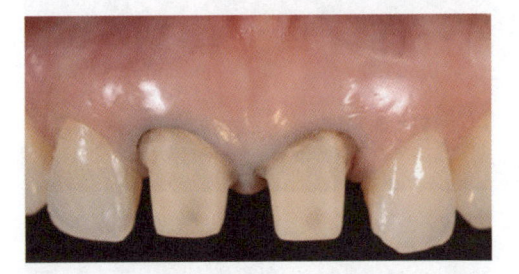

图 12-32

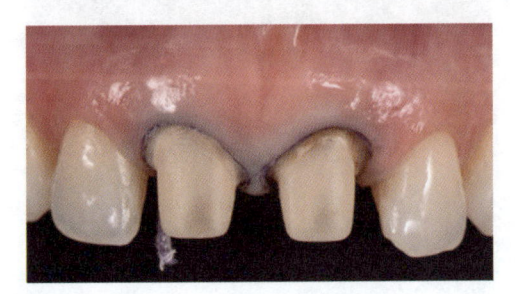

图 12-33
图 12-31、12-32、12-33　双排龈

256　根管治疗后的牙体修复

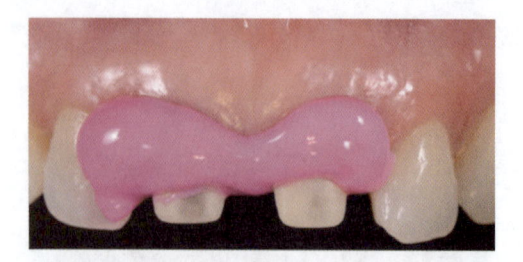

图 12-34

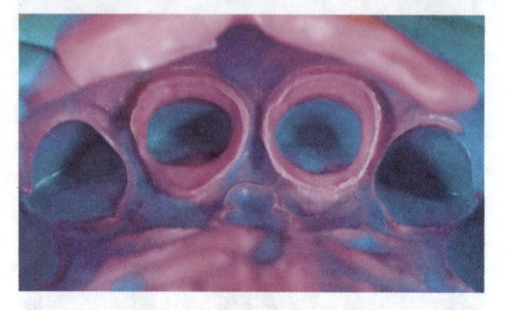

图 12-35
图 12-34、12-35　取印模使用 Imprint 4 Penta 重体和 Imprint 4 轻体常规套装（3M ESPE）

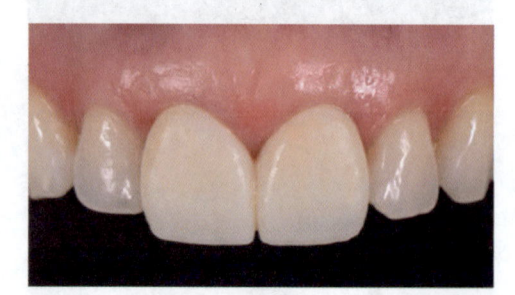

图 12-36

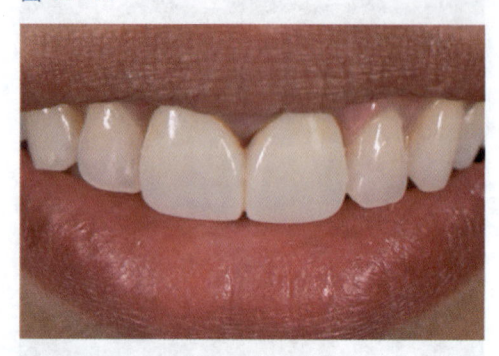

图 12-37
图 12-36、12-37　临时修复体进行了调整并重新黏固

12 临床过程

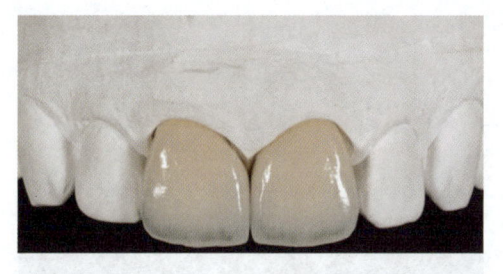

图 12-38

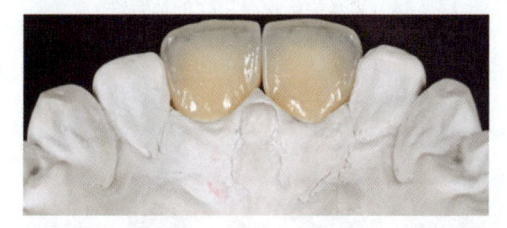

图 12-39

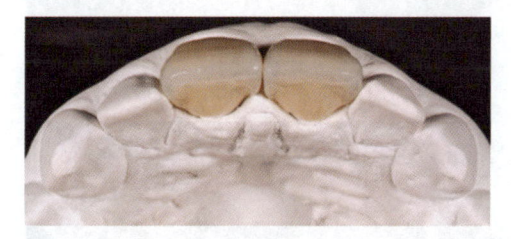

图 12-40

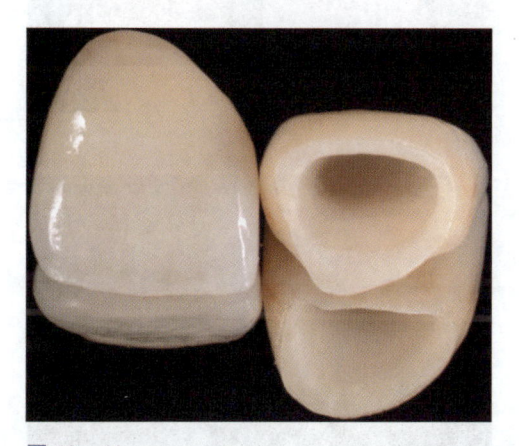

图 12-41
图 12-38、12-39、12-40、12-41 最终的修复体-顶端氧化锆（Lava Plus-高透明度，3M ESPE）贴面 IPS e.max Ceram（Ivoclar Vivadent）。这两种材料具有相似的热膨胀系数。

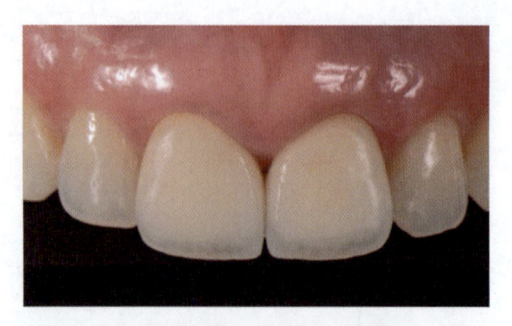

图 12-42 用水尝试检查边缘的适合性

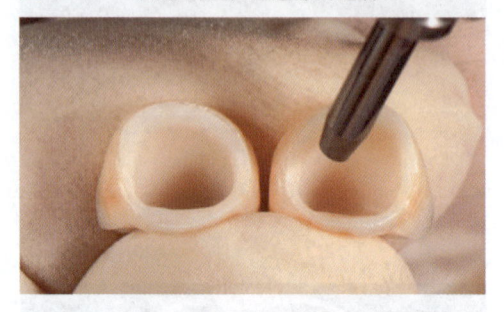

图 12-43 修复体被视为临床上可以接受后,凹面用氧化铝颗粒喷砂(≤50 μm,2 bar)。

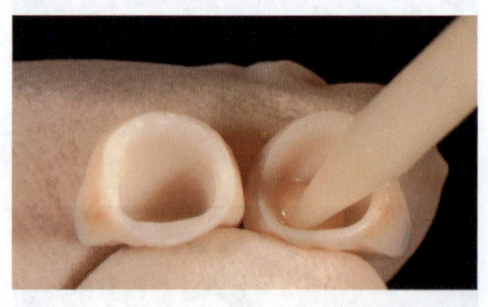

图 12-44

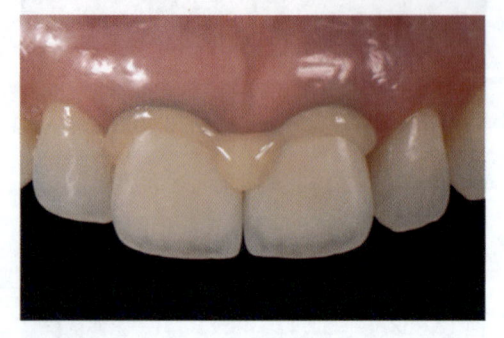

图 12-45

图 12-44、12-45 自黏结树脂水门汀(RelyX Unicem 2,3M ESPE)用于黏结封闭修复体

12 临床过程

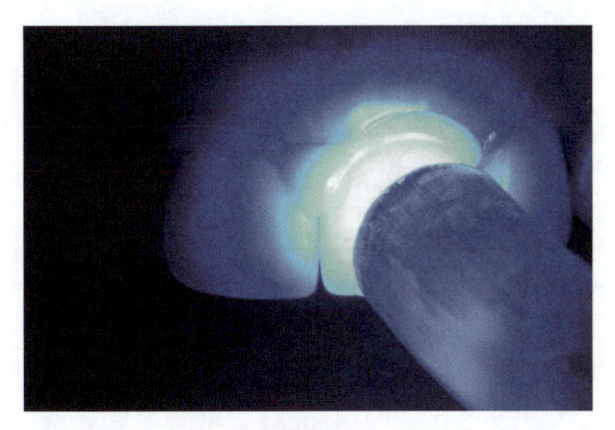

图 12-46 水门汀点固化 2 秒

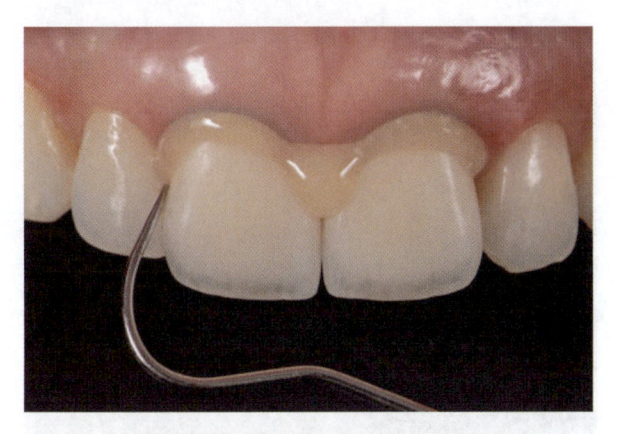

图 12-47 多余材料呈完整的一片被去除

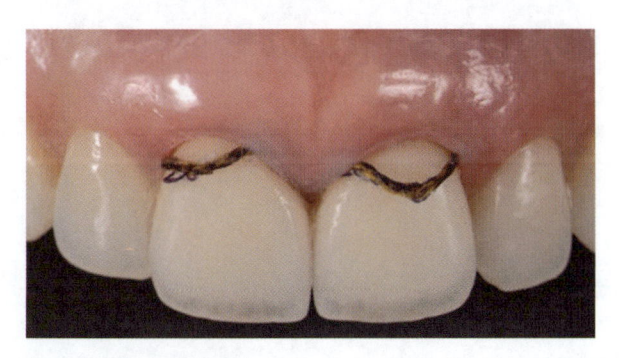

图 12-48 拆除排龈线

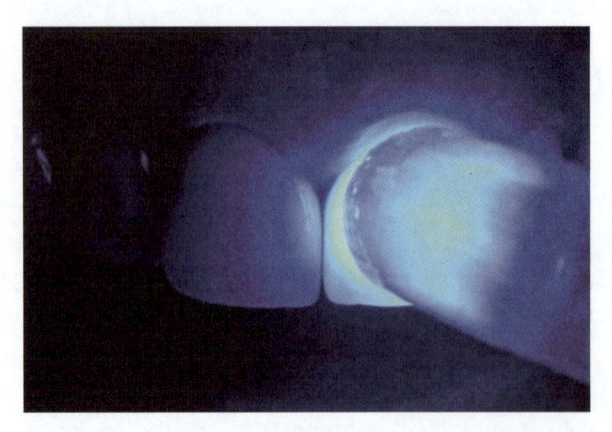

图 12-49 边缘用 LED 光固化灯照射以增强树脂水门汀在黏固操作后的转化程度

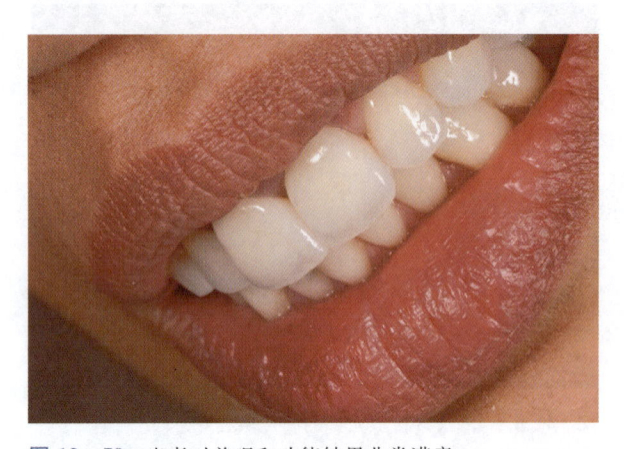

图 12-50 患者对美观和功能结果非常满意

（孙喆 译）